Gems of Ophthal
RETINA

Gems of Ophthalmology
RETINA

Editors

HV Nema MS
Formerly, Professor and Head
Department of Ophthalmology
Institute of Medical Sciences
Banaras Hindu University
Varanasi, Uttar Pradesh, India

Nitin Nema MS DNB
Professor
Department of Ophthalmology
Sri Aurobindo Institute of Medical Sciences
Indore, Madhya Pradesh, India

JAYPEE *The Health Sciences Publisher*

New Delhi | London | Panama

Jaypee Brothers Medical Publishers (P) Ltd

Headquarters

Jaypee Brothers Medical Publishers (P) Ltd
4838/24, Ansari Road, Daryaganj
New Delhi 110 002, India
Phone: +91-11-43574357
Fax: +91-11-43574314
Email: jaypee@jaypeebrothers.com

Overseas Offices

J.P. Medical Ltd
83 Victoria Street, London
SW1H 0HW (UK)
Phone: +44-20 317 08910
Fax: +44 (0)20 3008 6180
Email: info@jpmedpub.com

Jaypee Brothers Medical Publishers (P) Ltd
17/1-B Babar Road, Block-B, Shyamoli
Mohammadpur, Dhaka-1207
Bangladesh
Mobile: +08801912003485
Email: jaypeedhaka@gmail.com

Jaypee-Highlights Medical Publishers Inc
City of Knowledge, Bld. 235, 2nd floor, Clayton
Panama City, Panama
Phone: +1 507-301-0496
Fax: +1 507-301-0499
Email: cservice@jphmedical.com

Jaypee Brothers Medical Publishers (P) Ltd
Bhotahity, Kathmandu, Nepal
Phone: +977-9741283608
Email: Kathmandu@jaypeebrothers.com

Website: www.jaypeebrothers.com
Website: www.jaypeedigital.com

Gems of Ophthalmology—Retina

First Edition: **2018**

ISBN 978-93-5270-402-6

Printed at: Samrat Offset Pvt. Ltd.

Contributors

Abhinav Dhami MS
Shri Mahavir Vitreoretinal Service
Medical Research Foundation
Sankara Nethralaya
Chennai, Tamil Nadu, India

Ajit Majjhi MD
Consultant
Vitreoretinal Service
Centre for Sight
Hyderabad, Telangana, India

Aljoscha Steffen Neubauer MD
Consultant
Department of Ophthalmology
Ludwig-Maximilans University
Munich, Germany

Anand Rajendran FRCS DNB
Senior Consultant and Professor
Retina – Vitreous Service
Aravind Eye Hospital and
Postgraduate Institute of Ophthalmology
Madurai, Tamil Nadu, India

Anjali Hussain MS
Medical Retina and ROP Specialist
Al Zahara Hospital
Sharjah, UAE

Arup Chakrabarti MS
Founder Director
Chakrabarti Eye Care Center
Thiruvananthapuram, Kerala, India

Bhavya G MBBS
Resident
RP Centre of Ophthalmic Sciences
All India Institute of Medical Sciences
New Delhi, India

Deependra Vikram Singh MD
Consultant Vitreoretinal Surgeon
DRS Northex, Eye Institute
New Delhi, India

Dhananjay Shukla MD
Director
Retina Vitreous Service
Ratan Jyoti Nethralaya
Gwalior, Madhya Pradesh, India

Dhanashree Ratra MS
Consultant
Shri Mahavir Vitreoretinal
Service
Medical Research Foundation
Sankara Nethralaya
Chennai, Tamil Nadu, India

Fairooz Manjandavida MS
Consultant
Department of
Ocular Oncology
Narayan Nethralaya
Bengaluru, Karanataka, India

James A Eadie MD
Consultant
Department of Ophthalmology and
Visual Sciences
University of Wisconsin School of
Medicine and Public Health
Madison, Wisconsin, USA

Karobi Lahari Coutinho MS
Consultant Vitreoretinal Surgeon
Bombay Hospital, Institute of
Medical Sciences
Mumbai, Maharashtra, India

Lingam Gopal MS FRCS
Associate Professor and
Consultant
University Health System
Singapore
Shri Mahavir Vitreoretinal Service
Medical Research Foundation
Sankara Nethralaya
Chennai, Tamil Nadu, India

Mahesh Shanmugam DO FRCS PhD
Head
Department of Vitreoretinal and
Ocular Oncology Services
Sankara Eye Hospital
Bengaluru, Karnataka, India

Mayuri Bhargava MS
Senior Resident
Department of Ophthalmology
National University Hospital
Singapore

Meena Chakrabarti MS
Senior Consultant
Chakrabarti Eye Care Center
Thiruvananthapuram, Kerala, India

Michael M Altaweel MD
Consultant
Department of Ophthalmology and
Visual Sciences
University of Wisconsin School of
Medicine and Public Health
Madison, Wisconsin, USA

Mohammed Naseer MD
Consultant
Department of Ophthalmology
Salmaniya Medical Complex
Kingdom of Bahrain

Nazimul Hussain MS DNB
Consultant Ophthalmologist
Vitreoretinal Specialist
Al Zahara Hospital
Sharjah, UAE

Neha Sinha MBBS PG
Retina Service
King George's Medical University
Lucknow, Uttar Pradesh, India

Nidhi Relhan MS
Fellow
Srimati Kannuri Santhamma Centre for
Vitreoretinal Diseases
LV Prasad Eye Institute
Hyderabad, Telangana, India

Parijat Chandra MD
Associate Professor
Vitreoretinal Service
RP Centre for Ophthalmic Sciences
All India Institute of Medical Sciences
New Delhi, India

Peter N Youssef MD
Consultant
Department of Ophthalmology and
Visual Sciences
University of Wisconsin School of
Medicine and Public Health
Madison, Wisconsin, USA

Pradeep Sagar BK
Fellow
Department of Vitreoretinal and
Ocular Oncology Services
Sankara Eye Hospital
Bengaluru, Karnataka, India

Pradeep Venkatesh MD
Professor
Uvea and Retina Service
RP Centre for Ophthalmic Sciences
All India Institute of Medical Sciences
New Delhi, India

Pukhraj Rishi MS
Consultant
Shri Mahavir Vitreoretinal Service
Medical Research Foundation
Sankara Nethralaya
Chennai, Tamil Nadu, India

Rajesh Ramanjulu MS
Consultant
Department of Vitreoretinal and
Ocular Oncology Services
Sankara Eye Hospital
Bengaluru, Karnatata, India

Rajni Sharma MD
Assistant Professor
Department of Pediatrics
All India Institute of Medical Sciences
New Delhi, India

Rajvardhan Azad MD
Formerly, Chief
RP Centre for Ophthalmic Sciences
All India Institute of Medical Sciences
New Delhi, India

Richard E Appen MD
Consultant
Department of Ophthalmology and
Visual Sciences
University of Wisconsin School of
Medicine and Public Health
Madison, Wisconsin, USA

Sandeep Saxena MS FRCS
Professor
Retina Service
King George's Medical University
Lucknow, Uttar Pradesh, India

Santosh G Honavar MD FACS
Director
Department of Ocular Oncology
Centre for Sight
Hyderabad, Telangana, India

Shreyas Temkar MD
Senior Resident
RP Centre of Ophthalmic Sciences
All India Institute of Medical Sciences
New Delhi, India

Soman Nair MD
Senior Resident
RP Centre for Ophthalmic Sciences
All India Institute of Medical Sciences
New Delhi, India

Sonia S John MS
Consultant
Chakrabarti Eye Care Center
Thiruvananthapuram, Kerala, India

Subhadra Jalali MS
Associate Director
Srimati Kannuri Santhamma
Centre for Vitreoretinal Diseases
LV Prasad Eye Institute
Hyderabad, Telangana, India

Supriya Dabir MD
Associate Consultant
Aditya Jyoti Eye Hospital
Mumbai, Maharashtra, India

Suresh R Chandra MD
Professor
Department of Ophthalmology and
Visual Sciences
University of Wisconsin School of
Medicine and Public Health
Madison, Wisconsin, USA

Su Xinyi MMed PhD
Consultant
Department of Ophthalmology
National University Hospital
Singapore

Tarun Sharma MS
Director
Shri Mahavir Vitreoretinal Service
Medical Research Foundation
Sankara Nethralaya
Chennai, Tamil Nadu, India

Tengku Ain Kamalden MD
Senior Lecturer
Department of Ophthalmology
Faculty of Medicine
University of Malaya
Malaysia

Vinay PG MS
Fellow, Retina – Vitreous Service
Aravind Eye Hospital and
Postgraduate Institute of Ophthalmology
Madurai, Tamil Nadu, India

Vishal MY MS
Fellow, Retina – Vitreous Service
Aravind Eye Hospital and
Postgraduate Institute of Ophthalmology
Madurai, Tamil Nadu, India

Yog Raj Sharma MD
Formerly, Chief
RP Centre for Ophthalmic Sciences
All India Institute of Medical Sciences
New Delhi, India

Preface

Retina is a photosensitive layer of eyeball that conveys electrical impulses to the brain. A healthy retina is essential for the normal vision. An array of diseases can affect the retina which may often impair vision. They include retinitis, retinopathies, vascular occlusions, retinal detachment and degenerations.

The book *Gems of Ophthalmology—Retina* covers a wide range of retinal diseases. Initial chapters have been devoted to the diagnostic procedures pertaining to the retinal diseases. Ophthalmoscopy, fluorescein angiography, indocyanine green angiography, and fundus autofluorescence are helpful in reaching to a correct diagnosis of retinal disorders. Choroidal imaging, with enhanced depth imaging and swept source optical coherence tomography, is a new modality for measuring the thickness of choroid, is being increasingly used in clinical practice.

Diabetic retinopathy, hypertensive retinopathy and retinal vein occlusions are frequently encountered retinal disorders. The pathomechanism of diabetic macular edema (the most common cause of visual loss in diabetic retinopathy) and central serous chorioretinopathy are critically described. Hussain and coauthors discussed the management of age-related macular degeneration including stem cell and gene therapies.

Surgical aspects of retina are also covered in the book. These include surgical management of macular hole, giant retinal tears, rhegmatogenous retinal detachment, and retinal cysts, and advances in microincision vitreoretinal surgery.

Since the book is multi-authored, repetition could not be avoided; perhaps it is in readers' interest. However, there is no ambiguity.

The editors assure the readers that the major part of the work presented in this book comes from the Recent Advances in Ophthalmology series edited by Dr HV Nema and Dr Nitin Nema. In each chapter, author/s has provided references to the published work of their own group as well as relevant references from other experts for the benefit of readers who want to read the topic in detail.

Hopefully, the book will help postgraduates, residents, and general ophthalmologists to understand the diseases of retina in a better way and enable to manage them in an efficient manner to prevent blindness.

HV Nema
Nitin Nema

Acknowledgments

We wish to record our grateful thanks to all authors of chapters for their spontaneity, cooperation and hard work. Some of them have revised their chapters. Our special thanks go to Dr Dananjaya Shukla, Dr Pradeep Venkatesh, Dr Dhanshree Ratra, Dr Tarun Sharma, and Dr Lingam Gopal, for contributing their chapters on a short notice.

Credit goes to Shri Jitendar P Vij, Group Chairman, M/s Jaypee Brothers Medical Publishers (P) Ltd, New Delhi, India, who has agreed to start a new series—*Gems of Ophthalmology.* "*Retina*" is the fourth book of this series.

Ms Ritika Chandna, Developing Editor, M/s Jaypee Brothers Medical Publishers (P) Ltd, deserves our appreciation for her continued interest in refining the chapters.

Contents

CHAPTER 1

Ophthalmoscopy

Pukhraj Rishi, Tarun Sharma

INTRODUCTION

A comprehensive eye examination is a must for a complete assessment of the anterior and posterior segments of the eye—be it a diagnostic or preoperative evaluation. Although there are several methods of eye examination, viz. slit-lamp biomicroscopy, gonioscopy, perimetry, tonometry, and ultrasonography but ophthalmoscopy remains an important tool for a complete evaluation of the posterior segment of the eye. In December 1850, Helmholtz announced the invention of an "eye-mirror," which was the original ophthalmoscope. It was mounted with a holder for one lens, and lenses had to be changed constantly for eyes of different refraction. Rekoss introduced a revolving disk carrying a series of lenses.

PRINCIPLES OF OPHTHALMOSCOPY

Direct Ophthalmoscopy

The basic principle of ophthalmoscopy is shown in Figure 1.1. If the patient's eye is emmetropic, a light ray emanating from a point in the fundus emerges as a parallel beam. If this beam enters the pupil of an emmetropic observer, the rays are focused on the retina and an image is formed. This is called direct ophthalmoscopy.

The fundus can be seen only when the observed and the illuminated areas of the fundus overlap. In the emmetropic eye this can happen only if the light source and the observer's pupil are optically aligned. Under normal conditions this does not happen, hence the pupil normally appears dark (Fig. 1.2).

The illuminating and the observing beams are aligned using a semi-reflecting mirror or a prism allowing fundal view (Fig. 1.3).

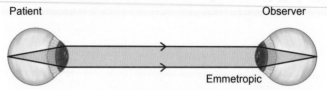

Fig. 1.1: Optics of image formation in an emmetropic eye.

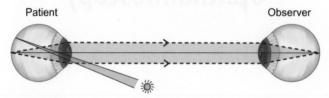

Fig. 1.2: The light source and the observer's pupil are not optically aligned.

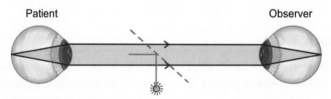

Fig. 1.3: The light source and the observer's pupil are optically aligned.

Indirect Ophthalmoscopy

Ruete introduced indirect ophthalmoscopy in 1852. There are several types of indirect ophthalmoscopes available. One must understand the optical principles of indirect ophthalmoscopy to carry out an ocular examination (including fundus angioscopy). The indirect ophthalmoscope can be used in the treatment of disorders of the posterior segment (Fig. 1.4).

There are five indirect ophthalmoscopy techniques. These are—(1) slit-lamp indirect, (2) head-mounted indirect, (3) monocular indirect, (4) modified monocular indirect, and (5) penlight ophthalmoscopy. Indirect ophthalmoscopy is carried out in a dark room with fully dilated pupils.

The equipment required for slit-lamp indirect ophthalmoscopy includes a slit-lamp and a condensing lens. The condensing lens may be either noncontact or contact lens.

Noncontact lenses: They are plus powered with two convex aspheric surfaces. The +60D version has the greatest magnification and is best used for the disk and macula. The +78D version is a commonly used diagnostic lens and the +90D is good for small pupils. They are available in clear or blue-free, "yellow retina protector glass." They are comfortable to the patient and minimize the risk of phototoxic retinal damage due to prolonged exposure to the focused beam.

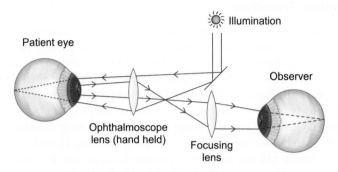

Fig. 1.4: Optics of indirect ophthalmoscope.

Lens	Field of view	Image magnification	Laser spot	Working distance
Super Quad 160®	160°/165°	0.5X	2.0X	Contact
Equator Plus®	114°/137°	0.44X	2.27X	Contact
Quad Pediatric	100°/120°	0.55X	1.82X	Contact
QuadrAspheric®	120°/144°	0.51X	1.97X	Contact
PDT Laser	115°/137°	0.67X	1.5X	Contact
Trans Equator®	110°/132°	0.7X	1.44X	Contact
Area Centralis®	70°/84°	1.06X	0.94X	Contact
Super Macula® 2.2	60°/78°	1.49X	0.67X	Contact

TABLE 1.1: Field of view and image magnification obtained by different contact lenses.

(PDT: photodynamic therapy)

Contact lenses: Goldman, Mainster, SuperQuad, Equator Plus, Area Centralis, Super Macula lenses are often used. The field of view and image magnification obtained by these lenses are listed in Table 1.1.

METHOD OF EXAMINATION

For examination, minimal slit-lamp intensity can be used in a dark room. Always focus the oculars to accommodate any examiner refractive error, then set the pupillary distance, remove all filters and keep the magnification to the lowest setting, usually X6–X10. The illumination of the slit-lamp should be adjusted for an intermediate slit height and a 2 mm width, and then placed in the straight ahead position between the oculars (0° or coaxial). Before examination, ensure that the condensing lens surfaces are clean. Hold the lens vertically between the thumb and index finger of the left hand to examine the patient's right eye and vice versa.

Examination Procedure

Instruct the patient to fixate straight ahead, to stare wide and to blink normally. Center the beam in the patient's pupil and focus on the cornea. Now the lens is placed in front of the patient's eye, directly in front of the cornea so the back surface just clears the lashes. The examiner's fingers may be placed on either the brow bar or the patient's forehead. Using the joystick, focus on the fundus image by slowly moving away from the cornea, keeping the beam centered in the pupil. Once the retinal image is focused, the magnification may be increased. Scan across the entire lens keeping it steady. In order to view the peripheral retina, ask the patient to change fixation into the nine cardinal positions of gaze. The lens is realigned and the slit-lamp refocused as necessary. To reduce interfering reflections, tilt the lens or move the illumination arm up to 10° on either side, once the fundus has been focused. For fine-tuning the fundus view, lateral and longitudinal adjustments of the lens may be made to optimize the field of view. When viewing finer fundus details, the intensity and magnification of the slit-lamp should be increased.

Head-Mounted Binocular Indirect Ophthalmoscopy

Binocular indirect ophthalmoscopy (BIO) is a technique used to evaluate the entire ocular fundus (Fig. 1.5). It provides for stereoscopic, wide-angled, high-resolution views of the entire fundus and the overlying vitreous. Its optical principles and illumination options allow for the visualization of the fundus regardless of high ametropia or hazy ocular media.

Light beams directed into the patient's eye produce reflected observation beams from the retina. These beams are focused to a viewable, aerial image following the placement of a high plus-powered condensing lens at its focal

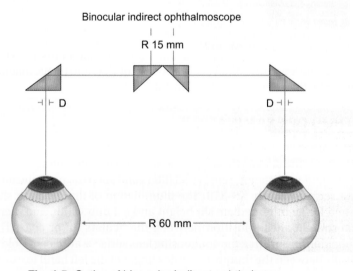

Fig. 1.5: Optics of binocular indirect ophthalmoscopy.

distance in front of the patient's eye. The resultant image is real, inverted, magnified, laterally reversed, and located between the examiner and the condensing lens. The observer views this image through the oculars of the head-borne indirect ophthalmoscope.

An indirect ophthalmoscope (Fig. 1.6) consists of a headband for comfortable placement, a light source with variable illumination and an adjustable mirrored surface in the main housing, and knobs to align the low plus powered eyepieces (+2.00D to +2.50D) with the examiner's interpupillary distance. A 20D condensing lens (Fig. 1.7A), a pair of scleral depressors (Fig. 1.7B) and a fundus drawing sheet (Fig. 1.7C) are need for proper indirect ophthalmoscopy and documentation.

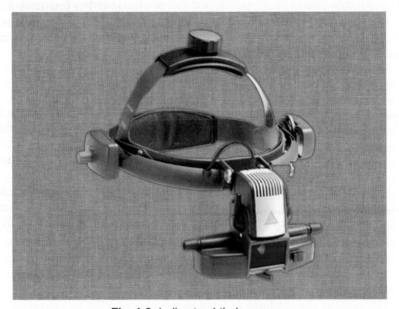

Fig. 1.6: Indirect ophthalmoscope.

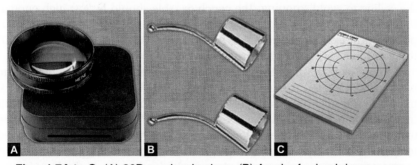

Figs. 1.7A to C: (A) 20D condensing lens; (B) A pair of scleral depressors; (C) Fundus drawing sheet.

Examination Procedure

Proper placement and adjustment of the BIO is an important step in the examination. Place the loose BIO onto the head and position the bottom of the front headband one index finger-width above the eyebrows. Tighten the crown strap until this headband position begins to stabilize, then position the back head strap on or below the occipital notch and tighten until secured. Now the knobs that control the instrument's main housing (oculars and light tower) should be loosened. The oculars should be as close to the examiner's eyes as possible and lie perpendicular or slightly angled downward from examiner's line of sight. The light source is adjusted in the upper half of examiner's field of view. This maximizes the observer's visual field and minimizes horizontal diplopia. Horizontally align each ocular by closing one eye and fixating the centrally positioned thumb of an outstretched hand. Turn on the light source and fixate straight ahead on a wall at 40–50 cm looking at the projected light source. Use the mirror knob to vertically place the light source at the upper one-half to one-third of the field.

The headset is adjusted and the voltage set to mid-range (occasionally the sneeze reflex may start from the periphery first). The choice of condensing lens depends upon the need for a panoramic view or detail; a 30D provides a panoramic view while fundus details can be obtained with 14D. Stereopsis is important and depends on the choice of lens. A full stereopsis is obtained with 14D, three-fourths with 20D and one-half stereopsis with 30D. A 30D lens can be used to get a view of the fundus in patients with a small pupil. The condensing lens should be held between the tip of the flexed index finger and the ball of the extended thumb of the nondominant hand and the scleral depressor with the dominant hand. The extended third finger acts as the pivot. The more convex surface should be toward the observer and the white-ringed edge closest to the patient so as to avoid bothersome light reflexes. These reflexes can be made to move in opposite directions from each other by slightly tilting the lens. Condensing lenses have their surfaces coated to reduce such flexes. The lens must be smudge free.

The patient should have at least some idea of what to expect in the examination. Although the patient may be examined in either sitting or supine position, it is best to recline the patient on a couch with the face directed towards the ceiling to avoid stooping. The couch or table should be just high enough to reach the examiner's hips. The examiner stands opposite to the clock hour position to be examined. The patient is instructed to keep both the eyes open and fixate towards his outstretched hand which points to the meridian of interest.

From a working distance of 18–20 inches, direct the light beam into the pupil, producing a complete red pupillary reflex. Pull backward on the lens, maintaining the central position of the pupil reflex, until the entire lens fills with the fundus image. Fine adjustments are made in the lens tilt and vertex distance to produce a distortion-free full lens view. The patient must be repeatedly urged to open the fellow eye. Good cycloplegia is the single most important factor in getting cooperation in this regard. An eye with inadequate cycloplegia is very photophobic.

All the vital elements involved in the visualization of the fundus, namely the observer's macula, the eyepiece of the scope, the center of the condensing lens, the patient's pupil and the object observed in the fundus must be kept on an axis to maintain the fundal view. In order to develop and achieve a continuous sweeping picture of the fundus, a major retinal blood vessel must be picked out from the posterior pole and followed as anteriorly as possible by the observer's movements alone. This vessel should then be followed back to the optic disk. This maneuver needs constant practice to master.

The problem of orientation in the fundus may be solved by learning to accurately draw the image exactly as we see in the condensing lens. The drawing chart may be placed inverted over the patient's chest. Positioning 180° away from the area of interest, the observer must think in terms of anterior in the fundus or posterior in the fundus (or central and peripheral). Draw the image seen in the lens on that part of the fundus chart that is closest to the observer.

Since 30% of the retina lies anterior to the equator, failure to study this region will result in overlooking serious pathology in many cases. A scleral depression not only allows for an easy and complete view of the ora serrata and the pars plana but also allows a better evaluation of the retinal topography making lesions such as horseshoe tears or vitreoretinal traction more visible. It is of particular value in differentiating a retinal hemorrhage from a retinal break, in recognizing a raised from a depressed lesion and in detecting whether a foreign body lies on or anterior to the retina. The absence of an overhanging orbital margin superonasally makes initial attempts at scleral depression easier. The depressor is applied to the superior lid, without pressure, at the tarsal margin. The patient looks up and the depressor slides posteriorly parallel to the surface of the globe, as the lid retracts. The depressor is gently pressed against the globe at the equatorial region and a grayish mound is seen to come up in view from the inferior part of the fundus. In viewing the ora, it is sometimes necessary to tilt the condensing lens somewhat forward, into a plane more nearly parallel to the iris. It must be remembered that scleral depression is a dynamic technique.

FUNDUS DRAWING COLOR CODE (PETER MORSE)

Color Code: Red

Solid

- Retinal arterioles
- Neovascularization
- Vascular abnormalities or anomalies
- Vortex vein
- Attached retina
- Hemorrhages (preintra and subretinal)
- Open interior portion of retinal break (tears, holes)
- Normal foveola (drawn as a red dot).

Cross Lined

- Open portion of giant tears or large dialysis
- Inner portion of chorioretinal atrophy
- Open portion of retinal holes in inner layer of the retinoschisis
- Inner portion of the areas of the retina.

Color Code: Blue

Solid

- Detached retina (Fig. 1.8)
- Retinal veins
- Outlines of retinal breaks (tears, holes)
- Outline of ora serrata (dentate processes, ora bays)
- Meridional, radial, fixed star-shaped and circumferential folds
- Vitreoretinal traction tufts
- Retinal granular tags and tufts (cystic, noncystic)
- Outline of flat neovascularization
- Outline of lattice degeneration (inner chevrons or Xs)
- Outline of thin areas of the retina
- Intraretinal cysts (with overlying curvilinear stripes to show configuration).

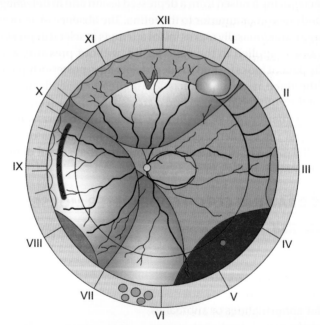

Fig. 1.8: A long-standing, partial, rhegmatogenous retinal detachment with demarcation lines and intraretinal macrocyst. A horse-shoe tear, lattice degeneration and a retinal dialysis are also seen. An improperly placed scleral buckle effect is made out. Pars plana is detached nasally. Retinoschisis with an inner-layer hole is seen in the inferotemporal periphery. Pars plana cysts are seen inferiorly.

Cross Lines

- Inner layer of retinoschisis
- White with or without pressure
- Detached pars plana epithelium anterior to the separation of ora
- Outer surface of the retina seen in rolled edge of retinal tears, inverted flap of giant retinal tear.

Stippled or Circles

Cystoid degeneration.

Interrupted Lines

Outline of change in area or folds of detached retina because of shifting fluid.

Color Code: Green

Solid

- Opacities in the media (cornea, anterior chamber, lens, vitreous)
- Vitreous hemorrhage
- Vitreous membranes
- Hyaloid ring
- Intraocular foreign bodies
- Retinal opercula
- Cotton wool patches
- Ora serrata pearls
- Outline of elevated neovascularization.

Stippled or Dotted

- Asteroid hyalosis
- Frosting or snowflakes on cystoid, retinoschisis, lattice degeneration.

Color Code: Brown

Solid

- Uveal tissues
- Pars plana cysts
- Ciliary processes (pars plicata)
- Striae ciliaris
- Pigment beneath detached retina
- Subretinal fibrosis demarcation lines
- Choroidal nevi
- Malignant choroidal melanomas
- Metastatic and other choroidal tumors
- Choroidal detachment.

Outline

- Chorioretinal atrophy beneath a detached retina
- Posterior staphyloma
- Edge of the buckle beneath a detached retina.

Color Code: Yellow

Solid

- Intraretinal edema
- Intraretinal or subretinal hard yellow exudates
- Deposits in the retinal pigment epithelium (RPE)
- Detached maculae in some retinal separations
- Retinal edema as a result of photocoagulation, cryotherapy or diathermy
- Long and short posterior ciliary nerves
- Retinoblastoma.

Stippled or Dotted

Drusen.

Color Code: Black

Solid

- Pigment within the detached retina (lattice, flap of horse-shoe tear, paravascular pigmentation)
- Pigment in choroid or pigmented epithelial hyperpigmentation in areas of attached retina
- Pigmented demarcation lines at the attached margin of the detached retina or within the detached retina
- Hyperpigmentation as a result of previous treatment with cryotherapy, photocoagulation or diathermy
- Completely sheathed retinal vessels.

Outline

- Partially sheathed vessels (lattices, retinoschisis)
- Edge of the buckle beneath an attached retina
- Long posterior ciliary nerves and vessels (pigmented)
- Short posterior ciliary nerves and vessels
- Chorioretinal atrophy.

INDIRECT OPHTHALMOSCOPY IN OPERATING ROOM

Many problems may be encountered whilst operating and performing an indirect ophthalmoscopy. The fundus to be examined is usually a difficult one, with a retinal detachment and/or PVR. The cornea may become edematous or abraded during the course of surgery. Particular care must be taken in patients having undergone LASIK surgery to prevent dislocation of corneal flap. The fundus picture may change with each step in surgery. The advantages of indirect ophthalmoscopy in the operation room stem from its safe working distance from the sterile operating field, in accurate localization of all retinal breaks and other fundus landmarks by scleral depression. It helps in obtaining a fine needle aspiration biopsy and treatment of choroidal or retinal tumors.

Indirect ophthalmoscopy is a valuable tool in the examination of children and uncooperative adults. Since the field of view is much larger with an indirect ophthalmoscope, fundus examination is possible even in a moving eye. A quick comparison with the other eye is also possible. Children would generally react more favorably to the more impersonal distance of an indirect examination. It is also useful equipment in examining the anterior segment for rubeosis and tumor seedings in children with advanced retinoblastoma.

Fundus angioscopy, and transillumination (Fig. 1.9) can be performed using indirect ophthalmoscopy; which helps in differentiating various types of fundus mass lesions. Nystagmus, aniridia, albinotic fundus, partial vitreous hemorrhage, fundus coloboma, microphthalmos, and persistent hyperplastic primary vitreous can be diagnosed with the help of an indirect ophthalmoscope.

Monocular Indirect Ophthalmoscopy

Monocular indirect ophthalmoscopy (MIO) combines the advantages of increased field of view (indirect ophthalmoscopy) with erect real imaging (direct ophthalmoscopy). By collecting and redirecting peripheral fundus reflected illumination rays, which cannot be accomplished with the direct

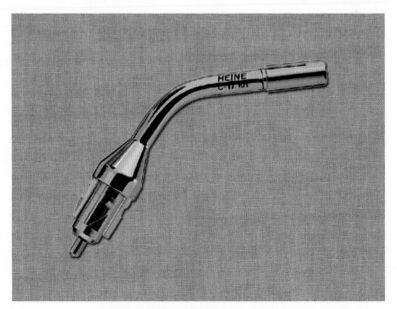

Fig. 1.9: Transillumination probe.

ophthalmoscope, the indirect ophthalmoscope (Fig. 1.10) extends the observer's field of view approximately four to five times. An internal lens system then reinverts the initially inverted image to a real erect one (Fig. 1.11), which is then magnified. This image is focusable using the focusing lever/eyepiece lever. It gives a field of view of approximately 30°, yet it is important that the

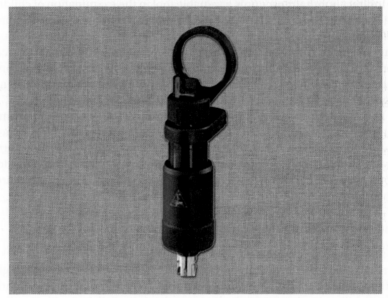

Fig. 1.10: Monocular indirect ophthalmoscope.

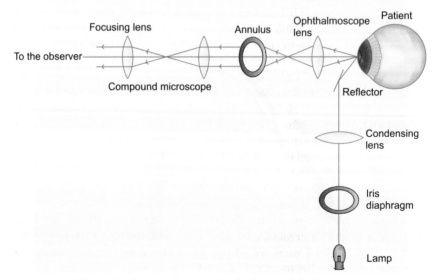

Fig. 1.11: Optics of monocular indirect ophthalmoscopy.

patient looks in six to eight different directions to see as much of the fundus as possible. The optical system of the MIO has a lens which erects the image and allows seeing things as they actually appear anatomically. It also gives a greater working distance from the patient, of 5–6 inches. The MIO has a yellow filter that allows one to see deeper details of the retina at about the level of the choroid. The cost of the MIO is nearly equal to that of a good BIO and of course it does not allow a stereoscopic view of the retina.

Examination Procedure

To examine the right eye, remove the patient's spectacle correction, stand to the patient's right side, and ask him to fixate straight ahead and level with the left eye. The observer should wear his refractive correction. The iris diaphragm lever is pushed fully to the left to maximally increase the aperture size. Center the red dot on the filter dial to open the aperture for normal viewing. The observers head should be against the forehead rest and the eye should be aligned through the instrument with the patient's right eye. Then position several inches in front of the patient and focus through the pupil onto the fundus using the thumb and focusing lever. Adjust the focus and iris diaphragm to produce a clear maximally illuminated fundus view. Continue to approach the patient until the observer's knuckle lightly touches the patient's cheek, as the working distance decreases, fundus magnification increases. Angle the light slightly nasally to illuminate and visualize the optic disk.

Modified Monocular Indirect Ophthalmoscopy

A thorough fundus examination is important and required in all young patients with strabismus or amblyopia in order to rule out organic causes of amblyopia prior to the initiation of the treatment. The patient cooperation obtained with the head-mounted BIO (using a 20D lens), and slit-lamp biomicroscope (using a 90D) is usually difficult or impossible on younger children. Also, the magnification of the fundus may be inadequate to allow accurate evaluation of posterior pole details. The direct ophthalmoscope is often the best available instrument for detailed retinal examination in young patients.

However, children often become frightened as the examiner approaches closely, as is necessary with the direct ophthalmoscope and cooperation is lost. Additionally, children often fix the ophthalmoscope light and track it as the examiner moves it, allowing examination of the macula but not of the disk. The field of view is small and the magnification is more than is usually necessary. This will prevent the examiner from seeing the large area of fundus. To avoid these difficulties, the direct ophthalmoscope can be used in conjunction with a 20D condensing lens. This combination provides a moderately magnified and wider angle view of the posterior pole. This avoids the close proximity between the patient and examiner required when using a direct ophthalmoscope alone. The technique is called *modified monocular indirect ophthalmoscopy* and has been noted for its ability to provide a good view of the retina through a small pupil.

Examination Procedure

To begin the examination a red reflex is visualized through the direct ophthalmoscope held approximately 18 cm from the patient's eye. A 20D lens is then placed 3–5 cm in front of the patient's eye in the path of the ophthalmoscope light beam, and the examiner then needs to move slightly toward or away from the patient until a clear image of the retina is observed.

An inverted, aerial image of the retina is produced, located between the observer and the lens. The apparent magnification will gradually increase as the examiner moves closer to this image (i.e. closer to the patient), allowing a more detailed examination. Moving closer to the image obtains a magnification of X4–X5. As the examiner moves closer, additional lenses in the ophthalmoscope are needed, to keep the image clear depending on the accommodative needs of the examiner. A viewing distance of approximately 18 cm from the patient is optimal, providing suitable magnification and a wide field of view.

A disadvantage of the technique, as with conventional direct ophthalmoscopy is the lack of a true stereoscopic view. However, lateral movement and the rotation of the direct ophthalmoscope during the examination gives good parallax clues to depth.

Penlight Ophthalmoscopy

This is a very old, basically bedside technique that originally utilized a penlight and a high plus lens. The patient must be dilated to get a large field of view and as much binocularity as possible. The ophthalmoscope is held just below the eyes and its light directed into the patient's eye. The patient's eye is viewed from over the top of the ophthalmoscope while a 20D lens is placed approximately 3–4 cm from the patient's eye. The light leaving the condensing lens must come to focus within the pupil allowing the fullest field of view of the retina, approximately 30°. The image is inverted and laterally reversed and located between the ophthalmoscope and the condensing lens. The degree of stereopsis depends on how fully the pupil is dilated and one's ability to converge and accommodate on the image. It still gives a larger field of view than an MIO, though less magnification. This is an alternative method to examine small infants. Should the bulb burn out in a BIO, one has an alternative means to get a good view of the peripheral fundus. Do not put hands on the patient's shoulder or head. Instead, use the back of the chair to steady yourself.

DIRECT OPHTHALMOSCOPY

Direct ophthalmoscope (Fig. 1.12) is most commonly used instrument in ophthalmic practice. The ophthalmologist must familiarize oneself with the use of the direct ophthalmoscope in an appropriate manner.

Before being able to recognize the abnormalities in fundus, one must know what normal looks like. It is advisable to examine as many of your colleagues as possible both inside and outside clinic hours. Good observational and recording skills can be developed with practice.

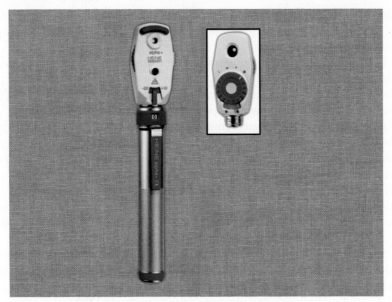

Fig. 1.12: Direct ophthalmoscope.

Examination Procedure

Direct ophthalmoscopy is best carried out in a dark room, with fully dilated pupils. One must be familiar with the color coding of the lens wheel and the various apertures and filters. Instruct the patient to look at a distant target (the white spot light on the vision chart) and to "pretend" to still see it even if obscured with your head. The patient may blink as required. Your left eye and left hand should be used to examine the patient's left eye. The field of view of the fundus is increased when the examiner goes closer to the patient's eye. When patients with low myopes or low hyperopes are to be examined, it is better to remove their glasses. However, for myopes and hyperopes above ±3.00DSph, and for astigmats above 2.50DCyl, it is advisable to keep the glasses on in order to overcome problems associated with magnification, minification and distortion. The extra reflexes produced by the spectacle lenses will at first prove distracting but can be overcome with practice.

Using a large diameter aperture, examine the external features of the eye, including the pupils. With a +1 or +2D lens in the ophthalmoscope, view the pupils at a distance of 40–66 cm from the patient. Look for media opacities. To find the location of the opacity, note the movement of the opacity with relation to the movement of the ophthalmoscope, using the pupillary plane as a reference point. If the opacity moves in the same direction as the ophthalmoscope, the opacity is located behind the iris. If the opacity moves in the opposite direction to the ophthalmoscope, the opacity is located in front of the iris.

Using the ophthalmoscope as a light source, which is held tangential to the iris one looks for any shadow that appears on the nasal side. If the nasal iridocorneal angle has no shadow, it denotes a wide-open angle. However, as this shadow increases in width relative to the overall cornea size, the angle seems narrow.

Dial up +10DSph lens in the lens wheel and observe the eye from a distance of 10 cm. Study the red reflex to detect any media opacity. The position of opacity can be inferred from its parallax with respect to the pupil. When the patient looks up and the opacity appears to move in the same direction within the red-reflex, then it is located anterior to the pupil plane (i.e. in the cornea or in the anterior chamber). Opacity that remains stationary lies in the plane of the pupil, but when it moves in the opposite direction to that of the patient's gaze it lies posterior to the pupil plane (i.e. the posterior lens or vitreous). It may be easier to move yourself slightly from side to side rather than ask the patient to move his eye to achieve the same effect. During ophthalmoscopy it is advisable to keep both eyes open and suppress the image from the other eye. It may take some practice to accomplish this.

It is better to move closer to the patient and gradually reduce the power of the lens in the wheel and focus on the crystalline lens, the vitreous, and finally the fundus. The power of the lens necessary to focus on the fundus will depend on patient's and observer's uncompensated refractive error and accommodation. Once a blood vessel on the fundus is located, move along it and locate the point at which it branches. Then move your field of view in the direction in which the apex of the branch is pointing till you reach the optic disk.

If one controls his accommodation, it allows for an estimation of the patient's refractive error by focusing the optic disk. Retinal blood vessels should be examined in each quadrant after locating the disk. Artery to vein ratio (A/V), arteriolar light reflex (ALR), branching of vessels to all four quadrants, and the crossing phenomenon must be assessed.

Once again focus the disk and move nasally to view the macula. In this position, you may obscure the fixation target, cause the pupil to constrict, dazzle the patient and notice some troublesome corneal reflections. These factors make the macula a difficult area to visualize. It may be useful to use a smaller aperture beam. The patient should not be asked to look into the light when viewing the macula through an undilated pupil. The patient will accommodate, and this together with the bright light from the ophthalmoscope will make the pupil even smaller reducing the ability to view the whole macular area.

Finally, ask the patient to look in the eight cardinal directions to view the peripheral fundus. You will need to adjust the lens in the wheel slightly as the periphery is closer to you than the optic disk, requiring more focusing power (plus lens). The red-free filter makes small macroaneurysms and small hemorrhages standout more clearly. It can also be helpful in estimating the C/D ratio. It is also used to differentiate between retinal nevus and choroidal nevus. The retinal blood supply and its RPE act like a red filter. Therefore, a nevus that lies behind the retina and located in the choroid will not be seen when viewed with the red-free filter. On the other hand, a nevus located on or in the retina will still be seen with the red free-filter in place. A cobalt-blue filter is useful in detection of nerve fiber drop out.

The direct ophthalmoscope gives a magnification of approximately 15X and a field of view of 6.5–10°. The formula M = 60D/4 holds well for up to ±10Ds of refractive error.

Hruby Lens Direct Ophthalmoscopy

The use of the slit-lamp biomicroscope allows a stereoscopic view of the retina. The auxiliary lenses provide high magnification with excellent resolution. The Hruby lens (-55D) produces an upright virtual image that is not laterally reversed.

Examination Procedure

Patient cooperation can be enhanced with attention to comfort and the use of a fixation device. Once the illuminated slit is imaged in the patient's pupil, the Hruby lens is introduced in front of the patient's eye as close as possible without contacting the cornea or lashes.

This mode of direct ophthalmoscopy can provide a very high level of magnification, even greater than that of the monocular hand-held direct ophthalmoscope. The actual level of magnification depends on that available through the slit-lamp. Stereopsis is provided to a greater degree than all other examination techniques.

The main disadvantage of this technique is the field of view. It is smaller than all other examination methods with the exception of direct monocular ophthalmoscopy (less than two disk diameters for an emmetropic patient). More dilation is required than in other binocular techniques. The quality of the image is easily degraded by media opacities; however, increasing the slit-lamp illumination can reduce this problem. As the magnification is so high, small movements of the observer, lens, or patient have an immediately noticeable effect on image quality.

WIDE ANGLE VIEWING SYSTEM

RetCam

The RetCam has a 3CCD chip video camera (Fig. 1.13). It is lightweight, easy to position and has a long cable for easy patient access. It has five changeable lenses: 130°, 120°, 80°, 30°, and Portrait. It has a large LCD display with 20 seconds of real time video per clip and a frame-by-frame or real time video review. It has a lighted control panel, a dual DVD-RAM for easy back-up, multi-image data recall and display, side by side image comparison, high resolution 24-bit color image, instant-digital image capture and is US FDA approved. It provides a 130° view for easy screening for retinopathy of prematurity (Figs. 1.14 and 1.15), integrated image and patient management capabilities, comprehensive photodocumentation, fluorescein angiography and built-in software for reporting, storage and archiving.

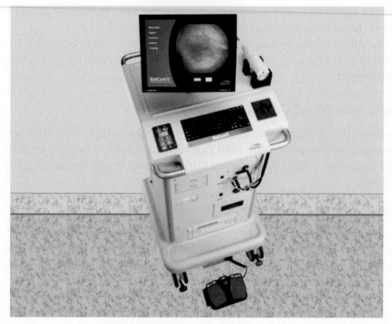

Fig. 1.13: RetCam viewing system.

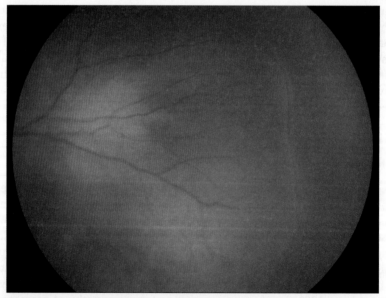

Fig. 1.14: Wide-angle fundus photograph (RetCam) of a premature infant showing retinopathy of prematurity with a demarcation ridge clearly made out.

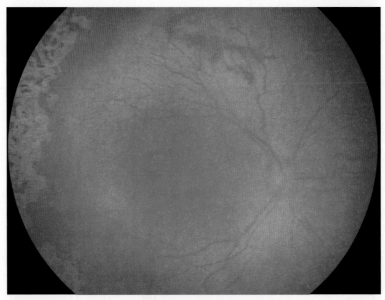

Fig. 1.15: Fundus photograph (RetCam) of a premature infant showing retinopathy of prematurity with laser photocoagulation marks. Preretinal hemorrhage is seen beyond the superotemporal vascular arcade.

Panoret

Panoret (Fig. 1.16) is a high-resolution, wide-angle retinal camera based on an innovative transscleral illumination concept using a fiber optic bundle, where no pupillary dilatation is necessary. Coverage angles are 50° and 100° with interchangeable front lens assembly. It is computer assisted in auto-light, auto-brightness and contrast control, along with auto disk storage. Fundus illumination may, however, be limited in heavily pigmented eyes. DVD recording is possible. DICOM 3.0 connectivity is available for telemedicine.

MII RetCam

Make in India Retinal Camera (MII RetCam) is a fundus imaging device that works on the principle of indirect ophthalmoscopy. However, it works as a fundus camera due to its ability to capture fundus images and record it. The device consists of a slot for a smartphone and a 20D lens (Fig. 1.17). It is specially designed for single-handed operation. This allows the other hand to be utilized either in indentation or to open the patient's eyelids. The device has been designed to fit any smartphone, either Android or IOS provided that the distance between cameras or flash light is close. The MII RetCam device needs a smartphone application (the MII RetCam app) while imaging. MII RetCam app allows the smartphone flashlight to be ON even in the still picture mode.

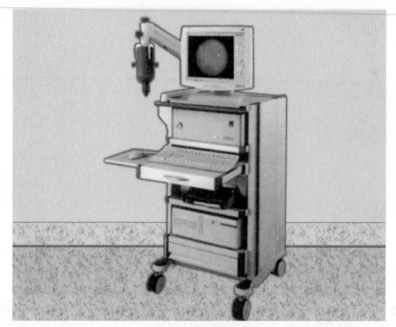

Fig. 1.16: Panoret.

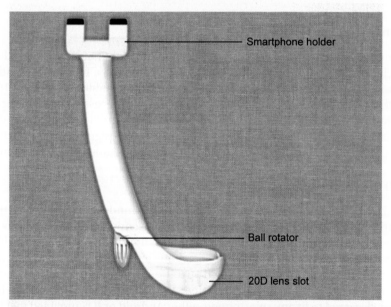

Fig. 1.17: Schematic diagram of MII RetCam with different components.

Furthermore, it allows patient data storage, which can be shared if required. The MII RetCam overcomes the imaging difficulties of traditional fundus cameras such as cost, portability, peripheral imaging, pediatric ocular imaging. The MII

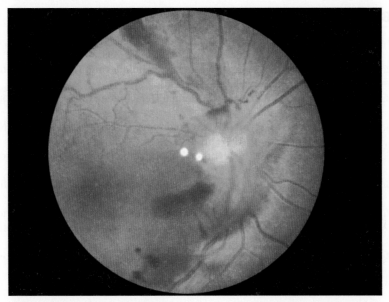

Fig. 1.18: Fundus photograph of the right eye using MII RetCam reveals features of proliferative diabetic retinopathy with considerable detail.

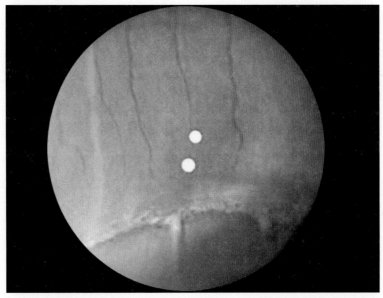

Fig. 1.19: Photograph of peripheral fundus using the MII RetCam reveals features of ora serrata including dentate processes and pars plana.

RetCam can also be utilized in diffuse light for anterior segment imaging. The MII RetCam needs a minimum of 5 mm pupil dilation for good quality images (Figs. 1.18 and 1.19).

BIBLIOGRAPHY

1. Benson WE, Regillo CD. Retinal detachment—Diagnosis and Management, 3rd edition. Philadelphia: Lippincott-Raven; 1998. pp. 75-99.
2. Havener WH, Gloekner S. Atlas of Diagnostic Techniques and Treatment of Retinal Detachment. St Louis: Mosby; 1967. pp. 1-51.
3. Michels RG, Rice TA, Wilkinson CP. Retinal Detachment, 2nd edition. St Louis: Mosby; 1997. pp. 347-70.
4. Regillo CD, Brown GC, Flynn Jr HW. Vitreoretinal Disease—The Essentials. New York: Thieme Publications; 1999. pp. 41-9.
5. Rosenthal ML, Fradin S. The technique of binocular indirect ophthalmoscopy. Highlights Ophthalmol. 1967;9:179-257.
6. Schepens CL, Hartnett ME, Hirose T. Schepens' Retinal Detachment and Allied Diseases, 2nd edition. Boston: Butterworth-Heinemann; 2000. pp. 99-129.
7. Sharma A, Subramaniam SD, Ramachandran KI, et al. Smartphone-based fundus camera device (MII Ret Cam) and technique with ability to image peripheral retina. Eur J Ophthalmol. 2016;26(2):142-4.
8. Yanoff M, Duker JS, Augsburger JJ, et al. Ophthalmology, 2nd edition. St. Louis: Mosby; 2004.

CHAPTER 2

Fundus Fluorescein Angiography

Pradeep Venkatesh

INTRODUCTION

Fluorescein angiography is a dynamic study of the retinochoroidal status following the administration of the dye sodium fluorescein. Despite the advent of several other technologies, fluorescein angiography continues to be the mainstay diagnostic modality to determine the health of the inner and outer blood retinal barriers. Although fluorescein angiography provides valuable additional information, it is not a substitute for meticulous clinical evaluation. The investigation has to be undertaken with specific objectives in mind and never as a test to reveal the cause of an unexplained loss of vision. In almost all cases wherein fluorescein angiography is necessary, the fundus already has changes discernible on ophthalmoscopy.

The retina depends for its survival on two circulations—the choroidal circulation and the central retinal arterial circulation. Fluorescein angiography helps us evaluate the retinal circulation but is unable to reveal the status of the choroidal circulation. Indocyanine green (ICG) angiography is necessary to study the choroidal vasculature.

The outer third of the retina is supplied by choroidal blood flow and the inner two-thirds by retinal blood flow. These two circulations complement each other. The retinal arteriolar vasculature is an end arterial system, and so lacks anastomoses (exception being the cilioretinal artery which is seen in about 20% of the population). The retinal arteriolar rami do not penetrate deeper than the inner nuclear layer and the capillaries have non-fenestrated endothelial cells. The endothelial cell-to-pericyte ratio is 1–2:1. Capillary density is maximum at the macula and absent at the extreme periphery, adjacent to the retinal vessels themselves and within the foveal avascular zone. The inner blood retinal barrier is constituted by the retinal capillary endothelium, and the outer blood retinal barrier is constituted by the retinal pigment epithelium

(RPE)–Bruch's membrane complex. The inner barrier is highly impermeable to passage of solutes and keeps the intravascular component from merging with the extravascular space (however minimal) within the retina. The Bruch's membrane is permeable to the passage of fluorescein dye. The impermeability of the outer blood retinal barrier is due to the tight intercellular junctions, the zonulae occludens, along the apical ends of the retinal pigment epithelial cells. The outer barrier keeps the choroidal compartment separate from the retinal layers.

Another feature of the ocular tissue that has a bearing on the appearance of the fluorescein angiogram is the presence of three important pigments: melanin (absorbs the entire visible wavelength), xanthophyll (absorbs blue wavelength), and hemoglobin (absorbs predominantly green wavelength). Melanin absorbs light rays over the entire visible spectrum. Owing to this absorption characteristics, melanin within the RPE prevents visualization of fluorescein dye that passes out easily through the choriocapillaris. As infrared light is not absorbed, ICG angiography enables visualization of the choroidal vasculature. Xanthophyll is a pigment that is unique to the macular region. Here, it is present within its deeper layers, particularly in the inner fiber of the cones (Henle's layer). Xanthophyll has the property of absorbing blue light and so acts like a blue minus filter. The exciter light used during fluorescein angiography is also blue. Hence, xanthophyll, by absorbing this blue light, contributes to the dark color of the macular region on a normal angiogram. Hemoglobin is the pigment that transports oxygen in the blood and so is usually confined to the intravascular compartment. Abnormally, however, it may reach the extravascular space whenever the vessels rupture from any cause. Hemoglobin has the property of absorbing light maximally at the green end of the visible spectrum. The emitted light by fluorescein sodium is also green. As a result, the concentration of hemoglobin within the bloodstream also has a bearing on the contrast of the angiogram. In fact, it may be near impossible to derive any useful information by undertaking angiography in a patient with severe polycythemia. In addition, blood that is present in the extravascular spaces prevents angiographic visualization of the underlying structures by acting as a physical, opaque barrier to the passage of light.

The permeability of a solute across different membrane barriers in the body is determined by the physiochemical properties of the solute (herein, sodium fluorescein), such as molecular weight, protein binding affinity, etc. and the nature of the junctional complexes (zonulae occludens, macula occludens, and zonulae occludens) across the cellular and acellular barriers. Fluorescein sodium is a xanthene derivative with a molecular weight that is "large" enough (376 kD) to prevent its passage across the tight barriers of the outer and inner blood retinal barriers. It has a high affinity for binding to the plasma proteins, mainly albumin (70–80% is normally protein bound). In addition, it also binds to the erythrocytes. Sodium fluorescein, bound or unbound does not normally pass across both the outer and inner blood retinal barriers. Although binding of fluorescein molecules reduces the amount of free fluorescein available for excitation, it facilitates the separation of the absorption (465 nm) and emission wavelengths (530 nm) by the filters more efficiently. Though mild-to-severe adverse events have been reported during fluorescein angiography, sodium fluorescein is a relatively inert dye. It is highly water soluble and is removed out of the body within 24–48 hours, mainly by the renal route.

PROCEDURE OF FUNDUS FLUORESCEIN ANGIOGRAPHY

As fluorescein angiography is an invasive procedure, written informed consent is mandatory before undertaking the test. Also, ensure that the emergency equipment is readily available in case of need. Inform the patient about why the test is being performed and the need for his cooperation to ensure quality images and information is gathered. The pupil must be well dilated and the patient must be seated comfortably at the fundus camera. At our center we inject 3 mL of sodium fluorescein 20% dye into the antecubital vein (preferred site for intravenous injection) using a 23 G needle (one may also inject the dye through a preplaced venflon or scalp vein). The timer is started as soon as injection of the dye commences; another click (which creates a blank image) is made at the end of the dye injection. This time interval indicates the injection time (ideally between 6 seconds and 8 seconds). To slow an injection creates poor image contrast while too rapid an injection may increase the risk of adverse events like nausea and vomiting. Then take sequential pictures so as to capture adequate frames during each of the four phases of the angiogram (read later). Capturing images every 1–2 seconds during the early phase was recommended during the era of analog fundus imaging (using film roll). In the current era of digital imaging, taking images so frequently is no longer a necessity because one gets real-time feedback about the quality of the image captured. Once the procedure is complete, the patient must be asked to be seated at the waiting area for about half an hour and inform the angiography team in case any rashes or itching develops. This and other adverse events must be managed adequately before releasing the patient from your observation. In case the patient develops significant side effects during the procedure, this must be written clearly in bold letters on the patient records and he/she must be advised to avoid getting the test again.

Fluorescein angiography can be performed using the blue filter on a direct or indirect ophthalmoscope but this method is not efficient and does not allow for documentation of the findings. Hence, the standard method for performing fluorescein angiography is through use of a fundus camera. The fundus camera, other than being able to capture color, red free images, etc. has the ability to capture fluorescein angiographic images because of special filters incorporated into the machine. These filters (a pair of barrier and exciter filters) become introduced into the optical pathway when angiography mode is activated. The exciter filter allows the passage of only blue light (465 nm) corresponding to the maximum absorption characteristics of fluorescein sodium. The barrier filter allows the passage of only green light (525 nm) corresponding to the maximum emission characteristic of the dye (Fig. 2.1). The quality of filters also shows a

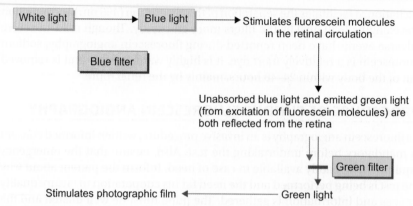

Fig. 2.1: Role of exciter and barrier filter in the optical pathway during fluorescein angiography.

tendency to deteriorate over a period of time. Whenever there is a mismatch or overlap between the exciter and barrier filters, the quality of the angiogram suffers. In fact, the phenomenon of pseudofluorescence results from the camera having a significant overlap of exciter and barrier filters wavelengths. In the non-digital era, analog cameras were used to capture the images and the results were read from film negatives or contact prints. The quality of images captured using analog cameras has superior resolution compared to most digital cameras. Despite this, they are no longer manufactured due to ergonomic reasons. Therefore, all fundus cameras currently in use are digital in nature and capture images using confocal or non-confocal pathways. Most digital cameras allow image capture up to 60°, unless special wide field lenses are used. Optos is a fundus camera that allows 200° ultra-wide field fluorescein angiography without any need for using special lenses.

INDICATIONS

Fluorescein angiography is normally undertaken if it is likely to change the diagnosis, likely to alter the treatment or to assess the progress and response to treatment, and also as a baseline in diseases that may change over a period of time. It is impossible to interpret the progress of a disease or to assess response to treatment by looking a single angiogram. The availability of a color photograph is also very useful for the proper interpretation of a fluorescein angiogram. Before making an attempt at interpretation, it would be prudent to note if the eye and the area on the angiographic pictures matches those of intended study, and whether all the phases of the angiographic study are present.

PHASES OF FUNDUS FLUORESCEIN ANGIOGRAPHY

Although there is a considerable overlap, four phases are recognized during fluorescein angiographic study. These phases are the prefilling, transit,

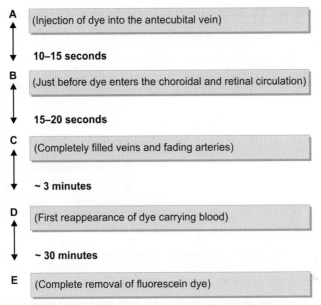

A (Injection of dye into the antecubital vein)

10–15 seconds

B (Just before dye enters the choroidal and retinal circulation)

15–20 seconds

C (Completely filled veins and fading arteries)

~ 3 minutes

D (First reappearance of dye carrying blood)

~ 30 minutes

E (Complete removal of fluorescein dye)

Fig. 2.2: Various phases of fluorescein angiography.

recirculation, and late phases. Each phase appears after an approximate interval following dye injection into the antecubital vein, and each phase has a certain importance as shown in Figure 2.2: In the prefilling phase (interval between A and B) one can recognize autofluorescence and early pseudofluorescence. Transit phase (interval between B and C) encompasses the arterial, arteriovenous (capillary), venous, peak, and late venous phase. The foveal avascular zone is best recognized in the peak phase when fluorescence in the choroidal and retinal vasculature (arteries and veins) is uniform. The staining of tissues is best appreciated in the recirculation phase (C, D) while the late phase (D, E) is important to diagnose angiographic cystoid macular edema and occult choroidal neovascular membranes. Late pseudofluorescence is also detected when present in the last phase of the angiogram.

INTERPRETATION OF FUNDUS FLUORESCEIN ANGIOGRAPHY

On interpretation, the functional integrity of the retinochoroidal layers may be classified into the following categories: normal, variant of normal, and abnormal. An abnormal angiogram may reveal areas of hyperfluorescence, hypofluorescence or a combination of the two (Flowchart 2.1). One must be careful not to interpret artifacts as abnormalities in the retina. For the accurate classification of an angiogram, the early, mid, and late phases must be viewed in sequence. Any attempt at making a diagnosis based on a single frame of the angiographic study may prove to be erroneous. As a generalization, it may be said that on an angiographic picture any "white" lesion is indicative

Flowchart 2.1: Interpretation of fundus fluorescein angiography.

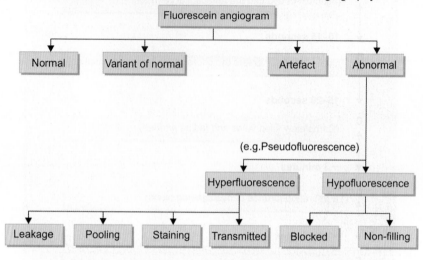

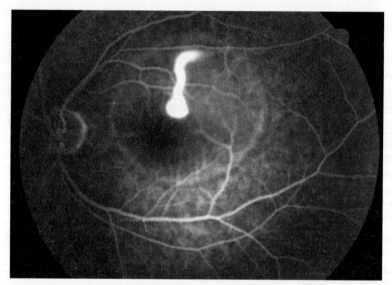

Fig. 2.3: Smoke stack leak in a central serous chorioretinopathy due to a focal defect in the outer blood-retinal barrier.

of hyperfluorescence, and any "dark" lesion, of hypofluorescence. The cause of hyperfluorescence is the leakage of fluorescein dye by a breach in the outer (e.g. central serous retinopathy; Fig. 2.3) and/or inner [e.g. neovascularization on the disk (NVD), neovascularization elsewhere (NVE), vasculitis; Fig. 2.4] blood-retinal barrier. When the hyperfluorescence is frank and increases from

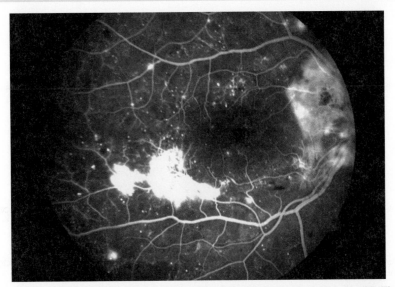

Fig. 2.4: Leakage from new vessels at the disk (NVD) and elsewhere (NVE) on the retina; this is indicative of an immature inner blood-retinal barrier within these abnormal vessels.

the early to the late phase in both size and intensity, it is known as a leakage as in cases of CSR and neovascularization. When the hyperfluorescence increases in intensity and the size remains constant on looking at the various phases, then it is called pooling (e.g. pigment epithelial detachment; Figs. 2.5A and B). Hyperfluorescence that is minimal in the early and midphases, but which becomes marked in the late phases is likely to be due to staining. In some cases (e.g. APMPPE, active choroiditis), a black lesion (hypofluorescent) in the early phases may become a whiter lesion (hyperfluorescent) in the late phases. A mottled hyperfluorescence that appears very early and remains unchanged in the later phases is most likely to be due to a "window defect" which is otherwise called transmitted hyperfluorescence.

A dark lesion (hypofluorescence) that remains constant through all the phases is indicative of a blocked hypofluorescence. A hypofluorescence that is most prominent in the AV phase of the angiogram, and which is associated with the nonfilling of the dye due to a functional or anatomical closure of the retinal vessels is indicative of capillary non-perfusion (Fig. 2.6). It is necessary to note that blocked fluorescence can imply a blocked choroidal background fluorescence or a blocked retinal and choroidal fluorescence. The former is indicative of a subretinal pathology while the latter of a preretinal/sub-hyaloid hemorrhage. The most common cause of blocked fluorescence is a preretinal/subretinal hemorrhage. Rarely, it is caused by pigment epithelial hyperplasia and hypertrophy. Peripheral lesions are best studied using wide-field angiography (Fig. 2.7).

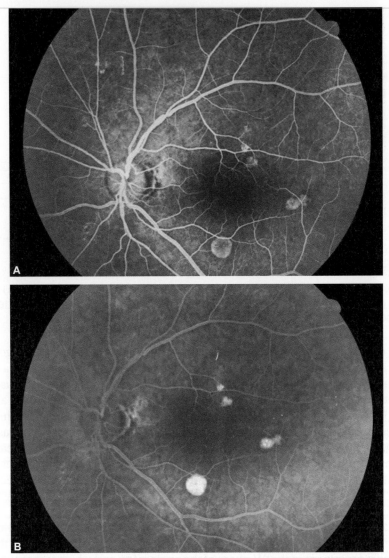

Figs. 2.5A and B: The early and late phases of an angiogram showing focal hyperfluorescence which increases in intensity but not in size; it results from the pooling of dye within the retinal pigment epithelial detachment.

CONCLUSION

In conclusion, it may be said that the interpretation of an angiogram is likely to be more accurate and fruitful if we seek answers to each of the following questions:

1. Is it normal or abnormal? If abnormal,
2. Is the abnormality black or white or mixed?
3. What is the time-characteristics of the abnormality?

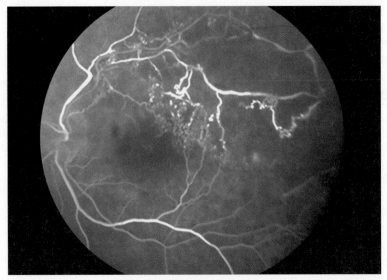

Fig. 2.6: Extensive capillary nonperfusion in the superotemporal retina of a patient with branch-retinal vein occlusion.

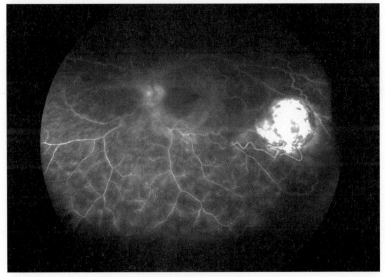

Fig. 2.7: Wide field fluorescein angiographic image of a patient with a vasoproliferative tumor of the retina.

4. Are all the retinal vessels filling normally?
5. What happens to the size of the abnormality in the various phases of the angiogram (constant/increases/decreases)?
6. What happens to the intensity of the color in the late phases compared to the mid and early phases (becomes more white/no change)?

7. How is the distribution of the abnormal fluorescence (patchy/homogenous)?
8. How are the margins of the abnormality, poor or clearly defined?
9. How do answers to the above correlate with the fundus picture?

BIBLIOGRAPHY

1. Rabb MF, Burton TC, Schatz H, et al. Fluorescein angiography of the fundus-a systematic approach to interpretation. Surv Ophthalmol. 1978;28:387-403.
2. Venkatesh P, Garg S, Azad RV. Retinal Imaging. New Delhi: Jaypee Brothers Medical Publishers (P) Ltd; 2008.
3. Venkatesh P, Garg S, Verma L, et al. Step by step fundus fluorescein and Indocyanine green angiography. New Delhi: Jaypee Brothers Medical Publishers (P) Ltd.; 2007.

CHAPTER 3

Indocyanine Green Angiography

Rajesh Ramanjulu, Mahesh Shanmugam, Pradeep Sagar BK

INTRODUCTION

Indocyanine green angiography (ICGA) allows the study of choroidal circulation and hence is specifically suited for studying sub-retinal pigment epithelial (RPE) diseases, such as occult choroidal neovascularization, idiopathic polypoidal choroidal vasculopathy (IPCV), and retinal central serous chorioretinopathy (CSC).

HISTORY

The entry of ICG into medicine came about in the mid-1950s. Irwin Fox, who was in search of a biocompatible dye that could be detected in blood, was the first to recognize the dye at Eastman Kodak laboratories. ICG exhibited sharply defined peak absorption of near-infrared light at 805 nm; this is the same wavelength at which the optical densities of oxygenated and reduced hemoglobin in blood are approximately equal. This relationship made it possible to measure ICG concentration in blood in terms of its optical density at 805 nm, regardless of oxygen saturation.

As the dye was unstable in aqueous solution, it was referred to Hynson Westcott and Dunning, a small Baltimore pharmaceutical company, for development into the stable lyophilized form that remains in use today.

The first medical use of ICG was in 1956 in cardiology for measuring the time-varying dilution of ICG in whole blood. From this, cardiac output could be determined and valvular septal defects could be characterized. The dye is excreted exclusively by the liver and this subsequently led to its application for measuring hepatic function and blood flow.

The first attempt at using ICG for angiography was made by Kogure et al. when they demonstrated the infrared absorption angiography of the canine brain vasculature. In 1971, Bernie Hochheimer demonstrated in cats that the infrared absorption angiography method could be simplified. He illuminated the fundus with a narrow band of near-infrared wavelengths and used Kodak high-speed infrared black and white films. Importantly, the ICG dye in the vessels could be imaged after filtering light from a standard fundus camera. This suggested that the technique might be used in human subjects. It took considerable effort to produce the first intravenously injected ICG fluorescence angiogram image in 1972. This was the first-ever published human ICG fluorescence angiogram.

Indocyanine green is a tricarbocyanine dye with both hydrophilic and lipophilic properties.[1] The empirical formula of ICG is $C_{43}H_{47}N_2NaO_6S_2$. The molecular weight is 775 D. When dissolved in saline solution, ICG tends to form polymers if the solution concentration is high; and, monomers, if the concentration is low. For this reason, the dye is dissolved in water for intravenous injections. ICG is stimulated with near-infrared wavelength light at 810 nm, and the emission spectrum is at 830 nm. The ICG molecule can be considered active at a wavelength between 790 nm and 830 nm.

Following intravenous administration, ICG binds to blood lipoproteins (fundamentally phospholipids) in a proportion that can reach 98%.[2-4] The emitted fluorescence intensity increases as a result of such binding. ICG is weakly fluorescent and exhibits only 4% of the fluorescence exhibited by fluorescein angiography. Elimination takes place in the liver, with secretion in the bile.

The ICG molecule has biophysical properties that make it useful for visualizing the choroidal circulation. The dye is excited by light close to infrared (longer operating wavelength), thereby increasing its ability to fluoresce better through pigment, fluid, lipid, and hemorrhage than fluorescein dye. ICG circulates almost entirely bound to plasma proteins, and gradually diffuses across the choriocapillaris; this retention of ICG in the choroidal circulation, coupled with low permeability, allows better visualization of the choroidal circulation. These properties make it possible to visualize choroidal neovascularization beneath blood layers, exudates or retinal pigment epithelial detachments (PEDs)[5,6] by differentiating (in the latter case) between the hypofluorescent serous component and the hyperfluorescent vascular component.

Indocyanine green is also useful in delineating the abnormal aneurysmal outpouchings of the inner choroidal vascular network seen in IPCV and the focal areas of choroidal hyperpermeability in central serous chorioretinopathy. It is an additional aid in differentiating abnormal vasculature in intraocular tumors, and in distinguishing the abnormal fluorescence patterns seen in choroidal inflammatory conditions such as serpiginous choroidopathy, acute multifocal placoid pigment epitheliopathy (AMPPE), to mention a few.

PHASES OF INDOCYANINE GREEN ANGIOGRAPHY

Indocyanine green angiography is typically divided into three phases—the arterial (initial dye filling pattern), venous phase and late stage:

1. *Arterial phase*: Choroidal hyperfluorescence usually begins in the subfoveal region and progresses in a radial fashion towards the periphery. A vertical watershed passing through the disk is well defined in this phase.
2. *Venous phase*: Choroidal veins become delineated in ICGA by 15–20 seconds after the injection of the dye. Approximately 25% of the individuals demonstrate a classic horizontal watershed area passing through the disk and fovea. The draining veins are arranged in a symmetrical fashion and divided into upper and lower beds, thus defining the watershed level (Fig. 3.1). An interesting fact is that 75% of the venous drainage is preferential for ST area and the remaining 25% in the IT and SN areas.
3. *Late phase*: ICG images several minutes into the late phases do not change much. The ability to discern choroidal vessels decreases with extravasation of dye, dye dilution and its clearance.

The ICG dye disappears from the circulation quickly and its retention rate at 15 minutes is less than 10%. Late phase ICGA pictures are obtained 15–20 minutes later, the persistence of the dye shows anomalous vasculature.

ADVERSE REACTIONS

Adverse reactions are similar to those observed with fluorescein, but are less frequent.[1] The dye should not be used in patients with shellfish or iodine allergies, liver disease, and end-stage renal disease. No studies in animal models have been made regarding the use of the dye in pregnancy. However, current practice patterns regarding the use of ICG angiography in pregnant patients may be unnecessarily restrictive.[7]

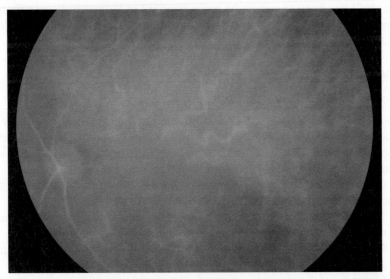

Fig. 3.1: One of early phases in indocyanine green angiography (ICGA) showing horizontal watershed demarcation, bisecting the disk and running along the macular area.

APPLICATIONS IN OPHTHALMOLOGY

Let us consider the advantages of ICG angiography over fluorescein angiography before discussing its clinical application:

- *Hazy media*: ICGA can be performed in conditions where the media preclude fundus fluorescein angiography (FFA). This is due to the Rayleigh scatter (A phenomenon seen when the scattering particles are smaller than the incident wavelengths, scatter intensity being larger or shorter wavelengths).
- Indocyanine green angiography can be performed even in the presence of vitreous hemorrhage, due to the phenomenon of Mie or forward scatter.
- Infrared light used is barely visible and so photophobic patients tolerate it.
- It measures the occult choroidal neovascular membrane (CNVM) more precisely as compared to FFA, which might under/overestimate.

DIAGNOSTICS APPLICATIONS

Nonexudative (Dry) Age-related Macular Degeneration

Indocyanine green angiography has been used to facilitate the diagnosis of basal laminar drusen and the associated subretinal deposits, and to differentiate them from reticular pseudodrusen. However, ICGA is not routinely used to study dry age-related macular degeneration (AMD) except in cases of drusenoid PED to confirm the absence of CNV.

Recently, ICGA has been reported to be useful for evaluating the atrophic areas present in Stargardt disease, in comparison with the atrophy of dry AMD.[8] The hypofluorescence evidenced by ICGA in the atrophic areas ("dark atrophy") has been shown to be more frequent in Stargardt disease than in atrophic AMD, suggesting a possible selective damage of the choriocapillaris in Stargardt disease.

Exudative (Wet) Age-related Macular Degeneration

Classic Choroidal Neovascularization

Classic CNV or type II CNVM is clearly defined by fluorescein angiography.[9,10] ICGA does not offer relevant supplementary information unless associated large PED/occult CNV is present. A classic CNVM may be seen much less distinctly in ICGA as compared with FFA (Figs. 3.2A to D).

Occult CNVMs (Type 1—beneath the RPE) demonstrate one of the following features on ICG angiography:

- Hot spot (<1 disk diameter area)—a well-defined leakage increasing in its size and intensity into the later phases
- Plaque (>1 disk diameter area)—a leakage with borders partly obscured and or ill defined.
- Mixture—of the above two patterns in a single or contiguous lesion.

Plaque was found to be the most common type (61% of the cases) and had a poor visual prognosis, whereas the focal spots or "hotspots" (29%) had a better

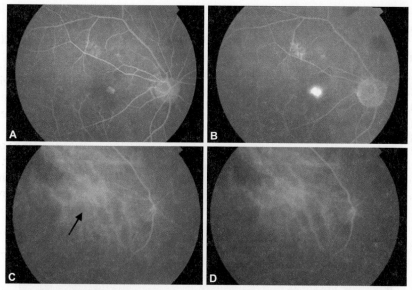

Figs. 3.2A to D: (A and B) Fundus fluorescein angiography (FFA) shows defined hyperfluorescent lesion increasing in intensity and size in the later phases stage of classic choroidal neovascular membrane (CNVM). (C and D) Indocyanine green angiography (ICGA) in this condition shows the same leakage area and so does not add much to our knowledge.

prognosis, and they were considered to be potentially treatable by ICG-guided laser photocoagulation.[11,12]

The term "occult" refers to a type of CNV that is difficult to visualize, analyze, and localize on FA.[13] The fundamental advantage of ICGA is that it allows early detection and localization of occult CNV.

Occult CNV can be grouped into two main types:

1. *Occult CNV without serous PED*: Fibrovascular PED (fibrovascular pigment epithelium detachment with irregular and poorly demarcated hyperfluorescence on FFA) (Figs. 3.3A to D). FA shows irregular and poorly delimited hyperfluorescence with late phase ill-defined leakage. This complemented with the OCT is sufficient in confirming the diagnosis and evaluating its activity.

2. *Occult CNV associated with serous PED*: Serous PED may be avascular or vascular, and fluorescein angiography fails to delineate the area of the underlying neovascular complex. This is primarily due to the hyperfluorescence of the PED, which masks the underlying CNV complex (Figs. 3.4A to D). When ICGA is used, the PED appears as a hypofluorescent lesion in all phases of the angiogram. In rare situations, it may appear iso- or at minimum hyperfluorescent in comparison to its surrounding and the underlying CNVM complex can be discerned as a hotspot or a plaque.

A type III variant, more popularly termed as RAP (retinal angiomatous proliferation) was identified by Yannuzzi et al. (2001).[14,15]

On the basis of the FA, RAP mimics the angiographic signature of the occult or minimally classic CNV and not typically of a vascularized PED.[16]

Some groups have described five different patterns of ICG angiograms in RAP, during the transit phase of high-speed ICG.[17] These are:

1. Focal hyperfluorescence (Figs. 3.5A to F)
2. Irregular hyperfluorescence
3. Circular hyperfluorescence (Figs. 3.6A to E)
4. Multifocal hyperfluorescence, and
5. Combined hyperfluorescence

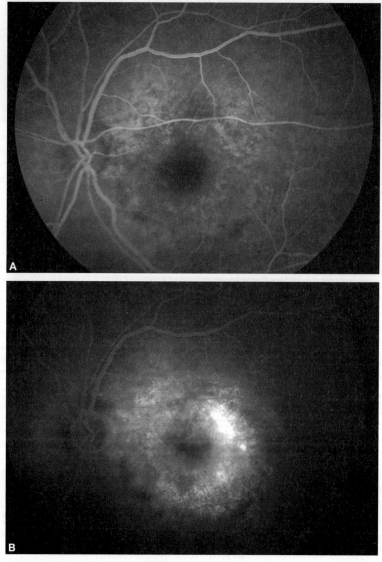

Figs. 3.3A and B

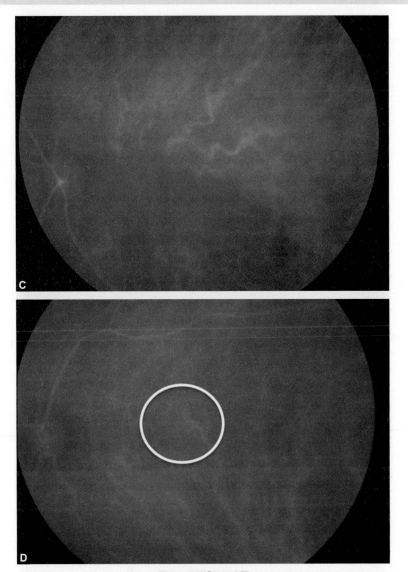

Figs. 3.3C and D

Figs. 3.3A to D: (A and B) Fundus fluorescein angiography (FFA) shows late leakage of undetermined source with a pigment epithelium detachment (PED) (fibrovascular). (C and D) Indocyanine green angiography (ICGA) shows a plaque leakage at the site of stippled leakage (on FFA).

POLYPOIDAL CHOROIDAL VASCULOPATHY

Polypoidal choroidal vasculopathy is a primary abnormality of the choroidal circulation characterized by an inner choroidal vascular network of vessels ending in an aneurysmal bulge or outward projection. Clinically, it is visible as a reddish-orange, spheroid and polyp-like structure.[18] The disorder is

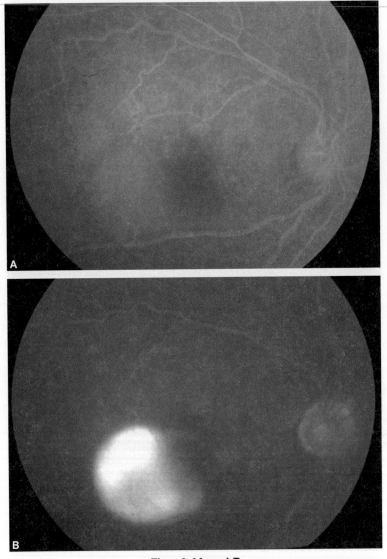

Figs. 3.4A and B

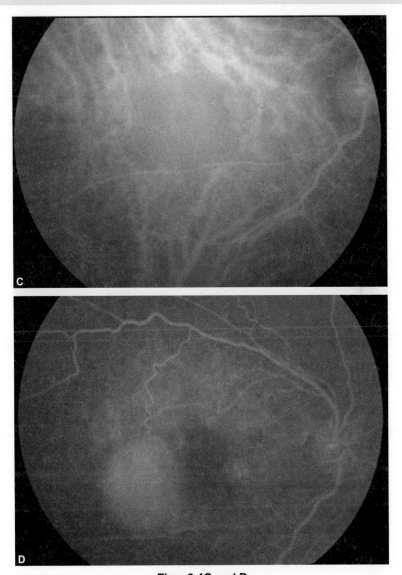

Figs. 3.4C and D

Figs. 3.4A to D: (A and B) Fundus fluorescein angiography (FFA) images of pigment epithelium detachment (PED). There is early hyperfluorescence which increases in intensity in later phases. (C and D) Indocyanine green angiography (ICGA) images of the same PED. Appears hypo in the early and late phases without any activity in the choroid. Thus ICGA helps us in showing the presence/absence of choroidal abnormality.

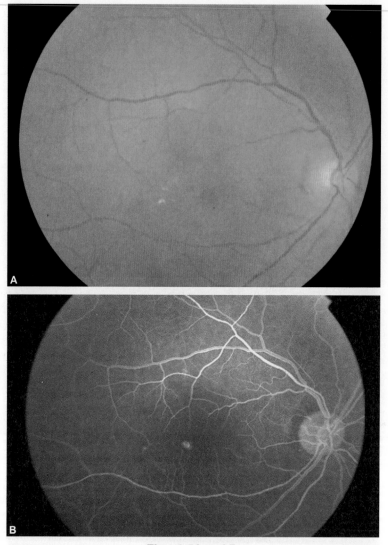

Figs. 3.5A and B

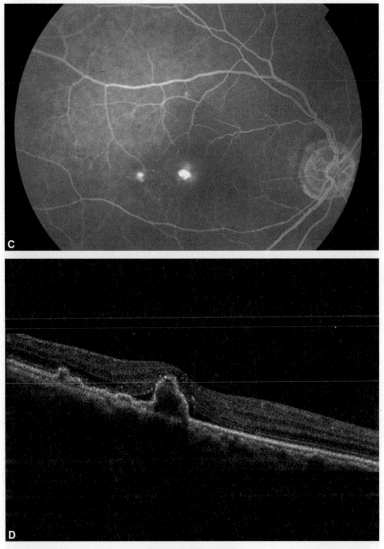

Figs. 3.5C and D

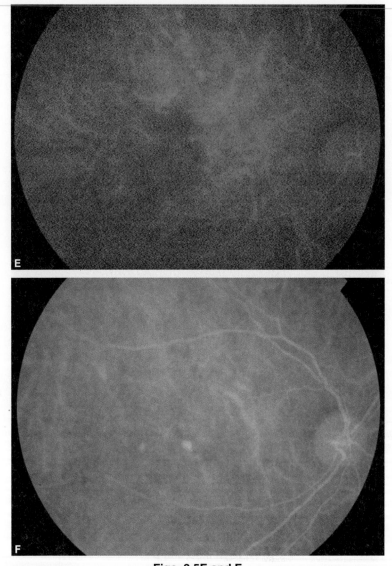

Figs. 3.5E and F

Figs. 3.5A to F: (A to C) CP and fundus fluorescein angiography (FFA) of a patient with retinal angiomatous proliferation (RAP). Early hyperfluorescence, as early as the beginning of the arterial phase with leakage in later phases stage of RAP. (D) OCT shows PED, intraretinal fluid and exudates. (E and F) Indocyanine green angiography (ICGA) corresponds to the finding of RAP and further confirming the diagnosis.

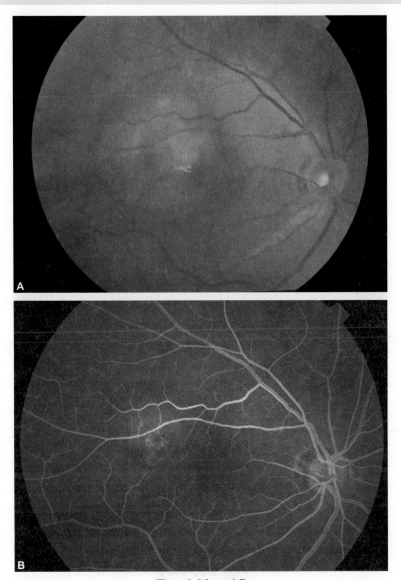

Figs. 3.6A and B

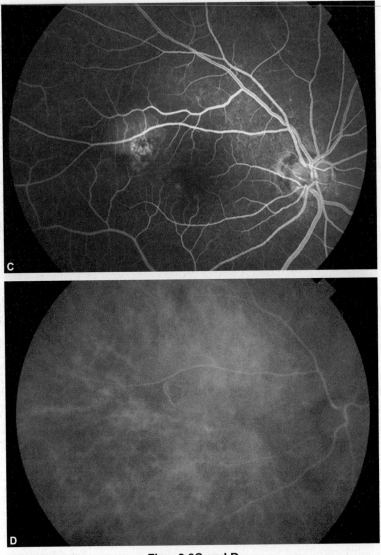

Figs. 3.6C and D

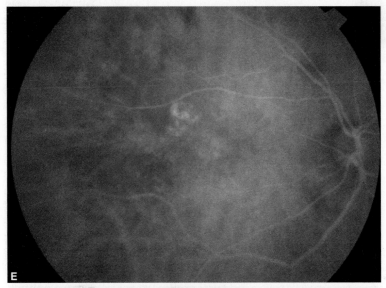

Fig. 3.6E

Figs. 3.6A to E: (A to C) A retino-retinal anastomosis well demonstrated on the ICGA. (D and E) Thereby diagnosing the condition as retinal angiomatous proliferation (RAP).

associated with multiple, recurrent, serosanguineous detachments of the RPE and neurosensory retina, secondary to leakage and bleeding from the peculiar choroidal vascular abnormality.[19] Although FA, sometimes, can establish the diagnosis of PCV when the vascular elements are large and located beneath atrophic RPE, ICG angiography is the first choice for imaging this entity. It can detect and characterize the polyps or the branching vascular network with enhanced sensitivity and specificity.[19,20]

The early phase of ICG angiogram shows a distinct network of vessels within the choroid, which are usually prominent in their size in comparison to the surrounding choroidal vessels. Shortly after the network is identified, small hyperfluorescent polyps become visible within the choroid (Figs. 3.7A to D). These polypoidal structures may correspond to the reddish-orange choroidal excrescence seen clinically, but the clinical examination typically does not show all the polyps, whereas the ICGA does. In the later phase of the angiogram, there is a uniform disappearance of the dye ("washout") from the bulging polypoidal lesions. The particular late ICG staining of occult CNV is not seen in the PCV.[19]

Indocyanine green angiography has led to the early discovery of polyps in the peripapillary, the macular and the extramacular areas.[21] Identification of the polyps would allow treatment with laser photocoagulation if extrafoveal, and with photodynamic therapy (PDT) or anti-VEGF agents.

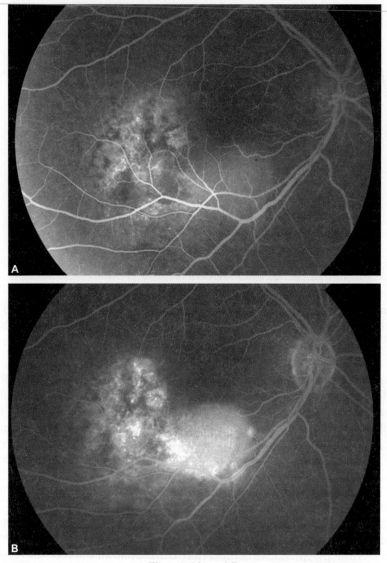

Figs. 3.7A and B

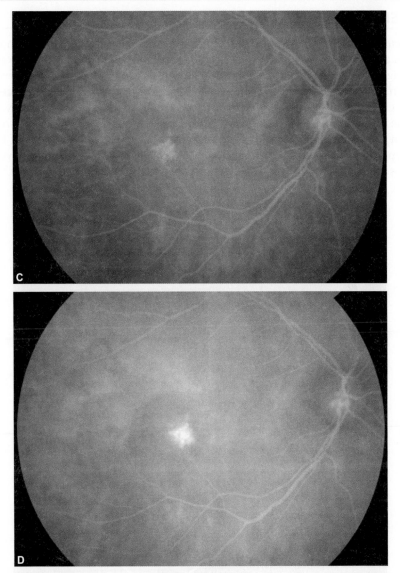

Figs. 3.7C and D

Figs. 3.7A to D: (A and B) Fundus fluorescein angiography (FFA) images demonstrating mottled hyperfluorescence with a large subfoveal pigment epithelium detachment (PED). FFA fails to recognize the etiology of the underlying leakage. (C and D) Indocyanine green angiography (ICGA), on the other hand, easily demonstrates a bunch of polyps confirming the diagnosis of polypoidal choroidal vasculopathy (PCV).

CENTRAL SEROUS CHORIORETINOPATHY

Acute phase: The leaking point of central serous chorioretinopathy seen on FA appears as a localized hypofluorescent area around the point of leakage (Figs. 3.8A to D). These hypofluorescent areas are continuously observed throughout dye passage. In these regions, biomicroscopy and fluorescein angiography showed no abnormalities such as RPE detachment or atrophy. In the late phase ICG angiogram (when the intravascular dye had been washed out), abnormal choroidal hyperfluorescence may be seen. The sizes of the hyperfluorescent areas can range from 0.5 to 3.0 disk diameters and they were observed surrounding the leakage point seen in fluorescein angiography.[22]

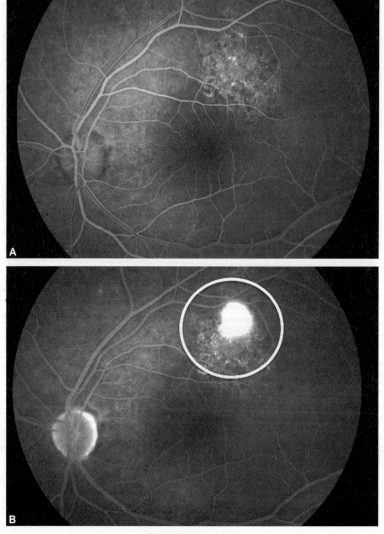

Figs. 3.8A and B

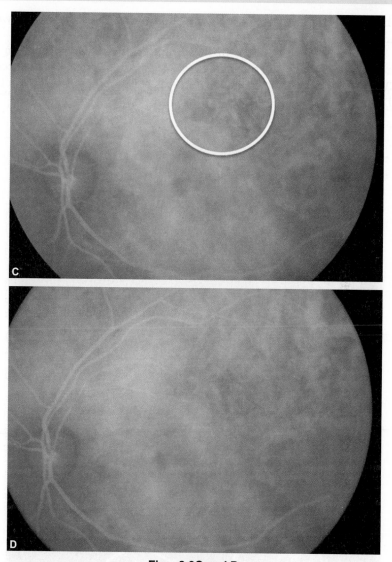

Figs. 3.8C and D

Figs. 3.8A to D: (A and B) Acute on chronic central serous chorioretinopathy (CSC). Fundus fluorescein angiography (FFA) images in the early phase shows window defects corresponding to the retinal pigment epithelial (RPE) changes in the chronic CSC. A hyperfluorescent spot shows up a bit late and increases in size and intensity showing leakage. (C and D) Viewed on indocyanine green angiography (ICGA) shows epicentral hypo and surrounding hyper and much larger areas of RPE alteration missed out on FFA.

Chronic phase: In patients with a long-standing disease, when choroidal hyperfluorescence fades, hypofluorescent spots became increasingly evident, revealing pigment epithelial alterations not shown by fluorescein angiography. RPE atrophic tracts can be well visualized and appear hyperfluorescent in cases with minimal amount of RPE atrophy and more hypofluorescent in cases with marked RPE atrophy (Figs. 3.9A to D).

Another great advantage of ICG angiography is the detection of concomitant/complicated secondary CNVM. A distinct leakage of the occult CNVM can be easily detected among the focal leakage point of the CSC or the PED.

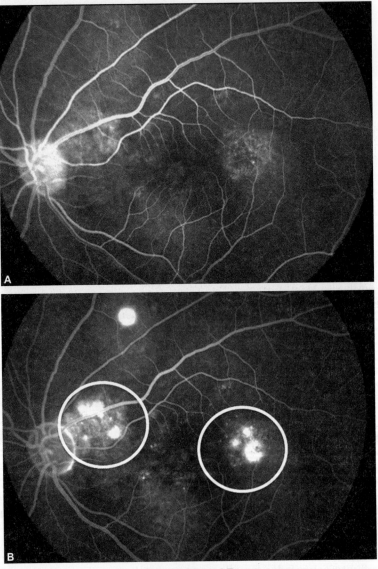

Figs. 3.9A and B

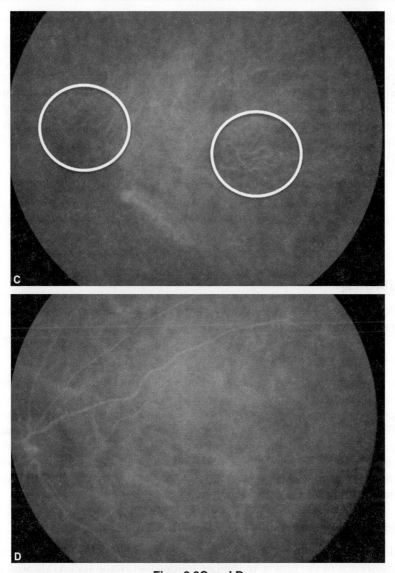

Figs. 3.9C and D

Figs. 3.9A to D: (A and B) Fundus fluorescein angiography (FFA) images of the LE, in the early and late phases in a patient with multifocal chronic central serous chorioretinopathy (CSC). The circled areas show epicenters of leakage. Indocyanine green angiography (ICGA) reveals interesting points as enumerated in the text. Early phases show hypofluorescence in the epicenter of the leakage (marked with the circles) with mild hyperfluorescence in the surrounding area. In the later phases, it achieves a ground glass appearance.

INFLAMMATORY LESIONS OF THE CHOROID

The most common finding on FA that corresponds to areas of active choroiditis is of early hypofluorescence with late hyperfluorescence; whereas in ICGA, they appear as hypofluorescent spots showing more extensive areas of involvement than seen on FA. In inflammatory disorders less information is obtained from the analysis of early phases as against the altered pattern of filling in intermediate and late phases of the ICGA. ICG angiography per se provides very limited information about the activity of the disease and to interpret the ICGA images, clinical and FA correlation is very essential.

To mention a few lesions and their ICGA findings:
- *Serpiginous choroiditis*: Hypofluorescent dots in all phases
- *Multifocal choroiditis*: Large irregular spots of hypofluorescence and many more in number as compared to those seen in FFA. Late homogeneous background fluorescence.
- *APMPPE*: Well-demarcated, hypofluorescent lesions in all phases.

TUMORS

Indocyanine green angiography has been described in four basic lesions of the choroid.

Melanoma and Nevus

The patterns of ICG videoangiography are varied, depending on the degree of tumor pigmentation, thickness, and vascularity. Pigmented melanoma shows hypofluorescence in the early phases, while the less pigmented ones may demonstrate even the intrinsic choroidal vasculature. Late phase angiograms usually show mild hyperfluorescence due to the leakage from underlying vessels. Rarely, a three-ring pattern can be appreciated in some melanomas during the later phases: a central region of dense hypofluorescence, a ring of mild hyperfluorescence, and a peripheral ring of hypofluorescence.[23]

Choroidal Metastasis

Indocyanine green angiography shows a pattern of subtle diffuse homogeneous fluorescence of the tumor. In the late frames metastatic lesions showed ill-defined isofluorescence without hyperfluorescence, and in the late frames they were hypofluorescent overall.[24]

Choroidal Hemangioma

A lacy diffuse hyperintense pattern with a filling of the peripheral portion of the hemangioma first, and then the central portion as imaged with rapid sequence photography is observed in ICGA. The normal choroidal pattern is obscured by the vascular channels of the tumor. The fluorescence clears at variable rates leaving traces of fluorescence in the vascular channels giving the silhouettes of the vascular channels.[24]

Choroidal Osteoma

As one can anticipate, it shows an overall hypofluorescence as compared to the surrounding choroid.[24]

THERAPEUTIC APPLICATION

- Indocyanine green angiography with the confocal SLO, capturing at the rate of 10 frames per second can identify choroidal feeder vessels supplying CNVM. A laser treatment to such extrafoveal feeder vessels, particularly in membranes that are large or subfoveal, may be effective in closing the feeder vessel and CNVM with the preservation of the fovea and central vision.[25]
- Indocyanine green enhances the efficacy of transpupillary thermotherapy (TTT), as the peak absorption spectrum of ICG is the same as the peak emission of the diode laser. This allows selective ablation of the chorioretinal lesions using ICG-augmented TTT. ICG-enhanced TTT to effectively treat retinoblastoma refractory to conventional focal treatments without deleterious ocular side effects has been reported.[26]

CONCLUSION

Indocyanine green angiography allows visualization of choroidal vascular pathology, being particularly useful in the diagnosis of polypoidal choroidal vasculopathy and occult CNVMs. It has helped in expanding the knowledge of certain disease such as CSC, wherein ICGA shows more extensive choroidal vascular pathology than what can be seen on FA. ICGA is seldom seen in isolation but along with FA, and currently the OCT. It also aids in selectively identifying and treating the feeder vessels of resistant CNVM.

REFERENCES

1. Hope-Ross M, Yannuzzi LA, Gragoudas ES, et al. Adverse reactions due to indocyanine green. Ophthalmology. 1994;101:529-33.
2. Cherrick GR, Stein SW, Leevy CM, et al. Indocyanine green: observations on its physical properties, plasma decay, and hepatic extraction. J Clin Invest. 1960;39:592-600.
3. Baker KJ. Binding of sulfobromophthalein (BSP) sodium and indocyanine green (ICG) by plasma alpha-1 lipoproteins. Proc Soc Exp Biol Med. 1966;122(4):957-63.
4. Brown N, Strong R. Infrared fundus angiography. Br J Ophthalmol. 1973;57(10):797-802.
5. Guyer DR, Yannuzzi LA. Occult choroidal neovascularization. In: Yannuzzi LA, Flower RW, Slakter JS (Eds). Indocyanine green angiography. St. Louis, Missouri: Mosby; 1997. pp. 157-80.
6. Guyer DR, Puliafito CA, Mones JM, et al. Digital indocyanine-green angiography in chorioretinal disorders. Ophthalmology. 1992;99(2):287-91.
7. Fineman MS, Maguire JI, Fineman SW, et al. Safety of indocyanine green angiography during pregnancy. Arch Ophthalmol. 2001;119:353-5.

8. Giani A, Pellegrini M, Carini E, et al. The dark atrophy with indocyanine green angiography in Stargardt disease. Invest Ophthalmol Vis Sci. 2012;53(7):3999-4004.

9. Hoang QV, Gallego-Pinazo R, Yannuzzi LA. Long-term follow-up of acute zonal occult outer retinopathy. Retina. 2013;33(7):1325-7.

10. Sorenson JA, Yannuzzi LA, Slakter JS, et al. A pilot study of digital indocyanine green videoangiography for recurrent occult choroidal neovascularization in age-related macular degeneration. Arch Ophthalmol. 1994;112(4):473-9.

11. Guyer DR, Yannuzzi LA, Slakter JS, et al. Classification of choroidal neovascularizaton by digital indocyanine green videoangiography. Ophthalmology. 1996;103:2054-60.

12. Guyer DR, Yannuzzi LA, Ladas I, et al. Indocyanine green-guided laser photocoagulation of focal spots at the edge of plaques of choroidal neovascularization. Arch Ophthalmol. 1996;114:693-7.

13. Coscas G. Age-related Macular Degeneration. In: Coscas G (Ed). Atlas of indocyanine green angiography fluorescein angiography, ICG angiography and OCT correlations. Philadelphia: Elsevier; 2005. pp. 118.

14. Yannuzzi LA, Freund KB, Takahashi BS. Review of retinal angiomatous proliferation or type 3 neovascularization. Retina. 2008;28 (3):375-84.

15. Gass JD. Serous retinal pigment epithelial detachment with a notch. A sign of occult choroidal neovascularization. Retina. 1984;4:205-20.

16. Rouvas AA, Papakostas TD, Ntouraki A, et al. Angiographic and OCT features of retinal angiomatous proliferation. Eye (Lond). 2010;24(11):1633-42.

17. Yannuzzi LA, Sorenson JS, Spaide RF, et al. Idiopathic polypoidal choroidal vasculopathy. Retina. 1990;10:1-8.

18. Spaide RF, Yannuzzi LA, Slakter JS, et al. Indocyanine green videoangiography of idiopathic polypoidal choroidal vasculopathy. Retina. 1995;15:100-10.

19. Yannuzzi LA, Ciardella AP, Spaide RF, et al. The expanding clinical spectrum of idiopathic polypoidal choroidal vasculopathy. Arch Ophthalmol. 1999;115:478-85.

20. Yannuzzi LA, Wong DW, Sforzolini BS, et al. Polypoidal choroidal vasculopathy and neovascularized age-related macular degeneration. Arch Ophthalmol. 1999;117:1503-10.

21. Yannuzzi LA, Nogueira FB, Spaide RF, et al. Idiopathic polypoidal choroidal vasculopathy: A peripheral lesion. Arch Ophthalmol. 1998;116:382-3.

22. Kitaya N, Nagaoka T, Hikichi T, et al. Features of abnormal choroidal circulation in central serous chorioretinopathy. Br J Ophthalmol. 2003;87(6):709-12.

23. Atmaca LS, Lu FB, Atmaca P. Fluorescein and indocyanine green videoangiography of choroidal melanomas. Jpn J Ophthalmol. 1999;43:25-30.

24. Shields CL, Shields JA, De Potter P. Patterns of indocyanine green videoangiography of choroidal tumours. Br J Ophthalmol. 1995;79:237-45.

25. Lee WK, Kim HK. Feeder vessel laser photocoagulation of subfoveal choroidal neovascularization. Korean J Ophthalmol. 2000;14(2):60-8.

26. Francis JH, Abramson DH, Brodie SE, et al. Indocyanine green enhanced transpupillary thermotherapy in combination with ophthalmic artery chemosurgery for retinoblastoma. Br J Ophthalmol. 2013;97(2):164-8.

CHAPTER 4

Fundus Autofluorescence: Overview and Applications in Retinal Practice

Anand Rajendran, Vinay PG, Vishal MY

INTRODUCTION

The phenomenon of autofluorescence, emanating from the lipofuscin-laden retinal pigment epithelium (RPE) cells has been known and studied for a few decades now. In the RPE, lipofuscin originates chiefly from phagocytosed photoreceptor outer segments (OS), whereas in many other cell types, it originates internally through autodigestion.[1,2] Phagocytosis of the tips of the photoreceptor outer segments, and their subsequent lysosomal digestion is one of the key functions of the RPE.[1-3] Although, the digestion of these outer segments is nearly complete, a miniscule portion remains undigested—the lipofuscin. The aggregation of fluorescent material in the RPE reflects the level of metabolic activity, which is largely determined by the quantity of photoreceptor OS renewal. Above the age of 70, about 20–33% of the cytoplasmic volume may be constituted by lipofuscin and melanofuscin granules.

The AF imaging is, essentially, a topographic "metabolic mapping" of the lipofuscin in the RPE and other fluorophores in the outer retina and subretinal space. This retinal autofluorescence is understood to reflect a balance between the accumulation and removal of lipofuscin in the RPE. The lipofuscin in the RPE cells is extraordinary, as this is largely formed as a result of the light energy trapping function of the retina. The lipofuscin is most concentrated in the RPE of the central retina, the area having the largest concentration of visual pigment as well as receiving the highest amount of light. These retinoid-derived fluorophores have an exhaustive system of conjugated double bonds which explains the long wavelength fluorescence emission from the lipofuscin.[4]

DEMONSTRATION OF FUNDUS AUTOFLUORESCENCE

Vitreous fluorophotometry gave us the first *in vivo* evidence of fundus autofluorescence (FAF). A distinct "retinal" peak was noted in the preinjection scans, whose magnitude increased with age, in keeping with the known properties of lipofuscin fluorescence.[5,6] These studies led to the development of a fundus spectrofluorometer,[7,8] created to evaluate, specifically, the excitation and emission spectra of the autofluorescence from small retinal foci (2° diameter) of the fundus and to permit absolute measurements of the emanated fluorescence.

FUNDUS AUTOFLUORESCENCE IMAGING MODALITIES

The Confocal Scanning Laser Ophthalmoscope

Although originally developed by Webb et al., it was in 1995 that von Ruckmann et al. first described FAF imaging with the confocal scanning laser ophthalmoscope (cSLO).[9,10]

The FAF signal has, compared to fundus reflectance or fluorescence angiography, a very low intensity. In order to enhance image contrast and reduce background noise, several single FAF images are recorded in series.[9,11-14] The mean image (of 4–16 frames) is then calculated, and the pixel values are normalized. The high rate of up to 16 frames per second and the high sensitivity of the cSLO allows FAF imaging to be recorded in rapidly and at minimal excitation energies.[15]

Three different cSLO systems have thus far been developed for creating FAF images: Heidelberg Retina Angiograph (HRA classic, HRA 2, and Spectralis HRA, Heidelberg Engineering, Heidelberg, Germany], Rodenstock cSLO (RcSLO; Rodenstock, Weco, Dusseldorf, Germany), and Zeiss prototype SM 30 4024 (ZcSLO; Zeiss, Oberkochen, Germany). Only the former is commercially available. These instruments use an excitation wavelength of 488 nm generated by an argon or solid-state laser for FAF imaging.

An additional development of the cSLO [Spectralis HRA + optical coherence tomography (OCT), Heidelberg Engineering, Heidelberg, Germany] is combination with spectral-domain OCT in the same instrument. This permits simultaneous cSLO and OCT recordings. With the cSLO system, any lateral eye movement can be detected in real time and input into the scanning system of the OCT modality, facilitating a very accurate registration of the OCT A-scans.

Another key feature is that, with the use of any of the cSLO imaging modes (reflectance, FAF, or angiography) as the reference image, retinal locations on the fundus image can be mapped to cross-sectional OCT findings with precision. The extremely high resolution of these images is like "optical biopsies" of the retina.

The Fundus Camera

The lipofuscin can be stimulated, by direct illumination, to fluoresce and has a wide emission band ranging from about 500 nm to 750 nm.[16] However, other structures in the eye in front of the retina also fluoresce, the crystalline lens being one of the foremost. In order to obtain clear and good quality autofluorescence images, the instrument has to be able to either reject or circumvent the fluorescence from the lens.

Scanning laser ophthalmoscopes have a confocal capability in which only the conjugate points on the fundus are imaged. Points not lying on the conjugate planes are rejected. This allows cSLOs to use excitation and barrier wavelengths similar to those used in fluorescein angiography to obtain autofluorescence photographs.

While the initial camera-based systems were restricted by lower contrast and narrower fields of view, the next generations involved shifting the excitation and emission wavelengths towards the red end of the spectrum to preclude autofluorescence from lens.[17,18] Image quality was enhanced using a new set of filters. A band-pass filter centered at about 580 nm for excitation and another centered at about 695 nm as a barrier filter were used. The nuclear sclerosis of the lens does not attenuate these. Additionally, as the lens fluorescence occurs with wavelengths shorter than the upper cutoff of the barrier filter, lens autofluorescence rarely is a problem with moderate degrees of nuclear sclerosis. The limitations of this system for autofluorescence include all those associated with a typical fundus camera especially, for patients with small pupils.

Differences between the Autofluorescence Images Taken with a cSLO and a Fundus Camera

The wavelengths used with the commercially available cSLO are absorbed more by blood as compared to the wavelengths in the modified fundus camera. This makes the contrast between the vessels and background higher in cSLO images than in images from the fundus camera. This possibly is the reason why the optic nerve often shows more fluorescence with a fundus camera system than with the cSLO. Light scattering affects fundus camera systems more than cSLO systems. All these factors may lead to a lower ability of the fundus camera system to discern smaller retinal vessels as compared to the cSLO. Macular pigments or fluorescein do not absorb the wavelengths used in the fundus camera. Fundus cameras utilize a cone of light entering the eye, hence small pupillary apertures reduce the intensity of autofluorescence. Fundus camera images need manual removal of the excess lens autofluorescence in patients with advanced degrees of nuclear sclerosis.

ASSESSING THE FUNDUS AUTOFLUORESCENCE IMAGE

When an FAF image is being evaluated, any abnormal recording should be discerned, and a plausible cause should be investigated for. The characteristics of a normal FAF image, which need to be understood first, are as follows:

- The *optic nerve head* is devoid of the RPE and the autofluorescent lipofuscin and is hence characteristically dark. The *retinal vessels* are also dark because of absorption from blood constituents. The *macular area* has the FAF signal most markedly reduced at the fovea. Beginning from the foveal center, a faint yet discernable increase in the signal can be observed at about the margin of the fovea, with a further steady increment toward the outer macula. Beyond these areas with decrements in FAF intensity, the FAF signal appears evenly distributed (Figs. 4.1A and B).

- The quality of the recorded image determines the accuracy with which abnormalities in the FAF image are depicted. Any opacity in the cornea, vitreous, the lens, or the anterior chamber may affect the detection of pathologies at the level of the RPE and the neurosensory retina.

Causes for a Reduced Fundus Autofluorescence Signal

- Reduction in RPE lipofuscin density
  - Retinal pigment epithelium atrophy [such as geographic atrophy (GA)]
  - Hereditary retinal dystrophies (such as RPE65 mutations).
- Increased RPE melanin content
  - Retinal pigment epithelium hypertrophy.
- Absorption from extracellular material/cells/fluid anterior to the RPE
  - Intraretinal fluid (such as macular edema)
  - Migrated melanin-containing cells
  - Crystalline drusen or other crystal-like deposits
  - Fresh intraretinal and subretinal hemorrhages
  - Fibrosis, scar tissue, borders of laser scars
  - Retinal vessels
  - Luteal pigment (lutein and zeaxanthin)
  - Media opacities (vitreous, lens, anterior chamber, cornea).

Causes for an Increased Fundus Autofluorescence Signal

- Excessive RPE lipofuscin accumulation
  - Lipofuscinopathies, including Stargardt disease, best disease, pattern dystrophy, and adult vitelliform macular dystrophy

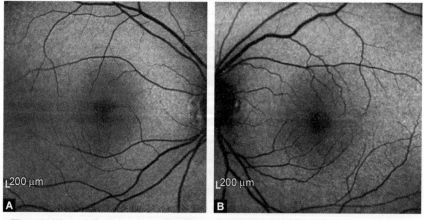

Figs. 4.1A and B: The normal fundus autofluorescence patterns. (A) The right eye. (B) The left eye of a patient.

- Age-related macular degeneration (AMD), such as RPE in the junctional zone preceding enlargement of the occurrence of GA.
- Occurrence of fluorophores anterior or posterior to the RPE cell monolayer
  - Intraretinal fluid (such as macular edema)
  - Subpigment epithelial fluid in pigment epithelial detachments
  - Drusen in the subpigment epithelial space
  - Migrated RPE cells or macrophages containing lipofuscin or melanolipofuscin (seen as pigment clumping or hyperpigmentation on funduscopy)
  - Older intraretinal and subretinal hemorrhages
  - Choroidal vessel in the presence of RPE and choriocapillaris atrophy, such as in the center of laser scars or within patches of RPE atrophy
  - Choroidal nevi and melanoma.
- Lack of absorbing material
  - Depletion of the luteal pigment, such as in idiopathic macular telangiectasia (IMT) type 2
  - Displacement of the luteal pigment, such as in cystoid macular edema.
- Optic nerve head drusen
  - Artifacts.

CLINICAL APPLICATIONS OF AUTOFLUORESCENCE

Macular and Retinal Dystrophies

In several macular and retinal dystrophies, autofluorescent material does aggregate in the RPE and the extracellular deposits in the neurosensory space may also be fluorescent. FAF imaging enables detection of the abnormal phenotype in some disorders when it is not otherwise evident (Figs. 4.2A to D).

Clinically discernable pale yellowish deposits at the level of the RPE/Bruch's membrane in Best's disease (Figs. 4.3A to D), adult vitelliform macular dystrophy, fundus albipunctatus (Figs. 4.4A to D), and Stargardt's macular dystrophy or fundus flavimaculatus are associated with markedly increased FAF intensities.[16,19] The focal flecks in Stargardt's disease are much more clearly highlighted on FAF images in comparison to fundus photographs. They show a bright FAF signal that may weaken as atrophy develops.

Age-related Macular Degeneration

Early Manifestation

Age-related macular degeneration, a complex disease with both genetic and environmental factors, has become the most common cause of legal blindness in industrialized countries.[20-23] A hallmark of ageing is the accumulation of lipofuscin (LF) granules in the cytoplasm of RPE cells (Figs. 4.5A and B).

Fundus autofluorescence as an imaging modality was used to map metabolic changes of RPE and LF accumulation *in vivo* and has been studied recently in patients with AMD. These help us to know the spatial correlation

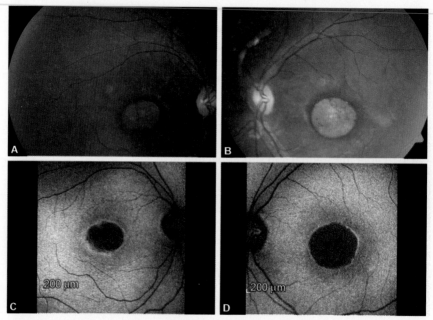

Figs. 4.2A to D: (A and B) A patient diagnosed with Stargardt's disease with the fundus photographs. (C and D) Fundus autofluorescence (FAF) images revealing central hypoautofluorescence reflecting the retinal pigment epithelium (RPE) atrophic pathology surrounded by the hyperautofluorescent ring.

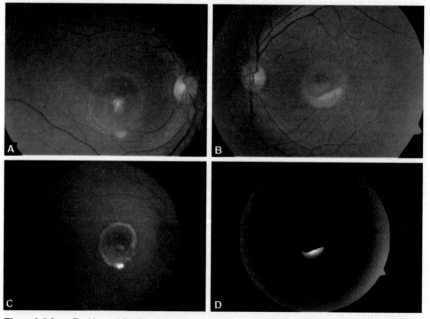

Figs. 4.3A to D: (A and B) The fundus pictures and (C and D) corresponding fundus autofluorescence (FAF) pictures of a patient with Best's disease demonstrating the hyperautofluorescence emanating from the accumulated lipofuscin-laden deposit in the neurosensory space.

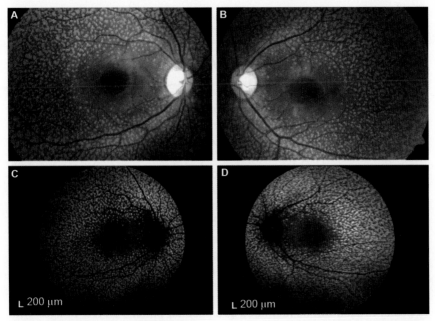

Figs. 4.4A to D: (A and B) A patient with fundus albipunctatus with fundus pictures. (C and D) Corresponding autofluorescence images showing the hyperautofluorescent specks.

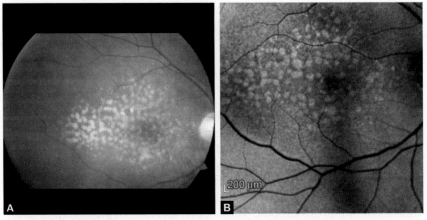

Figs. 4.5A and B: (A) The fundus picture autofluorescence image; (B) Highlighting the copious autofluorescence from the drusenoid material.

of FAF findings with established early AMD changes such as focal hypo- and hyperpigmentation and drusen.

One important observation in patients with early AMD is that alterations in the FAF signal are not necessarily associated with corresponding funduscopically or angiographically visible changes such as drusen and irregular hyper- or hypopigmentations.[18,23,24] This indicates that FAF findings may represent an independent measure of disease stage and activity.

CLASSIFICATION OF FUNDUS AUTOFLUORESCENCE PATTERNS IN EARLY AMD

Fundus autofluorescence findings in patients with early AMD were recently published by an international workshop on FAF phenotyping in early AMD.[3] Pooling data from several retinal centers developed a classification system with eight different FAF patterns.

It demonstrates the relatively poor correlation between visible alterations on fundus photography and notable FAF changes. Based on these results, it was speculated that FAF findings in early AMD may indicate more widespread abnormalities and diseased areas. These changes in FAF imaging at the RPE cell-level may precede the occurrence of visible lesions as the disease progresses.

Reticular Drusen

Reticular drusen can be identified as a peculiar pattern on FAF images, with multiple relatively uniform roundish or elongated spots with decreased intensities, and surrounded by an interlacing network of normal-appearing FAF signals.[23]

These are readily identified on FAF images and more easily detected than on funduscopy or fundus photographs. The exact anatomic location (i.e. sub-RPE, Bruch's membrane, choriocapillaris) and morphological pattern is not clearly understood.

Age-related Macular Degeneration—Geographic Atrophy

Geographic atrophy represents the atrophic late-stage manifestation of "dry" AMD, characterized by the development of atrophic patches that may initially occur in the parafoveal area.[25-27] During the natural course of the disease, the atrophy slowly enlarges over time, and there is foveal sparing until later. Due to the distinct changes in the topographic distribution of RPE lipofuscin, which is the dominant fluorophore for FAF imaging, the signal is markedly reduced over atrophic areas, while high-intensity FAF levels can be observed in the junctional zone surrounding the atrophic patches. FFA and fundus photography do not show any morphological changes at this stage.

Detection and Quantification of Atrophy

As FAF signal intensity is markedly reduced, areas of atrophy can be readily visualized on FAF images. In contrast to fluorescein angiography, FAF imaging represents a noninvasive imaging method and is less time consuming.

The advantages of FAF imaging in general atrophy have been used to detect and precisely quantify atrophic areas on FAF images using customized image analysis software.[28,29] This software allows the automated segmentation of atrophic areas by a region algorithm. Interfering retinal blood vessels that have a similar FAF intensity compared with atrophic areas are recognized by the software and can be excluded from the measurements.

Further developments include the alignment of FAF images at different examinations using retinal landmarks in order to correct for different scan angles and magnifications. This allows the accurate assessment of atrophy progression over time and can be used in longitudinal observations, including interventional trials.

Age-related Macular Degeneration—Pigment Epithelial Detachment

Retinal pigment epithelial detachments (PEDs) are a common feature of advanced AMD. Conventional imaging techniques such as fundus photography, fluorescein, or indocyanine green angiography cannot detect the variations in the area of PED which can be seen by FAF signal in that area.

Changes in FAF intensities in patients with PED secondary to AMD can be classified into four groups. Other dominant fluorophores with similar excitation and emission spectra inside the PED, such as extracellular fluid or degraded photoreceptors, may be present and contribute to typical patterns with abnormal FAF intensity (Figs. 4.6A and B). FAF phenotypes may reflect not only different stages in the evolution of a PED but also the heterogeneity on a cellular and molecular level in the disease process, and may thus be relevant for future molecular genetic analyses.

Age-related Macular Degeneration—Choroidal Neovascularization

Choroidal neovascularization (CNV) is a common cause of visual loss in patients with AMD and represents the growth of new subretinal vessels in the macular region.

Fundus Autofluorescence Findings in Early Choroidal Neovascularization

Eyes with "recent-onset" CNV were found to have patches of "continuous" or "normal" autofluorescence corresponding to areas of hyperfluorescence on the comparative fluorescein angiograms. This implied that RPE viability was preserved at least initially in CNV development. FAF imaging was able to delineate the edge of CNV lesions better than FFA and it was statistically larger.[31]

Fundus Autofluorescence Findings in Late-stage Choroidal Neovascularization

In eyes with long-standing CNV, decreased areas of AF were seen, implying nonviable RPE and lack of photoreceptor outer segment renewal. These

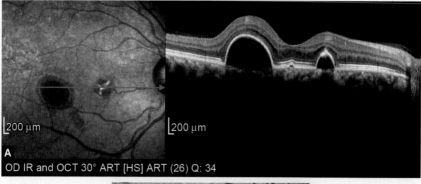

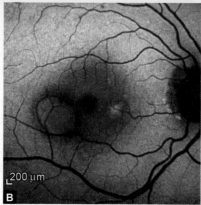

Figs. 4.6A and B: (A) The optical coherence tomography (OCT) picture and (B) Corresponding fundus autofluorescence image showing a large detachment of the retinal pigment epithelium with intermediate fundus autofluorescence (FAF) signal with surrounding well-defined less-autofluorescent halo delineating the entire border of the lesion.

represent areas of RPE atrophy beneath the CNV scars in the late stages of disease,[30] whereas areas of increased FAF seen inferior to lesions were thought to be due to a gravitational effect of fluid tracking under the retina, similar to that seen in central serous retinopathy.[31] Increased FAF signal has also been described around the edge of lesions that are thought to represent proliferation of RPE cells around the CNV.[30-32]

Classic Choroidal Neovascularization

Purely classic lesions showed low or decreased FAF signal at the site of the CNV, with a ring of increased FAF around some lesions (Figs. 4.7A and B).

Occult Choroidal Neovascularization

According to McBain et al. foci of decreased FAF were seen scattered within the lesion. These were felt to be due to small areas of RPE loss or damage caused

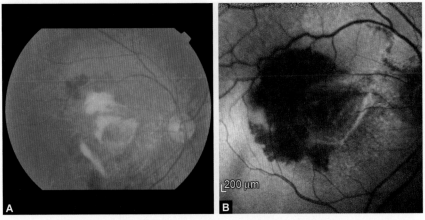

Figs. 4.7A and B: (A) Fundus picture and (B) Autofluorescence image showing the choroidal neovascular membrane (CNVM).

by the chronic, more indolent lesions growing underneath the RPE. Areas of increased FAF were less frequently associated with the edge of occult lesions compared with predominantly classic lesions.

RETINAL PIGMENT EPITHELIUM TEARS

Areas with RPE loss are characterized by a very low signal and intense hypo-autofluorescence because of a complete lack of RPE and loss of lipofuscin. They are sharply demarcated. The adjacent area with rolled-up RPE is characterized by the heterogeneous signal of distinct increased FAF. Thus, the exact location of the tear can be delineated in most cases (Figs. 4.8A and B).

IDIOPATHIC MACULAR TELANGIECTASIA

Idiopathic macular telangiectasia (or idiopathic parafoveal telangiectasis) is a descriptive term for different disease entities presenting with telangiectatic alterations of the juxtafoveolar capillary network with a predominant location temporal to the fovea (Figs. 4.9A and B).[32,33] It is usually classified as type I and type II.

Fundus Autofluorescence in Type 1 Idiopathic Macular Telangiectasia

Fundus autofluorescence imaging may show an increased signal that may be explained by a reduced macular pigment optical density (MPOD) due to retinal tissue defects in the area with cystoid changes. However, overall the distribution is normal, with the highest MPOD in the fovea and attenuation towards the periphery.

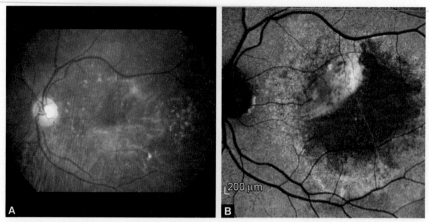

Figs. 4.8A and B: (A) Fundus picture and (B) Autofluorescence image showing a retinal pigment epithelium tear following the development of choroidal neovascularization secondary to age-related macular degeneration.

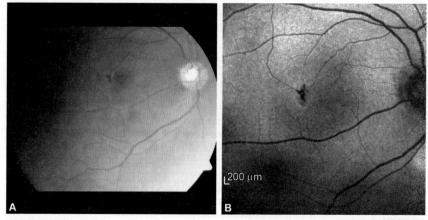

Figs. 4.9A and B: (A) Clinical picture of a patient with idiopathic juxtafoveal telangiectasia (IJT) and the (B) Fundus autofluorescence (FAF) image showing the intense hypoautofluorescence of the pigment deposits.

Fundus Autofluorescence in Type 2 Macular Telangiectasia

Macular pigment optical density is typically reduced in the macular area and the area of depletion largely corresponds to angiographic late-phase hyperfluorescence and increased confocal blue reflectance. In early stages, FAF shows minimal alteration whereas in late stages, it may be grossly abnormal. When intraretinal pigment clumping has occurred, FAF may show a reduced signal due to a blockade phenomenon.

CHORIORETINAL INFLAMMATORY DISORDERS

Autofluorescence photography complements other methods of imaging the ocular fundus. The amount of autofluorescence is governed by the amount of fluorophores in any given area in the fundus.

Choroidal neovascularization associated with intraocular inflammation is a common complication, and this secondary CNV produces characteristic autofluorescence findings. By observing autofluorescence characteristics, we can estimate the extent of damage, diagnose sequelae such as secondary CNV, learn more about the inflammatory process in question, and possibly anticipate future problems caused by the disease (Figs. 4.10A to D).

ACUTE POSTERIOR MULTIFOCAL PLACOID PIGMENT EPITHELIOPATHY

In the acute phases of acute posterior multifocal placoid pigment epitheliopathy (APMPPE), more lesions are visible by fluorescein angiography and ophthalmoscopy than those that are seen by autofluorescence photography.[34] The areas of decreased pigmentation with increased fluorescence and decreased autofluorescence suggest an atrophy or absence of functional RPE cells. Given the finding of increased pigmentation and autofluorescence

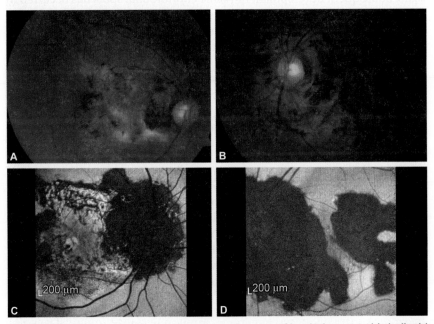

Figs. 4.10A to D: (A and B) Clinical picture of a case of healed geographic helicoid peripapillary choroidopathy (GHPC) with the fundus autofluorescence (FAF) images; (C and D) Images demonstrate the deep hypoautofluorescence of the scarred area and the neighboring mottled hyperautofluorescence.

centrally with a depigmented hypoautofluorescent surround, it is possible that with the healing of the lesions, there was a centripetal contraction of each placoid lesion with a retraction of the edges inward. The implication of these findings is that the RPE is affected secondarily to the choroidal changes.

ACUTE SYPHILITIC POSTERIOR PLACOID CHORIORETINITIS

Acute syphilitic posterior placoid chorioretinitis (ASPPC) shares similarities to APMPPE, as both conditions can cause yellowish plaque-like changes in the posterior pole.[35] There are important differences in appearance, and probably in pathophysiology. ASPPC usually causes a solitary yellow placoid lesion that has a more prominent color and opacification at its outer borders. The autofluorescence abnormalities are confined only to the placoid region.

MULTIFOCAL CHOROIDITIS AND PANUVEITIS

Autofluorescence photography of multifocal choroiditis and panuveitis (MCP) demonstrates clinically visible hypoautofluorescent chorioretinal scars.[36] However, autofluorescence photography often shows many more times the number of hypoautofluorescent spots than the number of chorioretinal scars. Subsequent development of visible chorioretinal spots has occurred in areas occupied by the hypoautofluorescent spots seen by autofluorescence imaging. Thus, autofluorescence appears to show areas of RPE damage from MCP that are more numerous and extensive than what the choroidal scars would indicate.

Secondary CNV is visible as a butterfly-shaped area of hyperautofluorescence. The borders of the autofluorescence show prominent attachments to hypoautofluorescent MCP scars. The hyperautofluorescence of past CNV persists despite subsequent treatment. Of interest is the finding of small hyperautofluorescent spots or rings in the vicinity of MCP scars.

ACUTE ZONAL OCCULT OUTER RETINOPATHY

The autofluorescent findings in acute zonal occult outer retinopathy (AZOOR) are limited largely because it is a rare disease. Autofluorescence photography showed that the outer border was intensely autofluorescent, consistent with the presence of lipofuscin, and that the central area of the lesion was hypoautofluorescent, consistent with atrophy of the RPE. The patient had visual field abnormalities consistent with the location and size of the autofluorescence abnormality.

BIRDSHOT CHORIORETINOPATHY

Autofluorescent abnormalities are usually associated with the depigmented lesions, while the early lesions do not necessarily cause autofluorescent abnormalities.

PERSPECTIVES IN IMAGING TECHNOLOGIES

After more than one decade of the first visualization of the topographic distribution of lipofuscin accumulation in the retinal areas using confocal scanning laser ophthalmoscopy (cSLO), FAF imaging is increasingly being used in research and in the clinical setting.[9] FAF findings also serve to identify high-risk features and rapid progress in an ongoing large interventional trial of patients with GA secondary to AMD. There are limitations to the currently used FAF imaging devices; these include resolution and quantification issues as well as the distinction of different underlying fluorophores according to spectral characteristics. Novel emerging imaging techniques offer new perspectives.

REFERENCES

1. Cuervo AM, Dice JR. When lysosomes get old. Exp Gerontol. 2000;35:119-31.
2. Sparrow JR, Boulton M. RPE lipofuscin and its role in retinal photobiology. Exp Eye Res. 2005;80:595-606.
3. Yin D. Biochemical basis of lipofuscin, ceroid, and age pigment-like fluorophores. Free Rad Biol Med. 1996;21:871-88.
4. Feeney-Burns L, Hilderbrand ES, Eldridge S. Aging human RPE: morphometric analysis of macular, equatorial, and peripheral cells. Invest Ophthalmol Vis Sci. 1984;25:195-200.
5. Delori, FC, Bursell, SE, Yoshida, A, et al. Vitreous fluorophotometry in diabetics: study of artifactual contributions. Graefe's Arch Clin Exp Ophthalmol. 1985;222:215-8.
6. Kitagawa, K, Nishida, S, Ogura, Y. In vivo quantification of autofluorescence in human retinal pigment epithelium. Ophthalmologica. 1989;199:116-21.
7. Delori FC. Fluorophotometer for noninvasive measurement of RPE lipofuscin. Noninvasive assessment of the visual system. OSA Technical Digest. 1992;1:164-7.
8. Delori FC. Spectrophotometer for noninvasive measurement of intrinsic fluorescence and reflectance of the ocular fundus. Appl Opt. 1994;33:7439-52.
9. von Ruckmann A, Fitzke FW, Bird AC. Distribution of fundus autofluorescence with a scanning laser ophthalmoscope. Br J Ophthalmol. 1995;79:407-12.
10. Webb RH, Hughes GW, Delori FC. Confocal scanning laser ophthalmoscope. Appl Opt. 1987;26:1492-9
11. Bellmann C, Holz FG, Schapp O, et al. Topography of fundus autofluorescence with a new confocal scanning laser ophthalmoscope. Ophthalmologe. 1997;94:385-91.
12. Bindewald A, Jorzik JJ, Roth F, et al. cSLO digital fundus autofluorescence imaging. Ophthalmologe. 2005;102:259-64.
13. Jorzik JJ, Bindewald A, Dithmar S, et al. Digital simultaneous fluorescein and indocyanine green angiography, autofluorescence, and red-free imaging with a solid-state laser-based confocal scanning laser ophthalmoscope. Retina. 2005;25:405-16.
14. Solbach U, Keilhauer C, Knabben H, et al. Imaging of retinal autofluorescence in patients with age-related macular degeneration. Retina. 1997;17:385-9.
15. American National Standards Institute. American national standard for the safe use of lasers: ANSI Z136.1. Orlando, FL: Laser Institute of America; 2000.
16. Delori FC, Dorey CK, Staurenghi G, et al. In vivo fluorescence of the ocular fundus exhibits retinal pigment epithelium lipofuscin characteristics. Invest Ophthalmol Vis Sci. 1995;36:718-29.

17. Delori FC, Fleckner MR, Goger DG, et al. Autofluorescence distribution associated with drusen in age-related macular degeneration. Invest Ophthalmol Vis Sci. 2000;41:496-504.

18. Spaide RF. Fundus autofluorescence and age-related macular degeneration. Ophthalmol. 2003;110:392-9.

19. von Rückmann A, Fitzke FW, Bird AC. In vivo fundus autofluorescence in macular dystrophies. Arch Ophthalmol. 1997;115:609-15.

20. Holz FG, Pauleikhoff D, Spaide RF, et al. Age-related macular degeneration. Berlin: Springer; 2004.

21. Holz FG, Pauleikhoff D, Klein R, et al. Pathogenesis of lesions in late age-related macular disease. Am J Ophthalmol. 2004;137:504-10.

22. Klein R, Klein BE, Tomany SC, et al. Ten-year incidence and progression of age-related maculopathy: the Beaver Dam eye study. Ophthalmology. 2002;109:1767-79.

23. Lois N, Owens SL, Coco R, et al. Fundus autofluorescence in patients with age-related macular degeneration and high risk of visual loss. Am J Ophthalmol. 2002;133:341-9.

24. Bindewald A, Bird AC, Dandekar SS, et al. Classification of fundus autofluorescence patterns in early age-related macular disease. Invest Ophthalmol Vis Sci. 2005;46:3309-14.

25. Blair CJ. Geographic atrophy of the retinal pigment epithelium. A manifestation of senile macular degeneration. Arch Ophthalmol. 1975;93:19-25.

26. Maguire P, Vine AK. Geographic atrophy of the retinal pigment epithelium. Am J Ophthalmol. 1986;102:621-5.

27. Schatz H, McDonald HR. Atrophic macular degeneration. Rate of spread of geographic atrophy and visual loss. Ophthalmology. 1989;96:1541-51.

28. Deckert A, Schmitz-Valckenberg S, Jorzik J, et al. Automated analysis of digital fundus autofluorescence images of geographic atrophy in advanced age-related macular degeneration using confocal scanning laser ophthalmoscopy (cSLO). BMC Ophthalmol. 2005;5:8.

29. Schmitz-Valckenberg S, Jorzik J, Unnebrink K, et al. Analysis of digital scanning laser ophthalmoscopy fundus autofluorescence images of geographic atrophy in advanced age-related macular degeneration. Graefes Arch Clin Exp Ophthalmol. 2002;240:73-8.

30. Dandekar SS, Jenkins SA, Peto T, et al. Autofluorescence imaging of choroidal neovascularization due to age-related macular degeneration. Arch Ophthalmol. 2005;123:1507-13.

31. Lafaut BA, Bartz-Schmidt KU, Vanden Broecke C, et al. Clinicopathological correlation in exudative age-related macular degeneration: histological differentiation between classic and occult choroidal neovascularization. Br J Ophthalmol. 2000;84:239-43.

32. Charbel Issa P, Scholl HPN, Helb HM, et al. Macular telangiectasia. In: Holz FG, Spaide RF (Eds). Medical retina. Heidelberg: Springer; 2007. pp. 183-97.

33. Helb HM, Charbel Issa P, Pauleikhoff D, et al. Macular pigment density and distribution in patients with macular telangiectasia. Invest Ophthalmol Vis Sci. 2006;28:808-15.

34. Spaide RF. Autofluorescence imaging of acute posterior multifocal placoid pigment epitheliopathy. Retina. 2006;26:479-842.

35. Matsumoto Y, Spaide RF. Autofluorescence imaging of acute syphilitic posterior placoid chorioretinitis. Retina. Retin Cases Brief Rep. 2007;1(3):123-7.

36. Haen SP, Spaide RF. Fundus autofluorescence in multifocal choroiditis and panuveitis. Am J Ophthalmol. 2008;145(5):847-53.

Choroidal Imaging with Enhanced Depth Imaging and Swept-source Optical Coherence Tomography

James A Eadie, Suresh R Chandra

INTRODUCTION

Optical coherence tomography (OCT) is a rapidly evolving imaging modality that has become a mainstay of the clinical and experimental ophthalmology practice. This technology uses light waves to generate a reflectivity versus depth profile of ocular structures.[1] The technology has evolved rapidly from the first-generation time domain (TD) OCT machines of the early 1990s to the high-resolution spectral-domain (SD) machines of today. Modern OCT technology allows for reliable imaging of the choroid. There are currently two predominate methodologies for imaging this tissue with OCT; enhanced-depth imaging (EDI) OCT,[2] and swept-source (SS) OCT.[3] Each method achieves the resolution of choroidal structures by different means.

Enhanced-depth imaging (EDI)-OCT was first described in 2008 by Spaide et al.[2] It is essentially a technique utilizing the existing SD-OCT technology in a way that maximizes the resolution of the choroid. SD-OCT uses broadband light, i.e. light containing a wide range of wavelengths to illuminate the retina.[4] The light interacts with, and is partially scattered by the tissue. The different wavelengths of the broadband light source will penetrate and be scattered by the tissue to different degrees. After interacting with the tissue, the light is reflected back to the OCT machine where is it combined with light from a reference arm. Merging these two light signals results in a complex interference pattern. Deeper tissues will generate a larger delay and will thus have a different interference profile when compared with more superficial tissues. This interference pattern can be decoded using complex mathematical models such as the Fourier domain transform, and can be used to reconstruct an image of the tissue with near-histological resolution.[5] The central wavelength, the median wavelength of the broad range of wavelengths contained in the light source, ranges between 800 nm and 850 nm. This is commonly referred to as the zero-delay. Resolution decreases with increasing distance from the zero-delay.[2] In the conventional SD-OCT, the zero-delay is located near the vitreoretinal interface. The retinal-pigment epithelium (RPE) scatters a significant amount of the signal in this modality. In EDI-OCT, the light source and detector are moved closer to the patient. This displaces the zero-delay posteriorly, thus essentially focusing the machine on the choroid at the expense of some inner retinal resolution. The resulting images allow for a reliable measurement of the choroidal thickness in a great majority of patients.[2]

In contrast to EDI-OCT, SS-OCT employs a new generation of OCT machines.[3] Instead of a broadband light source; these machines use a long-wavelength light source of a narrow band centered on 1050 nm. This 1050 nm wavelength maximizes the transmission efficiency in aqueous environments.[6] The light source in SS-OCT is tunable, meaning that the wavelength may be adjusted in a controlled manner to "sweep" across a specific spectrum. The tuning takes place over a range of approximately 100 nm, and obtains approximately 100,000 individual a-scans per second.[6,7] This technique yields a resolution of 8 μm.[7] Data from these a-scans is run through automated segmentation software and is reconstructed into an image of the anatomical structures. SS-OCT techniques minimize fringe artifacts, signal dispersion and improve signal efficiency.[6] The net result is a minimization of the scattering artifacts that can interfere with the effective resolution of choroidal structures in conventional SD-OCT.

The introduction of both EDI and SS-OCT, has led to a rapidly expanding understanding of the choroid in a growing number of disease and nondisease states. Fluctuations in choroidal thickness and changes to the morphological appearance of the choroid are being reported regularly. Choroidal imaging with OCT has led to an increased understanding of a wide array of diseases, including, but not limited to, a variety of neoplastic, inflammatory, and vascular processes. The clinical applications of these technologies continue to evolve, although its role at this point in time is primarily as a research tool.

IMAGING OF THE NORMAL CHOROID

As choroidal imaging with OCT becomes more widely available, a number of studies have emerged to establish the range of choroidal thickness in nonpathologic states (Fig. 5.1). Margolis and Spaide published the first such paper in 2009.[8] They imaged 30 patients with a mean age of 50.4 years who had no evidence of eye disease. They measured a mean subfoveal choroidal thickness (SFCT) of 287 μm with a standard deviation of ±76 μm. They also described a predictable topographical variation in thickness with the choroid nasal to the fovea being consistently thinner than the subfoveal choroid. Another interesting observation from this study was that subfoveal thickness tended to decrease with advancing age.[8] These findings were later reinforced by similar measurements found in subsequent studies.[9,10] The Beijing Eye Study performed EDI-OCT measurements on a much larger set of patients. In 2011 the study took EDI-OCT scans from 3233 patients in northern China.

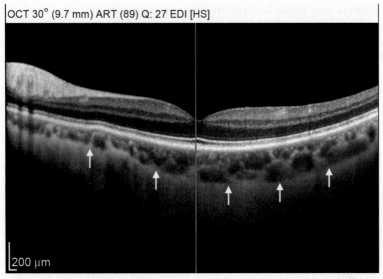

Fig. 5.1: Enhanced-depth imaging-optical coherence tomography (EDI-OCT) of a normal retina and choroid.

They found a mean choroidal thickness of 253.8 ± 107.4 μm in this population. Choroidal thickness decreased with age and increased with shorter axial length.[11] In this population SFCT decreased by an average of 15 μm for every 1 diopter of myopa.[11] They found no correlation between SFCT and blood pressure, ocular perfusion pressure, intraocular pressure (IOP), smoking, diabetes or hypertension.[11] A separate retrospective study that performed regression analysis on 123 normal eyes aged 15–84 (average 47 years old) also found a negative correlation between age and choroidal thickness. In their analysis, they saw a decrease in choroidal thickness of 3.14 μm for each year of age.[12]

The SFCT in children was measured with EDI-OCT in a large study out of Denmark.[13] In this cohort of 1,323 healthy children, the average SFCT was 369 ± 81 μm in girls and 348 ± 72 μm in boys ($p = 0.14$). Interestingly, this study showed that the increasing choroidal thickness was associated with later stages of puberty in girls.[13] Again, this study showed that SFCT decreased with increasing axial length.

Several studies have been published that examine the effects of medications and hydration on choroidal thickness in nonpathologic states. Mansouri et al. conducted a study that showed that choroidal thickness increased by a maximum of 5.7% after drinking 1,000 mL of water in 5 minutes.[14] Predictably sildenafil citrate was also shown to increase choroidal thickness by 12.7% at hours 1 and 3.[15] In contrast, choroidal thicknesses were observed to transiently decrease for a period of 4 hours following ingestion of coffee[16] and for several hours after smoking a cigarette.[17] These studies serve to illustrate the dynamic nature of choroidal tissue, not only over the course of a person's life but also on an hour-to-hour and perhaps minute-to-minute basis.

There is one published report that compares measurements of normal choroidal thickness in EDI-OCT to those taken with SS-OCT.[18] In this study the investigators were only able to image the entire choroid in 74.4% of patients with EDI-OCT versus 100% with SD-OCT.[18] For those patients whom imaging was obtained with both modalities there was excellent agreement between the two (average SFCT of 279 μm with EDI versus 285 μm with SS in 61 eyes). The eyes in which the EDI-OCT machine was not able to measure the entire choroid were more hyperopic with thicker choroids.

EDI AND SS-OCT IMAGING IN GLAUCOMA

There are currently two predominant threads in the medical literature surrounding EDI and SS-OCT in glaucoma. The first are reports of choroidal thickness variations in glaucoma. In a review paper, Banitt found nine reports that have been published describing choroidal thickness in glaucomatous eyes.[19] All of these studies focus on choroidal thickness in the macula. Six of the papers showed no statistically significant difference in choroidal thickness when compared with normal controls, while three reports show a connection between a thinning in the peripapillary region of the choroid and glaucoma.[20-28] More studies are needed to examine choroidal thickness in all of the various types of glaucoma before the role of choroidal tissue in these diseases can be appreciably understood.

Another subset of the medical literature examines the anatomy of the optic nerve complex in glaucoma. Using EDI-OCT, Park et al. were able to image the pores of the lamina cribrosa in 76% of patients.[29] Furthermore, they were able to image the subarachnoid space around the optic nerve in 23% of patients, as well as the central retinal artery and vein as it passes through the lamina cribrosa in a significant number of eyes. Lee et al. published an observational case series of 100 patients with open-angle glaucoma who had imaging of the lamina cribrosa before and after the introduction of IOP lowering agents. Patients were included if they achieved a 20% lowering of IOP on follow-up examination. The study reported a mean pre-treatment lamina cribrosa depth of 584.73 μm that decreased to 529.18 μm following a drop in IOP ($p < 0.001$).[30] This showed a reversal of bowing of the lamina cribrosa with treatment and provided a potential window into the pathological mechanisms of glaucoma.

CHOROIDAL IMAGING IN CENTRAL SEROUS CHORIORETINOPATHY

Central serous chorioretinopathy (CSC) is a condition characterized by serous detachments of the neurosensory retina, or in some cases, the RPE. It is typically self-limited but can be recurrent or bilateral in approximately one-third of cases.[31] The pathophysiology of CSC is poorly understood, although endogenous and exogenous steroids appear to play a role.[32,33] Choroidal hyperpermeability has been documented with indocyanine green angiography (ICGA) in eyes with CSC.[34] Choroidal imaging with EDI and SS-OCT has given practitioners a new window into the pathophysiology of this disease. The choroidal thickness is increased in patients with CSC (Fig. 5.2). Imamura et al. published the first paper documenting choroidal thickness with EDI-OCT in patients with CSC.[35] They reported an average choroidal thickness of 505 µm in 19 patients with CSC. This number was significantly higher than choroidal thickness measurements from previously reported normal subjects. Since this manuscript was published, numerous other papers have confirmed this finding to be a hallmark of the disease.[36-38] Jirarattanasopa et al. reported an average mean whole macular thickness of 329.3 µm in 34 patients with CSC and 23 µm in 17 normal controls.[38] They also observed greater choroidal thickness localized to areas of leakage on fluorescein angiography (FA).[38] Maruko et al. went on to show that SFCT in fellow eyes with angiographic evidence of choroidal hyperpermeability was also increased.[36] Yang et al. used EDI-OCT to document larger lumen diameter in the choroidal vasculature in patients with CSC than that which was observed in control eyes, suggesting vascular dilation is part of the disease process.[39] This finding was again demonstrated with images taken from an experimental, en face SS-OCT machine in a significant number of patients with CSC.[40]

Photodynamic therapy (PDT) with verteporfin has become the standard of care for the management of chronic CSC. Multiple reports have documented the effectiveness of this treatment in facilitating the resolution of angiographic leakage as well as subretinal fluid.[41-44] Maruko et al. examined SFCT with EDI-OCT in patients with CSC before and after treatment with either argon laser photocoagulation or half-dose PDT. Although the authors demonstrated the resolution of subfoveal fluid in both arms of the study, interestingly, choroidal

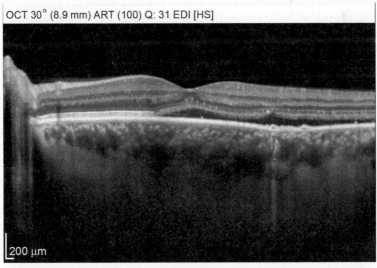

OCT 30° (8.9 mm) ART (100) Q: 31 EDI [HS]

200 µm

Fig. 5.2: Enhanced-depth imaging-optical coherence tomography of a patient with CSC showing thickened choroid. Note that the posterior edge of the choroid is beyond the resolving depth of the scanner.

thickness was reduced in the PDT group but not in the argon laser group.[37] The reduction in choroidal thickness following treatment has been shown to persist for 1 year following treatment with PDT.[45]

CHOROIDAL IMAGING IN UVEITIS

Imaging of the choroid with EDI and SS-OCT has been described in a limited number of uveitides. In a small series of 21 eyes with idiopathic panuveitis, choroidal thinning, as well as a correlation between visual acuity and the ratio of choroidal to retinal thickness has been described.[46] Two conflicting reports have been published on choroidal thickness in Behçet's uveitis. One study found that patients with bilateral disease displayed an average choroidal thickness of 398.77 µm in the active phase, defined by prominent vascular leakage on FA, and 356.72 µm in the quiescent phase ($P = 0.0004$).[47] Both of these numbers were significantly higher than choroidal thickness measurements taken from the age, sex, and spherical equivalent-matched controls (256.96 µm, $P < 0.0001$). Interestingly, the same report looked at 13 patients with unilateral Behçet's uveitis and found no difference in choroidal thickness between the involved and uninvolved eyes. They did however find a difference between uninvolved eyes in patients with Behçet's and eyes from normal matched controls.[47] In contrast, a second report was published that examined choroidal thickness in 35 patients with posterior uveitis from Behçet's disease. It showed thinner choroids in affected patients when compared with similarly matched controls.[48]

Vogt–Koyanagi–Harada disease (VKH) is the uveitic condition that has been examined most thoroughly with EDI and SS-OCT choroidal imaging. In 2011, Maruko et al. looked at 16 eyes from patients with VKH and showed an average choroidal thickness of over 800 microns.[49] This decreased to 341 in only 2 weeks of corticosteroid treatment. The resolution of increased choroidal thickness mirrored the resolution of exudative retinal detachment. In same patients, the recurrence of exudation was accompanied by a re-thickening of the choroid. This observation has implications for objective measurements of response to treatment.[49] Similar reports have subsequently been published that support these observations.[50-55] Another interesting finding in VKH that has recently been reported using SD and SS-OCT is the presence of a quantifiable undulation in the RPE and its correlation with choroidal thickness as a marker for acute disease.[54] In a study that followed 16 patients until the development of sunset glow fundus, investigators found that despite significantly thickened choroids in the initial and recurrent phases of the disease, choroids were ultimately significantly thinner than in age-matched controls.[51] Ultimate choroidal thinning in long-standing VKH was again observed in 30 eyes from 16 patients in a separate study.[52] One possible explanation for the eventual thinning of the choroid in VKH may be inferred from observations made by Fong et al. in 2011 with EDI-OCT. They reported a clear loss of focal hyper-reflectivity in the inner choroid in both the acute and convalescent phases of VKH, which they postulated might be indicative of permanent structural damage to the choroid.[53] A small series of 22 eyes recently showed a frank loss of the choriocapillaris to varying degrees in 50% of patients. This loss was associated with lower visual acuity and may be a marker for visual prognosis in the convalescent phase.[55]

Several cases and small reports have been published examining other uveitic entities with EDI and SS-OCT. These include descriptions of multiple evanescent white dot syndrome,[56] lymphoma,[57]and sarcoid granulomas.[58] Due to the limited number of patients in these reports, definitive conclusions regarding the choroid in these particular conditions cannot be drawn. There a large number of uveitic entities that have not been examined or described using this imaging modality.

CHOROIDAL IMAGING IN AGE-RELATED MACULAR DEGENERATION

Several reports have suggested that abnormalities in choroidal circulation are contributing factors in the severity of age-related macular degeneration (ARMD).[59-61] Choroidal assessment with OCT has provided another angle from which this concept may be explored. The first report of choroidal thickness measurements in patients with ARMD was published by Manjunath et al. in 2011. Using a Cirrus HD-OCT with software version 4.5 they imaged the choroid of 57 eyes from 47 patients. They found a range of choroidal thicknesses but were unable to statistically correlate choroidal thickness with disease stage or treatment.[62] Two other reports have been published that compare choroidal thickness measurements in patients with ARMD to those with polypoidal choroidal vasculopathy (PCV),[63] and CSC.[64] These studies both show that choroidal thickness is decreased in patients with ARMD when compared with those who have PCV. Interestingly, Jirarattanasopa et al. were able to show a connection between choroidal thickness and angiographic subtypes of neovascular ARMD.[63] As one would expect, subtypes displaying the features of choroidal hyperpermeability on angiography displayed thickened choroids when compared with classic angiographic subtypes of the disease.[63] However, it is difficult to draw broad conclusions as to a pattern of choroidal thickness in ARMD from these studies due to the limited number of patients examined and their comparison to other known retinal/choroidal diseases as opposed to age-matched controls. There is one study that examines the choroidal thickness in patients with retinal angiomatous proliferation (RAP) lesions specifically. It found an average choroidal thickness of 129.5 µm in patients with RAP lesions, and 201.3 µm in age-matched controls.[65]

Kang et al. retrospectively reviewed choroidal thickness measurements in 40 eyes with exudative ARMD taken with EDI-OCT and correlated choroidal thickness with response to anti-VEGF treatment. They found that patients who responded favorably to ranibizumab had thicker subfoveal choroids.[66] Although this was a limited number of patients, this finding suggests a potential clinical application for this technology in the setting of exudative ARMD.

CHOROIDAL CHANGES IN RETINAL VEIN OCCLUSIONS

There is very little in the current medical literature that examines the choroid in retinal vein occlusion. Tsuiki et al. published a retrospective observational study that measured the SFCT before and after treatment with bevacizumab.[67]Although the total number of patients in the series was limited to 36, there were two interesting findings that demonstrated statistical significance. First, eyes with central retinal vein occlusion (CRVO) had increased choroidal thickness when compared with the fellow eye. Perhaps more interestingly, treatment with bevacizumab markedly decreased this choroidal thickness, thus implying a possible VEGF-mediated effect on choroidal physiology.

CHOROIDAL IMAGING IN MYOPIC EYES

Multiple studies have demonstrated thinner choroids in myopic eyes (Fig. 5.3) using EDI and SS-OCT technology.[9-12,68-72] Fujiwara published the first study that looked specifically at choroidal thickness in highly myopic eyes with EDI-OCT in 2009.[6] In 55 eyes with a mean refractive error of –11.9 D they showed that the average SFCT was only 93.2 µm. This correlated negatively with both age and refractive error. In an examination of choroidal thickness maps generated with EDI-OCT, the choroid was found to be thickest centrally in control eyes while it was thickest in the outer superior quadrants of highly myopic eyes.[69] The significance of this finding is unclear. EDI-OCT has been used to successfully image and measure the scleral thickness in highly myopic eyes as well.[70] Hayashi et al. showed that the mean subfoveal scleral thickness in 75 eyes with eight or more diopters of myopia was 284 µm.

OCT 30° (10.2 mm) ART (100) Q: 34 EDI [HS]

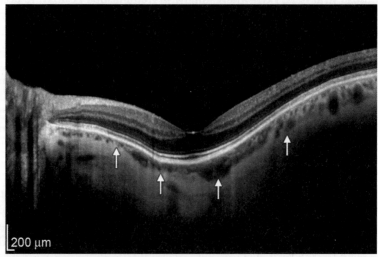

200 µm

Fig. 5.3: Enhanced-depth imaging-optical coherence tomography of an eye with high myopia displaying a thin choroid.

Perhaps of more clinical relevance, several papers have been published that show a relationship between choroidal thickness and visual acuity in highly myopic eyes.[71-73] Variations in choroidal thickness have been shown to predict which patients with myopic choroidal neovascularization (CNV) are more likely to respond favorably to anti-VEGF treatment.[74,75] Patients with thinner choroids in this clinical setting were shown to have a higher risk of recurrence as well as a lower rate of CNV resolution.[74] These studies strongly suggest a role of choroidal anatomy and processes in the pathogenesis of myopic degeneration and may help to steer further therapeutic research in this direction.

CHOROIDAL CHANGES IN INHERITED RETINAL DEGENERATIONS

The literature is sparse regarding choroidal anatomy in inherited retinal diseases. Two studies report variations in choroidal anatomy in association with retinitis pigmentosa (RP). Both papers show that the choroid is thinner in patients with RP than in age-matched controls.[76,77] One study shows a correlation between choroidal thickness and visual acuity[77] while the other does not.[76] In a separate paper out of Moorfields Eye Hospital 20 patients with a variety of inherited retinal diseases, including Stargardt macular dystrophy (Fig. 5.4), Best's disease, Bietti crystalline dystrophy and others, were imaged with EDI OCT. Across these conditions, there was no statistical correlation between choroidal thickness and visual acuity.[78]

OCT 30° (9.2 mm) ART (100) Q: 40 EDI [HS]

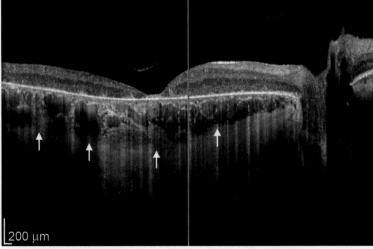

Fig. 5.4: Enhanced-depth imaging-optical coherence tomography of a patient with Stargardt macular dystrophy. Note the abnormal morphological structure of the choroidal vasculature.

RETINAL AND CHOROIDAL TUMORS IMAGED WITH OCT

Among the most intriguing clinical applications for EDI and SS-OCT is the capability to precisely measure and characterize ocular tumors. With thick tumors there are limitations to the depth that this technology can image. Accounts of the maximum reliable depth of imaging vary from 1.0 mm to 3.0 mm with EDI-OCT.[79-81] This parameter is yet to be established with SS-OCT. Shah et al. imaged 104 choroidal nevi with EDI-OCT and reported excellent image detail in 49%.[82] They observed a thinning of the choriocapillaris in the area of the nevus in 94% of cases. A shadowing effect deep to the nevus was seen in 59%; RPE atrophy and loss, IS-OS junction irregularities and photoreceptor loss were observed in 15–43% of cases.[82] Carol Shields published a series of 37 small melanomas (less than 3 mm thickness) followed with EDI-OCT. She showed that B-scan ultrasonography overestimated tumor thickness by an average of 55% when compared with OCT,[80] showing that this technology may be a more precise method for documenting growth in small, pigmented lesions. She went on to describe the EDI-OCT features of small choroidal melanomas (Figs. 5.5A to D) compared with choroidal nevi. Statistically significant features include increased tumor thickness, subretinal fluid, subretinal lipofuscin deposition, and retinal irregularities, including shaggy photoreceptors, and intraretinal edema. Perhaps most interestingly, elongated photoreceptors were

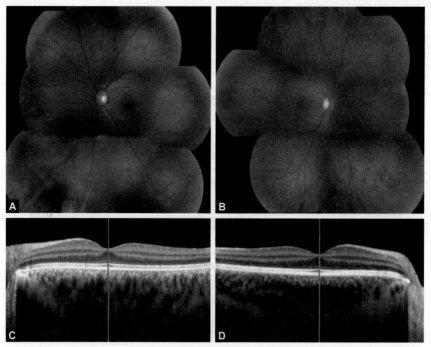

Figs. 5.5A to D: Montages of a patient with unilateral primary ocular melanocytosis displaying asymmetry of choroidal thickness. Color fundus photographs—(A) Left eye; (B) Right eye; and (C and D) EDI-OCT.

observed in the retina overlaying the lesion in 49% of cases of small ocular melanoma and in 0% of cases of choroidal nevus.[80]

The most common intraocular malignancy is choroidal metastasis. Demerci et al. imaged 24 metastatic tumors with EDI-OCT. As with the Shields study, the average tumor thickness as measured with EDI-OCT differed greatly from measurements taken with ultrasonography (average lesion depth 854 vs 2064 µm). Ultrasonography overestimated tumor depth by an average of 59%. They showed a dome-shaped configuration in 25% and a plateau-shaped configuration in 75% of cases. Thinning of the overlaying choriocapillaris was observed in 100% of the metastatic tumors. Shaggy photoreceptors overlaying the lesion and subretinal fluid with hyper-reflective speckles were seen in 79% and 75% of cases respectively.[81]

There are several small case series that describe other choroidal lesions. Pellegrini et al. published a series of 15 patients with unilateral choroidal melanocytosis and showed that the subfoveal choroid was 23% thicker in the involved eye.[83] In a separate study, circumscribed choroidal hemangiomas imaged with EDI-OCT appear as a low-medium reflective band with a homogenous signal and intrinsic spaces, which distinguishes them from the surrounding normal choroid.[79] A single case report of EDI-OCT used to image choroidal osteoma demonstrated a variety of reflectivity patterns.[84] Many other intraocular tumors have not yet been imaged with this technology and this remains an area of active research.

CONCLUSION

Enhanced-depth imaging and SS-OCT are new and exciting technologies. They are providing window into a great number of eye diseases and shedding light onto the role of the choroid in many of these processes. The role of this technology in clinical practice is yet to be firmly established, and is evolving as the medical literature generated by it continues to grow.

REFERENCES

1. Huang D, Swanson EA, Lin CP, et al. Optical coherence tomography. Science. 1991;254:1178-81.
2. Spaide RF, Koizumi H, Pozzoni MC. Enhanced depth imaging spectral-domian optical coherence tomography. Am J Ophthalmol. 2008;146(4):496-500.
3. Van Velthoven MEJ, Faber DJ, Verbraak FD, et al. Recent developments in optical coherence tomography for imaging the retina. Prog Retin Eye Res. 2007;26:57-77.
4. Brezinski M. Optical coherence tomography theory. In: Brezinski M (Ed). Optical Coherence Tomography. New York: Elsevier Inc; 2006. pp. 97-145.
5. De Boer JF, Cense B, Park BH, et al. Improved signal-to-noise ratio in spectral-domain compared with time-domain optical coherence tomography. Opt Lett. 2003;28:2067-9.
6. Postsaid B, Baumann B, Huang D, et al. Ultrahigh speed 1050 nm swept/source/ Fourier domain OCT retinal and anterior segment imaging at 100,000 to 400,00 axial scans per second. Opt Express. 2010;18(19):20029-48.

7. Mansouri K, Medeiros FA, Marchase N, et al. Assessment of choroidal thickness and volume during water drinking test by swept-source optical coherence tomography. Ophthalmology. 2013;l120(12):L2508-2516.
8. Margolis R, Spaide R. A pilot study of enhanced depth imaging optical coherence tomography of the choroid in normal eyes. Am J Ophthalmol. 2009;147:811-5.
9. McCourt E, Cadena B, Bernett C, et al. Measurement of subfoveal choroidal thickness using spectral domain optical coherence tomography. Ophthalmic Surg Lasers Imaging. 2010;41:S28-S33.
10. Joon W, Yong U, Byung R. Choroidal Thickness and volume mapping by a six radial scan protocol on spectral-domain optical coherence tomography. Ophthalmology. 2012;119:1017-23.
11. Wen B, Liang X, Jost J, et al. Subfoveal choroidal thickness: the Beijing Eye Study. Ophthalmology. 2013;120:175-80.
12. Erkul S, Kapran Z, Uyar M. Qunatitative analysis of subfoveal choroidal thickness using enhanced depth imaging optical coherence tomography in normal eyes. Int Ophthalmol. 2014;34(1):35-40.
13. Ziao Q, Jeppesen P, Larsen M, et al. Subfoveal choroidal thickness in 1323 children aged 11 to 12 years and association with puberty: the Copenhagen Child Cohort 2000 Eye Study. Invest Ophthalmol Vis Sci. 2014;55:550-5.
14. Mansouri K, Medeiros F, Marchase N, et al. Assessment of choroidal thickness and volume during water drinking test by swept-source optical coherence tomography. Ophthalmology. 2013;120(12):2508-16.
15. Vance S, Imamura Y, Freund K. The effects of sildenafil citrate on choroidal thickness as determined by enhanced depth imaging optical coherence tomography. Retina. 2011;31(2):332-5.
16. Vural A, Kara N, Sayin N. Choroidal thickness changes after a single administration of coffee in healthy subjects. Retina. 2014;34(6):1223-8.
17. Sizmaz S, Kucukerdonmez C, Pinarci E, et al. The effect of smoking on choroidal thickness measured by optical coherence tomography. Br J Ophthalmol. 2013;97(5):601-4.
18. Copete S, Flores-Moreno I, Montero J, et al. Direct comparison of spectral domain and swept-source OCT in measurement of choroidal thickness in normal eyes. Br J Ophthalmol. 2014;98:334-8.
19. Banitt M. The choroid in glaucoma. Curr Opin Ophthalmol. 2013;24:125-9.
20. Maul E, Friedman D, Chang D, et al. Choroidal thickness measured by spectral domain optical coherence tomography: factors affecting thickness in glaucoma patients. Ophthalmology. 2011;118:1571-9.
21. Mwanza J, Hochberg J, Banitt M, et al. Lack of association between glaucoma and macular choroidal thickness measured with enhanced depth imaging optical coherence tomography. Invest Ophthalmol Vis Sci. 2011;52:3430-5.
22. Mwaza J, Sayyad F, Budenz D. Choroidal thickness in unilateral advanced glaucoma. Invest Ophthalmol Vis Sci. 2012;53:6695-701.
23. Thew J, Kim Y, Choi K. Measurement of subfoveal choroidal thickness in normal-tension glaucoma in Korean patients. J Glaucoma. 2014;23(1):46-9.
24. Fenolland J, Giraud J, May F, et al. Evaluation de l'epaisseur choroidienne par tomographie en coherence optique (SD-OCT). Etude preliminaire dans le glaucome a angle ouvert. J Fr Ophthalmol. 2011;34:313-7.
25. McCourt E, Cadena B, Bernett C, et al. Measurement of subfoveal choroidal thickness using spectral domain optical coherence tomography. Ophthalmic Surg Lasers Imaging. 2010;41(Suppl.):S28-S33.

26. Roberts K, Artes P, O'Leary N, et al. Peripapillary choroidal thickness in healthy controls and patients with focal, diffuse and sclerotic glaucomatous optic disc damage. Arch Ophthalmol. 2012;130:980-9.

27. Hirooka K, Tenkumo K, Fujiwara A, et al. Evaluation of peripapillary choroidal thickness in patients with normal-tension glaucoma. BMC Ophthalmol. 2012:12:29.

28. Usui S, Ikuno Y, Miki A, et al. Evaluation of the choroidal thickness using high-penetration optical coherence tomography with long wavelength in highly myopic normal tension glaucoma. Am J Ophthalmol. 2012;153:10.e1-16e1.

29. Park S, De Moraes C, Teng C, et al. Enhanced depth imaging optical coherence tomography of deep optic nerve complex structures in glaucoma. Ophthalmology. 2012;119:3-9.

30. Lee J, Kim, T, Weinreb R, et al. Reversal of lamina cribosa displacement after intraocular pressure reduction in open-angle glaucoma. Ophthalmology. 2013;120:553-9.

31. Gilbert C, Owens S, Smith P, et al. Long-term follow-up of central serous chorioretinopathy. Br J Ophthalmol. 1984;68:515-20.

32. Bouzas E, Scott M, Mastorakos G, et al. Central Serous chorioretinopathy and glucocorticoids. Surv Ophthalmol. 2002;47:431-48.

33. Carvahalo-Recchia C, Yannuzzi L, Negrao S, et al. Corticosteroids and central serous chorioretinopathy. Ophthalmology. 2002;109:1834-7.

34. Iida T, Kishi S, Hagimura N, et al. Persistent and bilateral choroidal vascular abnormalities in central serous chorioretinopathy. Retina. 1999;19:508-12.

35. Imamura Y, Fujiwara T, Margolis R, et al. Enhanced depth imaging optical coherence tomography of the choroid in central serous chorioretinopathy. Retina. 2009;29:1469-73.

36. Maruko I, Iida T, Sugano Y, et al. Subfoveal choroidal thickness in fellow eyes of patients with central serous chorioretinopathy. Retina. 2011;31:1603-8.

37. Maruko I, Iida T, Sugano Y, et al. Subfoveal choroidal thickness after treatment of central serous chorioretinopathy. Ophthalmology. 2010;117:1792-9.

38. Jirarattanasopa P, Ooto S, Tsujikawa A, et al. Assessment of macular choroidal thickness by optical coherence tomography and angiographic changes in central serous chorioretinopathy. Ophthalmology. 2012;119:1666-78.

39. Yang L, Jonas J, Wei W. Choroidal vessel diameter in central serous chorioretinopathy. Acta Ophthalmol. 2013;91:e358-e362.

40. Ferrara D, Mohler K, Waheed N, et al. En face enhanced-depth swept-source optical coherence tomography features of chronic central serous chorioretinopathy. Ophthalmology. 2014;121:719-26.

41. Yannuzzi L, Slakter J, Gross N, et al. Indocyanine green angiography guided photodynamic therapy for treatment of chronic central serous chorioretinopathy: a pilot study. Retina. 2003;23:288-98.

42. Cardillo Piccolino F, Eandi C, Ventre L, et al. Photodynamic therapy for chronic central serous chorioretinopathy. Retina. 2003;23:752-63.

43. Chan W, Lai T, Lai R, et al. Half-dose vertoporfin photodynamic therapy for acute central serous chorioretinopathy: one-year results of a prospective study. Retina. 2008;115:1756-65.

44. Chan W, Lai T, Lai R, et al. Half-dose vertoporfin photodynamic therapy for chronic central serous chorioretinopathy: one-year results of a prospective study. Retina. 2008;28:85-93.

45. Maruko I, Iida T, Sugano Y, et al. One-year choroidal thickness results after photodynamic therapy for central serous chorioretinopathy. Retina. 2011;31:1921-7.

46. Karampelas M, Sim D, Keane P, et al. Choroidal assessment in idiopathic panuveitis using optical coherence tomography. Graefes Arch Clin Exp Ophthalmol. 2013;251(8):2029-36.

47. Kim M, Kim H, Known H, et al. Choroidal thickness in Bachet's uveitis: an enhacned depth imaging-ocular coherence tomography and its association with angiographic changes. Invest Ophthalmol Vis Sci. 2013;54:6033-9.

48. Coskun E, Gurler B, Pehlivan Y, et al. Enhanced depth imaging optical coherence tomography findings in Behçet's disease. Ocul Immunol Inflamm. 2013;21(6):440-5.

49. Maruko I, Iida T, Sugano Y, et al. Subfoveal choroidal thickness after treatment of Vogt-Koyanagi-Harada disease. Retina. 2011;31(3):501-7.

50. Nakayama M, Keino H, Okada AA, et al. Enhanced depth imaging optical coherence tomography of the choroid in Vogt-Koyanagi Harada disease. Retina. 2012;32(10):2061-9.

51. Nakai K, Gomi F, Ikuno Y, et al. Choroidal observations in Vogt-Koyanagi-Harada disease using high-penetration optical coherence tomography. Graefes Arch Clin Exp Ophthalmol. 2012;250(7):1089-95.

52. Da Silva F, Sakaata V, Nakashima A, et al. Enhanced depth imaging optical coherence tomography in long-standing Vogt-Koyanagi-Harada disease. Br J Ophthalmol. 2013;97(1):70-4.

53. Fong A, Li K, Fong D. Choroidal evaluation using enhanced depth imaging spectral-domain optical coherence tomography in Vogt-Koyanagi-Harada disease. Retina. 2011;31:502-9.

54. Hosoda Y, Uji A, Hangai M, et al. Relationship between retinal lesions and inward choroidal bulging in Vogt-Koyanagi-Harada disease. Am J Ophthalmol. 2014;157(5):1056-63..

55. Nazari H, Hariri A, Hu Z, et al. Choroidal atrophy and loss of choriocapillaris in convalescent stage of Vogt-Koyangai-Harada disease: in vivo documentation. J Ophthal Inflamm Infect. 2014;4:9.

56. Hua R, Chen K, Liu M, et al. Multi-modality imaging on multiple evanescent white dot syndrome—a Spectralis study. Int J Ophthalmol. 2012;5(5):644-7.

57. Arias J, Kumar N, Fulco E, et al. The seasick choroid: a finding on enhanced depth imaging spectral-domain optical coherence tomography of choroidal lymphoma. Retin Cases Brief Rep. 2013;7(1):19-22.

58. Rostaqui O, Quergues G, Haymann P, et al. Visualization of sarcoid granuloma by enhanced depth imaging optical coherence tomography. Occul Immunol Inflamm. 2014;22(3):239-41.

59. Grunwald J, Hariprasad S, DuPont J, et al. Foveolar choroidal blod flow in age-related macular degeneration. Invest Ophthalmol Vis Sci. 2005;46(3):1033-8.

60. Mullins R, Johnson M, Faidley E, et al. Choriocapillaris vascular dropout related to density of drusen in human eyes with early age-related macular degeneration. Invest Ophthalmol Vis Sci. 2011;52(3):1606-12.

61. Berenberg T, Metelitsina T, Meadow B, et al. The association between drusen extent and foveolar choroidal blood flow in age-related macular degeneration. Retina. 2012;32(1):25-31.

62. Manjunath V, Goren J, Fujimoto J, et al. Analysis of choroidal thickness in age-related macular degeneration using spectral domain optical coherence tomography. Am J Ophthalmol. 2011;125:663-8.

63. Jirarattanasopa P, Ooto S, Nakata I, et al. Choroidal thickness vascular hyperpermeability, and compliment factor H in age-related macular degeneration and polypoidal choroidal vasculopathy. Invest Ophthalmol Vis Sci. 2012;53:3663-72.

64. Kim S, Oh J, Kwon S, et al. Comparison of choroidal thickness among aptients with healthy eyes, early age-related maculopathy, neovascular age-related macular degeneration, central serous chorioretinopathy and polypoidal choroidal vasculopathy. Retina. 31:1904-11.
65. Yamakazi T, Koizumi H, Yamagishi T, et al. Subfoveal choroidal thickness in retinal angiomatous proliferation. Retina. 2014;34(7):1316-22.
66. Kang H, Kwon H, Yi J, et al. Subfoveal choroidal thickness as a potential predictor of visual outcome and treatment response after intravitreal ranibizumab injections for typical exudative age-related macular degeneration. Am J Ophthalmol. 2014;157(5):1013-21.
67. Tsuiki E, Kiyoshi S, Ryotaro U, et al. Enhanced depth imaging optical coherence tomography of the choroid in central retinal vein occlusion. Am J Ophthalmol. 2013;156:543-7.
68. Fujiwara T, Imamura Y, Margolis R, et al. Enhanced depth imaging optical coherence tomography of the choroid in highly myopic eyes. Am J Ophthalmol. 2009;148(3):445-50.
69. Ohsugi H, Ikuno Y, Oshima K, et al. 3-D choroidal thickness maps from EDI-OCT in highly myopic eyes. Optom Vis Sci. 2013;90(6):599-606.
70. Hayashi M, Ito Y, Takahashi A, et al. Scleral thickness in highly myopic eyes measured by enhanced depth imaging optical coherence tomography. Eye. 2013;27(3):410-7.
71. Flores-Moreno I, Ruiz-Medrano J, Duker JS, et al. The relationship between retinal and choroidal thickness and visual acuity on highly myopic eyes. Br J Ophthalmol. 2013;97(8):1010-3.
72. Nishida Y, Fujiwara T, Imamura Y, et al. Choroidal thickness and visual acuity in highly myopic eyes. Retina. 2012;32(7):1229-36.
73. Ho M, Liu DT, Chan VC, et al. Choroidal thickness measurement in myopic eyes by enhanced depth optical coherence tomography. Ophthalmology. 2013;120(9):1909-14.
74. Ahn S, Woo S, Kim K, et al. Association between choroidal morphology and anti-vascular endothelial growth factor treatment outcome in myopic choroidal neovascularization. Invest Ophthalmol Vis Sci. 2013;54(3):2115-22.
75. Yang HS, Kim J, Kim J, et al. Prognostic factors of eyes with naive subfoveal myopic choroidal neovascularization after intravitreal bevacizumab. Am J Ophthalmol. 2013;156(6):1201-10.
76. Dhoot D, Huo S, Yuan A, et al. Evaluation of choroidal thickness in retinitis pigmentosa using enhanced depth imaging optical coherence tomography. Br J Ophthalmol. 2013;97(1):66-9.
77. Ayton L, Guymer R, Luu C. Choroidal thickness profiles in retinitis pigmentosa. Clin Experiment Ophthalmol. 2013;41(4):369-403.
78. Yeoh J, Rahman W, Chen F, et al. Choroidal imaging in inherited retinal disease using the technique of enhanced depth imaging optical coherence tomography. Graefes Arch Clin Exp Ophthalmol. 2010;248(12):1719-28.
79. Torres V, Brungnoni N, Kaiser P, et al. Optical coherence tomography enhanced depth imaging of choroidal tumors. Am J Ophthalmol. 2011;151(4):586-93.
80. Shields CL, Kaliki S, Rojanaporn D, et al. Enhanced depth imaging optical coherence tomography of small choroidal melanoma comparison with choroidal nevus. Arch Ophthalmol. 2012;130(7): 850-6.
81. Demerci H, Cullen A, Sundstrom J. Enhanced depth imagingoptical coherence tomography of choroidal metastasis. Retina. 2013;34(7):1-6.

82. Shah S, Kaliki S, Rojanaporn D, et al. Enhanced depth imaging optical coherence tomography of choroidal nevus in 104 cases. Ophthalmology. 2012;119:1066-72.

83. Pellegrini M, Shields C, Arepalli S, et al. Choroidal melanocytosis evaluation with enhanced depth imaging optical coherence tomography. Ophthalmology. 2014;121: 257-61.

84. Erol M, Coban D, Ceran B, et al. Enhanced depth imaging optical coherence tomography and fundus autofluorescence findings in bilateral choroidal osteoma: a case report. Arq Bras Oftalmol. 2013;76(3):189-91.

CHAPTER 6

Diabetic Retinopathy: An Update

Dhananjay Shukla

DIABETES PANDEMIC: REPEATEDLY REVISING ESTIMATES

The global burden of diabetes mellitus is growing at such an alarming rate that the growth beats the periodic estimates and future projections by a wide margin with consistency. Sample the following projections: WHO estimated in 2002 that 177 million people worldwide suffered from diabetes, and by the year 2030, the number of people with diabetes would more than double to 370 million.[1] In 2009, this projection for 2030 was revised to 438 million.[2] In 2015, the estimate for 2030 was again upgraded (by 35%) to 592 million.[3] We do not know what the real figures would be 13 years from now, but the repeatedly surpassed projections and their implications appear ominous. Closer home, 1 in 12 Indian adults have diabetes, more than half of whom are undiagnosed.[3] This number (close to 70 million adults) is about the double of what was estimated (35 million) for today in 2003,[4] and constitutes about 17% of the current global diabetic population of 415 million.[3] Diabetic retinopathy (DR), the most common microvascular complication of diabetes,[5] is likely to be present in about a third of diabetic subjects at any given time, and eventually affects nearly all diabetics after two to three decades.[6,7] This exponential increase in systemic diabetes and concurrent retinopathy has projected DR as one of the leading causes of visual loss globally.[8]

PATHOGENESIS

Risk Factors Affecting Diabetic Retinopathy

Epidemiological Factors

In type 1 diabetes mellitus (DM), DR is rare before the age of 13 years. After this age, the prevalence and severity of retinopathy increase with increasing age. In type 2 diabetes, the severity of retinopathy is not related to age.[6,7] No significant predilection was seen for the male or female gender in Wisconsin Epidemiologic Study of Diabetic Retinopathy (WESDR).[6,7] Pima Indians have a higher risk of developing proliferative diabetic retinopathy (PDR) as compared to white Americans.[9] People of Indian origin, in India or abroad, have a particularly high predisposition for developing DM.[1]

Systemic Diabetes

Type 1 diabetics typically have a faster progression of DR and more commonly lose vision due to PDR. Type 2 diabetics, who outnumber type 1 patients 9:1, lose vision more commonly due to diabetic macular edema (DME). After 20 years of diabetes, 99% of type 1 and 60% of type 2 diabetics have retinopathy; and 53% of type 1 and 5% of type 2 patients have PDR.[6,7] Two major clinical trials proved that intensive control of diabetes [glycosylated hemoglobin (HbA1C) close to 7 g/dL] reduces both the incidence and progression of DR in spite of an early worsening of retinopathy. Tight control works best when applied at the earliest after detection of diabetes.[10,11]

Genetic Factors

A majority of type 1 diabetics have HLA – DR3 or DR4. A long-term follow-up of WESDR patients showed no effect of HLA type on the development and progression of DR.[12] The genetic transmission is low: only 3–6% of siblings and 8% of the offspring of the diabetic patient are prone to become diabetic. Type 2 DM has a stronger genetic predisposition in spite of no HLA association, and 30% of the offspring and 40% of siblings are affected.[13]

Other Systemic Diseases

Hypertension (HT) is extremely common in diabetics. The United Kingdom Prospective Diabetes Study (UKPDS) showed that tight blood pressure control reduced the progression of DR and the need for photocoagulation. Nephropathy worsens DR through rheological, platelet, and lipid abnormalities. It increases the risk of both macular edema and PDR.[14] Increased serum cholesterol causes an increase in hard exudates at macula with a subsequent visual compromise. This effect is additional to the increased risk of atherosclerosis and ischemic heart disease in diabetics.[15] Anemia aggravates retinal hypoxia by the decreased oxygen-carrying capacity of the blood and is an independent risk factor for high-risk PDR and severe visual loss. When hemoglobin falls below 12 g/dL, the risk of retinopathy has been reported to increase twofold.[14]

Physical Factors

The most important determinant of retinopathy is the duration of diabetes after the onset of puberty. The risk of retinopathy is the same in two adults of whom one developed diabetes at age 6, and the other, at age 12.[16] DR accelerates during pregnancy and needs to be strictly monitored and controlled. PDR is twice as likely in pregnant women. Severe NPDR is also a risk factor for congenital anomalies in the newborn.[9]

Socioeconomic Factors

Though the increasing incidence of diabetes has been linked to lifestyle changes and urbanization,[4] it is probably incorrect to call diabetes a disease of the rich. Neither hyperglycemia, nor DR has been found to be associated with socioeconomic status.[9,17] Though smoking has no association with DR and moderating drinking may be of some benefit in type 1 DM, (WESDR), it is prudent to advise against both, as smoking diabetics are twice as likely to die, and "moderate" drinking is rare in alcoholics.

Local Factors

While cataract occurs early in diabetic eyes, its removal poses an increased risk of anterior and posterior segment complications like uveitis, endophthalmitis, posterior capsular opacification and cystoid macular edema (CME). Contrary to the traditional belief that cataract surgery accelerates DR, there is currently no clear evidence that the current standard cataract surgery—phacoemulsification—causes the progression of DR or DME in controlled diabetes and mild-moderate NPDR (less severe retinopathy).[18] Caution should be exercised in the presence of severe NPDR or worse (more severe retinopathy) or preexisting DME, both of which should be treated before cataract surgery, especially in a poorly controlled diabetic subject.[18]

On the other hand, various degenerative and atrophic diseases of the retina (glaucoma, myopia, optic atrophy, retinitis pigmentosa) are associated with a dramatically reduced risk of the progression of DR. These conditions reduce the metabolic demand of retina and thereby substantially decrease the effect of hypoxia, the stimulus for new vessel formation.[19]

Biochemical Mechanisms[20-24]

Sorbitol Pathway

Excess glucose in a diabetic's bloodstream is channeled through alternative metabolic pathways, one of which is the sorbitol pathway. The enzyme aldose reductase converts excess glucose into an intermediate product, sorbitol, intracellularly. The stabilization of sorbitol as fructose sugar is a slow reaction and occurs extracellularly. Since sorbitol cannot be transported out of the cell rapidly and it is osmotically active, it accumulates water inside the cell. This is the main mechanism for pericyte loss; and also adversely effects photoreceptor function, retinal blood flow and vasodilatation. Besides cataracts, diabetic neuropathy also results from sorbitol pathway.

Nonenzymatic Glycation of Proteins

This is the mechanism of browning of meat when incubated with glucose. In diabetic eyes, there is a similar adhesion of glucose with proteins, which results in continued cross-linking, and the formation of advanced glycosylation (now called "glycation") end-products (AGE). Since this is a very slow process, it only affects tissues with a slow protein turnover like the basement membrane. Quick-turnover proteins like hemoglobin are not affected. Therefore, HbA1C, a glycosylated protein, only indicates diabetic control, without affecting the function of hemoglobin.

Protein Kinase C Pathway

Incomplete metabolism of excess glucose leads to the accumulation of intermediates like AGE proteins and diacyl glycerol (DAG). Elevated levels of DAG result in the increased activity of ubiquitous enzyme, protein kinase C (PKC), which decreases retinal blood flow. PKC is also activated by vascular endothelial growth factor (VEGF) and mediates its functions, mainly blood–retinal barrier (BRB) breakdown and neovascular proliferation.

Oxidative Stress

Accumulated glucose and AGE products undergo auto-oxidation resulting in free radical release. Free radicals are also contributed by the sorbitol pathway. Besides, glycated proteins also inactivate antioxidant enzyme systems, which remove excess free radicals.

Angiogenic Factors

Vascular endothelial growth factor is a peptide produced mainly by extravascular tissue: glia, retinal pigment epithelium (RPE), macrophages and T-cells; it is upregulated by hypoxia and is potently angiogenic. It is the major catalyst for both inner BRB breakdown (disruption of tight junctions) and new vessel formation (capillary endothelial proliferation) in the retina and the iris, in most occlusive vascular diseases. Besides hypoxia, it is also released in response to trauma and inflammation. Other growth factors like the fibroblast growth factor and the insulin-like growth factor, have only a synergistic, supportive or permissive role adjuvant to VEGF. Angiogenesis is kept in check by inhibitory factors like the pigment epithelium-derived factor and angiostatin, which appear to have a reciprocal relationship with VEGF.

Histopathological Changes[20,21,24]

Diabetic retinopathy has traditionally been considered a vascular disease, primarily a capillaropathy. Since only the inner half of retina is vascular, it is also presumed to be an inner retinal disease. The hallmark pathological changes in DR are tissue hypoxia and edema, primarily caused by microvascular occlusion and leakage. These nuggets of traditional wisdom have however been increasingly disputed over the past decade or so, with evidence of neuronal degeneration and inflammation in diabetic eye disease.

Thickening of Capillary Basement Membrane

The glycation of capillary basement membrane (CBM) collagen results in its thickening, directly and by decreased proteoglycan levels, which normally inhibit collagen production. There is also a concomitant vacuolization in CBM. These changes result in increased platelet adhesion, reduced diffusion of nutrients, and decreased binding (and therefore, decreased sequestration) of growth factors (e.g. fibroblast growth factor) which are subsequently released in the blood stream, free to induce angiogenesis.

Loss of Capillary Pericytes

Sorbitol accumulation, along with free radicals from various sources, destroys pericytes, which are the "muscles" of the capillaries, and maintain their tone. Pericyte loss not only results in microaneurysm formation by focal dilatations of the weakened capillaries, but also results in the thickening of CBM, normally inhibited by pericytes.

Endothelial Cell Damage

The accumulation of sorbitol, AGE products and glucose itself is toxic to the capillary endothelium. The damage is exacerbated by accelerated blood flow in the later stages of DR. This results in a leakage from the inner BRB, acellularity of the capillaries and also leukocytosis and leukocyte adhesion to the capillary wall.

Hematological Alterations

There are changes in blood cells—RBCs and WBCs become less deformable, the latter also become activated, and the platelets aggregate more easily. These cellular changes, accompanied by reduced blood flow, cause thrombus formation in the capillaries. The consequent capillary occlusion is prolonged by defective fibrinolytic mechanisms, resulting in widespread retinal ischemia.

Extravascular Changes in Diabetic Retinopathy[20,24]

Multiple studies have shown ample evidence of neurosensory dysfunction long before the earliest vascular changes appear. There is evidence of decreased blue–yellow color perception and contrast sensitivity, reduced oscillatory potentials on b-wave of the electroretinogram (ERG), and nerve fiber layer defects on red-free photography in this preclinical stage. Many of these changes are due to neuronal cell death caused by abnormal glutamate metabolism, which points at the malfunction of yet another extravascular tissue—Müller cells and astrocytes. Finally, VEGF, the central catalyst of the most important changes during the progression of DR, is released by nonvascular tissue.

Contribution of Outer Retina[5,24,25]

Retinal pigment epithelium is an important source of both angiogenic (VEGF) and angiostatic (PEDF) factors which have a central role in the pathogenesis of DR. The contribution of the RPE to the causation and persistence of DME has also been suspected; susceptibility of old diabetics to DME may partly be explained by a weaker RPE pump.

Rod photoreceptors, with their highest rate of metabolism, completely deplete the oxygen levels in the inner retina, precipitating tissue hypoxia. Rods are probably the reason why retina, which is an outpouching of the brain, gets affected by diabetes much earlier than brain, heart, major vessels, kidney, and peripheral nerves. The destruction/degeneration of rods and RPE (e.g. retinitis pigmentosa, scatter photocoagulation) is known to protect the retina from hypoxia and subsequent neovascularization.

Is Diabetic Retinopathy an Inflammatory Disease?[26]

This is a surprising, exciting, and fundamental question raised about the pathogenesis of DR. While DR has only two of the classic five macroscopic signs of inflammation (swelling and loss of function); it has *all* the microscopic attributes of inflammation: vasodilatation, altered blood flow, fluid and protein exudation, and leukocytosis. Leukocytes clog the capillaries more efficiently than RBC, because of their larger size and lower pliability. VEGF released by capillary shutdown and hypoxia is also released during inflammation. Other inflammatory mediators (ICAM-2, B-integrins) are also observed in DR. Therefore, there is now good evidence that DR may be a chronic, low-grade inflammation.

CLINICAL FEATURES OF DIABETIC RETINOPATHY[5,16,23,24]

Diabetic retinopathy is asymptomatic for a long-time in its course till advanced sight-threatening lesions (central macular edema and bleeding new vessels) develop, when it is generally too late to recover the lost vision. This aspect is important in proactive screening for DR, just like screening for retinopathy of prematurity in premature and underweight newborns. Since the symptoms are too late, it is imperative to recognize the signs early, and also to know which signs warrant close follow-up or early treatment.

Microaneurysms

Microaneurysms (MA) are the earliest clinical change and the hallmark of DR. Clinically seen as red dots, they appear mostly in the posterior pole, and may be difficult to distinguish from dot hemorrhages (*it is not mandatory to make this differentiation clinically, either*). They are formed either by pericyte loss in the capillary wall (patent MA, leak fluid and cause macular edema), or by endothelial proliferation (solid MA, typically bordering capillary dropouts do not leak).

Soft Exudates

This popular term is a misnomer; there is no exudation in these lesions: they are more appropriately called cotton–wool spots. They are nerve fiber layer infarcts, which appear white due to accumulation of axoplasmic debris in the neurons. They are a soft indicator for DR progression; but one should look for intraretinal microvascular abnormalities (IRMA, which are a strong predictor of progression) in their vicinity. Excessive soft exudates warrant a check for other comorbidities like hypertension, HIV, etc.

Hemorrhages

Dot and blot hemorrhages occur in deeper capillary plexuses (mainly the outer plexiform layer) and spread anteroposteriorly like a cylinder. The dot-like appearance is due to viewing this blood column head on. Blot hemorrhages are not merely larger bleeds; they are hemorrhagic infarcts of retina (arteriolar occlusion), and therefore a strong predictor of the progression of DR. On the other hand, when bleeds occur in the retinal nerve fiber layer, they assume a frayed splinter-like appearance following the distribution of nerve fibers: these are more common in hypertension.

Venous Caliber Alterations

Veins have been described as dilated, tortuous, reduplicated, looped or beaded in DR. Venous beading (localized constrictions and dilatations of venous wall) is the most important venous change, and a strong indicator of the progression of retinal hypoxia and DR (Fig. 6.1). This appearance is also called *sausaging* when the constrictions of venous wall appear at longer intervals.

Intraretinal Microvascular Abnormalities

This intentionally equivocal term, originally coined to describe irregularly dilated capillaries, is used to convey the dilemma about the nature of these vessels, arteriovenous shunts or intraretinal new vessels. Since new preretinal vessels are observed to arise from areas of IRMA, some authors believe they are indeed early new vessels, which do not bleed/leak significantly due to compact nature of the surrounding retina (Figs. 6.2A and B). They are the strongest predictors of the progression of DR.

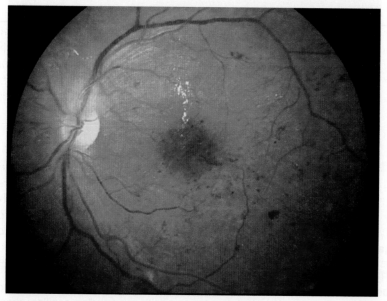

Fig. 6.1: Venous beading is a key prognostic sign of worsening of diabetic retinopathy (DR), when present in two or more quadrants. Beading is apparent in the superotemporal major vein after the first, second, and third arteriovenous crossings.

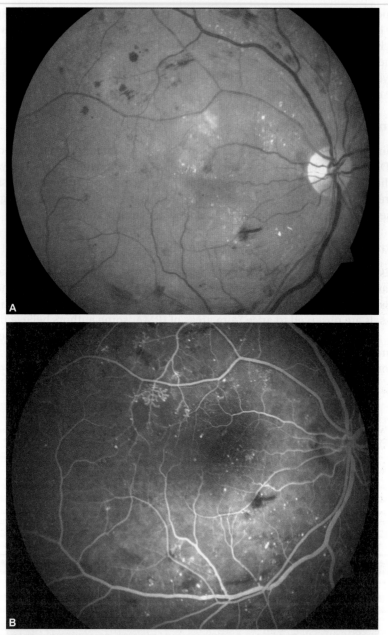

Figs. 6.2A and B: (A) Intraretinal microvascular abnormalities (IRMA) are the most important indicators of retinal hypoxia and progression of diabetic retinopathy (DR). IRMA is faintly visible arising from the second vertical branching of the superotemporal major artery. (B) Fluorescein angiography (FA) clearly shows the IRMA as a large telangiectatic structure with surrounding capillary dropout superotemporal to foveal avascular zone (FAZ).

New Vessels

When endothelial tubules, budding from the venous end of the capillary bed break through the internal limiting membrane (ILM) to lie on the inner retinal surface, they are called true new vessels. When present on or within a disk diameter (DD) from the optic disk, they are called neovascularization disks (NVD); elsewhere in the fundus, they are labeled as neovascularization elsewhere (NVE). An NVD indicates the ischemia of at least a quadrant of the retina. NVE are mostly seen with three DD of the arcades, and the preferential sites are temporal to the macula and the nasal to optic disk. An NVD is seen in nearly half of the eyes with PDR.

Macular Edema

Diabetic macular edema is the most frequent cause of visual impairment in diabetic patients. It may occur at any stage of DR but is more common in advanced stages (e.g. 70% of eyes with PDR). When edema occurs close to or at the center of the macula, it is called clinically significant macular edema (CSME). CSME can be focal (localized area of edema surrounded by hard exudate rings, with culprit microaneurysms in the center) or diffuse (generalized edema of two disk areas or more involving the foveal center). The hard exudates associated with DME are lipoprotein residues left behind as they are absorbed at a slower rate than the plasma component of edema. They indicate absorbing edema and not CSME per se. When excessive, they may cause substantial visual loss by subretinal fibrosis, and warrant an investigation for hyperlipidemia, hypertension or nephropathy.

NATURAL COURSE AND GRADING OF DIABETIC RETINOPATHY

Diabetic retinopathy progresses in a diabetic eye through discrete stages, which have been known and studied for over a century. Historically, the term *classification* has been used to designate the stages of progression of DR; however, *staging* or *grading* are more accurate descriptions of a study of the natural course of the disease, rather than its *types or subtypes*. The current gold standard system for grading was proposed by the Early Treatment for Diabetic Retinopathy Study (ETDRS) group in 1991.[27,28] This grading of DR (represented by a *severity scale*) is based on stereophotographs captured in seven standard fundus fields, and a comparison of the clinical features of DR in a given case against the standard stereopairs of ETDRS color slides to determine the severity of retinopathy.[27] The ETDRS retinopathy severity scale had 15 levels, from level 10 (no DR) to 90 (ungradable, beyond advanced PDR).[28] For practising physicians, this research-level grading has been collapsed into a more clinically acceptable five levels.[29] Nonproliferative diabetic retinopathy (NPDR) has been graded into four stages, which have discrete risks of progression (to PDR within 1 year); no DR; mild NPDR (5%), moderate NPDR (20%), and severe NPDR (50%). Severe NPDR is the watershed zone, and must

TABLE 6.1: Classification of diabetic retinopathy and follow-up schedule.

Disease severity level	Findings on dilated ophthalmoscopy	*Follow-up schedule
No apparent retinopathy	No abnormalities	Yearly
Mild NPDR	Microaneurysms only	Yearly
Moderate NPDR	More than just microaneurysms but less than severe nonproliferative diabetic retinopathy	6–12 months
Severe NPDR	Any of the following (4:2:1 rule): >20 intraretinal hemorrhages in each of four quadrants; definite venous beading in two quadrants; prominent IRMA in one quadrant	2–4 months
PDR	One or more of the following: neovascularization, vitreous/preretinal hemorrhage	Treat with panretinal photocoagulation

*Follow-up is shorter in the presence of uncontrolled disease, pregnancy, noncompliance, etc. (see text)
(NPDR: nonproliferative diabetic retinopathy; PDR: Proliferative diabetic retinopathy; IRMA: Intraretinal microvascular abnormalities)
Source: Adapted from American Academy of Ophthalmology. Preferred practice pattern: diabetic retinopathy. San Francisco: American Academy of Ophthalmology; 2016.

be carefully discriminated from the previous moderate stage. PDR is the stage where treatment is warranted (Table 6.1). The initially analogue (print-based) photography of 30° fields has now been largely replaced by digital imaging: Joslin Vision Network established the parity of nonmydriatic low-light digital imaging with the ETRDS gold standard; the former was much faster, easy to store and share, and preferred by the patients who did not require pupillary dilatation.[30] More recently, the same group and several others demonstrated that ultra-wide field photography (200° image) not only equaled ETRDRS analog imaging; but actually showed prognostically significant peripheral lesions in 9% cases, which were outside the ETDRS fields.[31,32]

DIFFERENTIAL DIAGNOSIS OF DIABETIC RETINOPATHY

Any retinopathy in a diabetic eye is presumed by default to be DR, and this presumption holds good in most of the cases. However, in a significant minority, DR can either look like other retinal diseases, or a coexisting disease can alter the fundus picture and management protocol substantially.

Diabetic retinopathy has traditionally been considered a disease of the posterior retina. A minority of patients however show DR more prominently in the fellow eye periphery, both on clinical examination and fluorescein angiography (FA) (Figs. 6.3A to D).[19,32] Peripheral examination is therefore now important in DR. Chronic ischemia in DR sometimes leads to neovascularization without the preceding preproliferative retinal lesions like venous beading, IRMA. This featureless neovascularization is deceptively subtle, but nonetheless associated with significant capillary dropouts on FFA. Two clues to suspect it are the sheathing of the retinal arterioles (not venules, as in Eales' disease) and asymmetric retinopathy between the two eyes.[19,24] Bilateral asymmetry in DR can also follow unilateral degenerative diseases like retinitis pigmentosa, high myopia, chorioretinal scarring following multifocal choroiditis (*which incidentally was the reason scatter photocoagulation was*

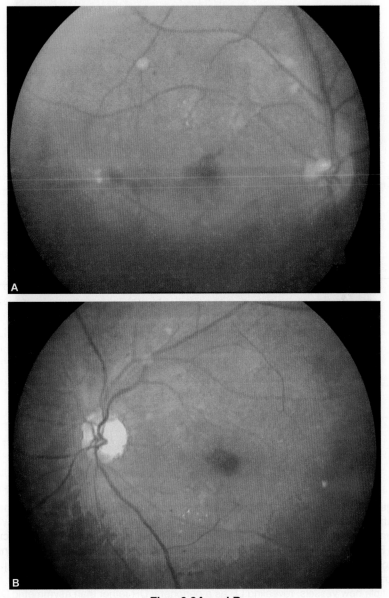

Figs. 6.3A and B

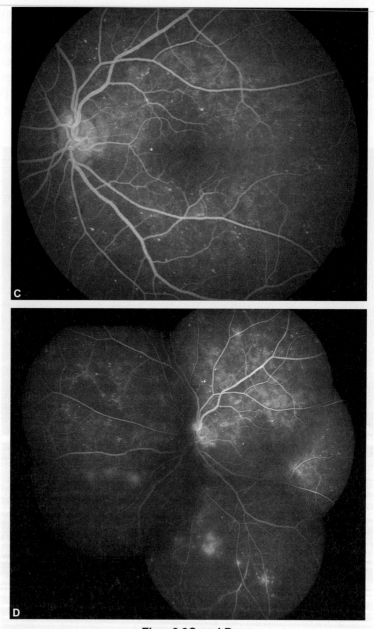

Figs. 6.3C and D

Figs. 6.3A to D: (A) Proliferative diabetic retinopathy (PDR) with vitreous hemorrhage in the right eye (RE). (B) Left eye (LE) of the same patient appears to show an asymmetrically mild DR, albeit with some horizontal retinal folds in the superior macula. (C) Fluorescein angiography (FA) of the posterior pole appears to endorse the clinical diagnosis of mild nonproliferative diabetic retinopathy (NPDR). (D) Peripheral FA captures (focusing on inferonasal quadrant) reveal extensive capillary dropouts and multiple new vessels, revealing LE as a peripheral DR rather than asymmetric DR.

attempted to treat PDR by inducing iatrogenic multifocal chorioretinal scars) or optic atrophy.[19,24,25] The most common cause of unilateral optic disk edema in a middle-aged person is nonarteritic anterior ischemic optic neuropathy (NAION), which should warrant a check for hypertension and visual fields. Malignant hypertension and intracranial space-occupying lesions should also be suspected when bilateral disk edema presents with DR. However, after these dangerous entities have been ruled out, one should remember that diabetes itself can cause mild and visually insignificant disk edema (more commonly bilateral, in a type 1 diabetic), called *diabetic papillopathy*.[19] Finally, diabetic subjects are likely to develop idiopathic macular telangiectasia (MacTel, type 2), which may mimic, and sometimes coexist with DME. FA can be misleading; optical coherence tomography (OCT) however clearly shows foveal atrophy rather than edema, avoiding unnecessary and harmful laser photocoagulation.[33]

The most common systemic comorbidity with diabetes is hypertension. Hypertensive retinopathy (HTR) has distinctive features like flame hemorrhages, arteriovenous crossing changes, serous macular detachment and later, disk edema. However, HTR shares features like hard and soft exudates with DR, and should be suspected when its classic features are present, even

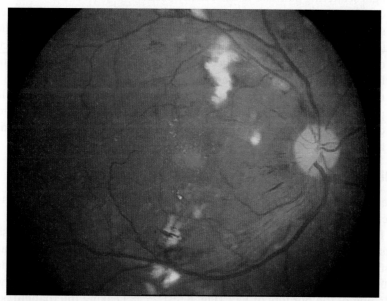

Fig. 6.4: This 25-year-old type 2 diabetics had a fundus picture suggestive of hypertensive retinopathy (flame hemorrhages and cotton-wool spots), but had no history of hypertension. Repeat blood pressure (BP) check revealed severe hypertension (180/110 mm Hg). While hypertension is extremely common in diabetics, several cases remain undiagnosed.

in young adults (Fig. 6.4). Similarly, when hard exudates are very prominent, serum lipid profile must be checked before treating macular edema.

IMAGING IN DIABETIC RETINOPATHY

Fundus Fluorescein Angiography

Fundus fluorescein angiography (FFA) is a crucial but often misused investigation for DR. The ETDRS study recommended FFA only for guiding treatment of CSME; and not for grading DR. However, there are several important indications of FFA, some of which were not addressed by the ETDRS:

- *Normal-looking fellow eye of severe NPDR/PDR (asymmetric DR)*: Many have PDR with peripheral new vessels or featureless retina (see above), which may be clinically missed (Figs. 6.3A to D). Asymmetric DR is very uncommon; subtle new vessels are not uncommon.[19]
- *Macular ischemia*: Clinically suspected by subnormal vision, sclerosed macular arterioles, blot hemorrhages or soft exudates in macula; macular ischemia can be confirmed by irregular or enlarged foveal avascular zone (FAZ) (Figs. 6.5A and B).[34]
- *Asteroid hyalosis*: When severe NPDR or worse is suspected (e.g. by examination of the fellow eye), FA easily reveals the capillary dropouts/ new vessels inaccessible to clinical examination due to the highly reflective light scattering particles of asteroid hyalosis.
- *Confusion between severe NPDR and PDR*: Severe grade IRMA can sometimes look like NVE, and the latter leak profusely on FA unlike IRMA (Figs. 6.2B and 3D). However, when extensive capillary dropout is detected on FA, even severe NPDR, especially in type 2 DM, becomes an indication for early scatter photocoagulation.[35]
- *Confusion between NVD, diabetic papillopathy and NAION*: In the late phases, NVD leaks profusely into vitreous cavity, whereas the leakage from diabetic papillopathy is intraretinal, and vascular filling defects in the disk and choroid are absent (unlike NAION).[19]

Salient Angiographic Findings in Diabetic Retinopathy

The two most important phases of FFA in a diabetic eye are the mid-arteriovenous (A-V) or capillary phase and the late venous phase.

In A-V phase, the key findings are the extent of capillary nonperfusion outside the arcades, and FAZ in the posterior pole. The latter, though variable in size, is about 500 μ in diameter; and considered abnormal when exceeding 1,000 μ. A more sensitive indicator of macular ischemia is the irregularity or notching of the borders of FAZ (Fig. 6.5B).[24,34,36] Leaking microaneurysms are also visible in this phase, many more than clinically evident; and can be differentiated from solid MA and dot hemorrhages, which are invisible.[24,37] IRMA and new vessels are seen at the borders of CNP areas; the former leak minimally; the latter profusely. In late phases of FA, intraretinal leaks from

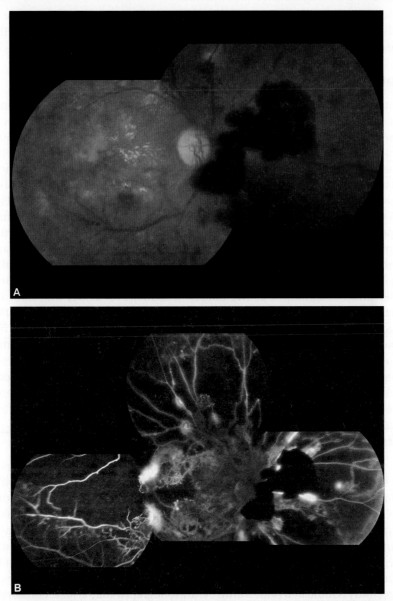

Figs. 6.5A and B: (A) This uncontrolled diabetic presented with a fulminant picture: besides the bleeding neovascularization disk (NVD), also note the venous beading of arcade vessels at 6:00 and 4:00 meridians. The macular edema had a pale hue, especially temporally, indicative of macular ischemia. (B) Fluorescein angiography (FA) is characterized by widespread ischemia, in the macula as well as midperiphery. Leaking new vessels emit cotton-ball hyperfluorescence.

microaneurysms and capillaries become prominent in macula, sometimes taking a honeycomb or petalloid pattern due to cystoid edema.[24,37] Preretinal, intravitreal leaks of NVD and NVE cause classic cotton ball hyperfluorescence, clouding the underlying tissue (Fig. 6.5B). The former can therefore be differentiated from the leak of diabetic papillopathy, which remains within the disk tissue, outlining the overlying empty telangiectatic vessels.[19,24,37]

Optical Coherence Tomography

Optical coherence tomography is based on the same principle as ultrasound except that it uses the reflection of infrared light (820 nm) rather than sound waves (laser interferometry). OCT is primarily a tool of macular assessment, which gives a high-resolution histopathological view of the macula in vivo. Due to its noninvasive nature and quick image acquisition, OCT has replaced FA as the default tool for the early diagnosis, need for treatment, prognosis of treatment (by the integrity of outer retinal layers), and follow-up of DME (Figs. 6.6A and B).[24,32] OCT is essential to detect clinically subtle vitreoretinal traction, especially in DME refractory to treatment. When significant macular traction is present, vitrectomy, rather than photocoagulation or pharmacotherapy, is the treatment of choice.[24,32] The importance of OCT skyrocketed after pharmacotherapy with corticosteroids, followed by anti-VEGF drugs, replaced laser photocoagulation as the default treatment for DME; and after the identification of center-involving DME replaced clinically significant DME (CSME) as the default target for treatment. OCT also showed, for the first time, that serous macular detachment does not always indicate central serous chorioretinopathy, and can coexist with DME, significantly affecting the visual prognosis in the natural course and after treatment.[38] However, it can only demonstrate the architecture of macula; it fails to assess functional parameters like macular ischemia and sites of leakage like FA.

Ultrasonography

B-scan ultrasound (USG) is an essential investigation in PDR with hazy media for surgery, most commonly due to vitreous hemorrhage (VH). The ultrasound informs about the status of the macula (the most important information), the nature and the extent of posterior vitreous detachment (PVD), areas of vitreoretinal traction, and the presence and nature of retinal detachment (Fig. 6.7). Tractional retinal detachment (TRD) is more common, and rhegmatogenous detachment (RRD), though rare, is an urgent indication for vitrectomy. B-scans are repeated at monthly intervals, till the VH subsides, or vitrectomy is indicated (vide infra).[24] Ultrasonography may also be considered for diabetic cataracts, with PDR in the fellow eye, to plan, if required, on concomitant photocoagulation or vitrectomy along with cataract surgery.

Electroretinogram

Abnormalities in the oscillatory potential of the ERG have been shown to precede vascular pathology in DR.[24,34] Multifocal ERG singles out individual responses from small areas of the retina (especially the posterior pole), unlike conventional Ganzfeld ERG, which is a summation response. The former is

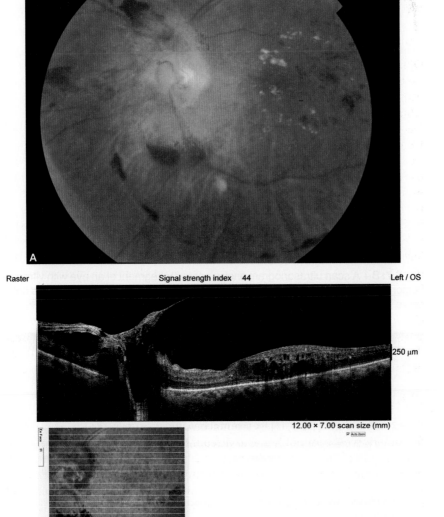

Figs. 6.6A and B: (A) This eye shows active proliferative diabetic retinopathy (PDR) with center-involving diabetic macular edema (DME); however, injecting antivascular endothelial growth factor (VEGF) drugs could result in presence of the extensive fibrous tissue at disk and inferiorly could boomerang into a tractional detachment. Even with optimum management using judicious scatter photocoagulation and intravitreal steroids, this case is at high risk for needing vitrectomy. (B) Optical coherence tomography (OCT) confirms the vigorous traction at the optic nerve, and none at macula.

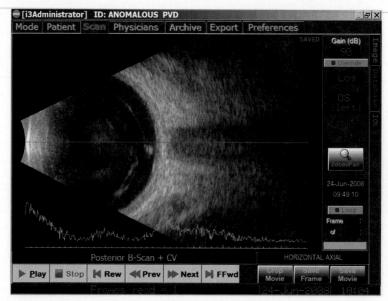

Fig. 6.7: B + A scan ultrasonogram shows posterior segment of an eye with vitreous hemorrhage, with subtotal posterior vitreous detachment (PVD) attached at the optic nerve head, and a splitting of vitreous layers (anomalous PVD).

TABLE 6.2: Screening schedule: Early detection of diabetic retinopathy.		
Type of diabetes mellitus	*Recommended initial eye examination*	**Routine follow-up*
Type 1	Five years after onset or during puberty	Yearly
Type 2	At the time of diagnosis	Yearly
Pregnancy with preexisting DM	Prior to pregnancy for counseling	Early in the first trimester Each trimester or more frequently as indicated 6 weeks postpartum

Abnormal findings will dictate more frequent follow-up examinations.
(DM: diabetes mellitus)
Source: Adapted from American Academy of Ophthalmology. Preferred practice pattern: diabetic retinopathy. San Francisco: American Academy of Ophthalmology; 2016.

useful in predicting retinal areas that would develop focal dysfunction (edema), especially in the presence of small pupils and nuclear sclerosis.[39] ERG, however, remains a research tool, not essential in the clinical management of DR.

SCREENING FOR DIABETIC RETINOPATHY

The traditional diagnostic methods are tuned to diagnose sight-threatening retinopathy. However, for the maximum impact of the pharmacological therapies, which prevent more than treat DR, earlier detection of DR is essential. The examination schedule for type 1 and 2 diabetic patients is shown in Table 6.2. The most popular current method for screening is clinical ophthalmoscopy. Though readily available, this method has inherently low sensitivity for critical lesions like venous beading, even in expert hands. For nonophthalmologists, a sensitivity of only 50% with direct ophthalmoscopy has been reported for detecting PDR. However, physicians caring for diabetics will probably use only the direct ophthalmoscope.

Dilated fundus photography is the most widely accepted standard for the screening, detection, and follow-up of DR. The gold standard for the detection and classification of DR is 30° stereoscopic fundus photography in seven standard fields, as defined by the ETDRS group.[27] However, expensive camera equipment, recurrent expenses of film processing and archiving, and need for expert photographers and graders limit its utility. Digital nonmydriatic wide-field (>45°) cameras are set to replace conventional film-based photography due to comparable sensitivity, lowered recurring costs, ease of use, scope for participation of non-ophthalmologists in screening, and feasibility for mass-screening by the telemedical transmission of images to a grading center.

Stereoscopic pictures are possible without mydriasis for the screening and referral of sight–threatening DR (moderate NPDR or above, suspected DME). AAO has reported that single-field (45°) nonstereofundus photography is also an acceptable alternative.[40]

It must be noted in conclusion that none of the above systems is an alternative to comprehensive examination by an ophthalmologist for the assessment of other ocular diseases and the patient as a whole. It should also be remembered that clinical examination by slit-lamp biomicroscopy remains the gold standard for detecting and in grading of DME. The above advances are therefore useful adjuncts, but not replacements, for clinical assessment by a trained ophthalmologist.

MEDICAL MANAGEMENT OF DIABETIC RETINOPATHY

Control of Diabetes and Associated Diseases

A self-evident but often neglected aspect of the management of DR is the fundamental truth that the eye is a part of the body. Unless systemic diabetes, and associated comorbidities like hypertension, dyslipidemia, renal disease, and anemia are strictly and consistently controlled, all the effort spent on the eye is bound to fail. Control of systemic morbidity also prevents, delays, and minimizes the occurrence and progression of DR.[9] So, the ophthalmologist managing DR needs to periodically check that the diabetic patients keeps their blood sugar, blood pressure, cholesterol, and hemoglobin within normal range, and no trace of protein in their urine.[14,41] These are simple, inexpensive tests, which are of great value in assessing and managing DR in a wholesome and comprehensive manner. Finally, a healthy diet and active lifestyle help reduce the incidence and complications of metabolic syndrome and diabetes, including DR.[42]

Photocoagulation

Beetham and Aiello first observed that retinopathy was markedly asymmetric in diabetics with unilateral disseminated chorioretinal scars, high myopia, or optic atrophy being minimal in the affected eye.[24] This observation led them to deduce that if multifocal chorioretinitis could be iatrogenically produced by scattered laser photocoagulation in an eye with PDR, it should regress. Thus scatter laser or panretinal photocoagulation (PRP) became the established treatment of PDR, standardized subsequently by two landmark trials, Diabetic Retinopathy Study (DRS) and ETDRS.[24,42] The latter also established the efficacy of laser photocoagulation in the treatment of DME.

Indications, Utility and Limitations of Laser Photocoagulation[24,42,43]

Diabetic Macular Edema

Almost all cases with CSME are candidates for laser photocoagulation, as it is clear from the ETDRS trial that the vision once reduced by CSME does not recover even with successful treatment. Visual prognosis after laser is worse if CSME is diffuse, or is associated with CME, heavy exudation or macular ischemia. Laser scar can also creep into the fovea in long-term, and therefore any subset of CSME that involves the center of the macula is a candidate for pharmacotherapy, preferably with anti-VEGF agents. For noncenter involving DME, laser photocoagulation remains the treatment of choice.

Proliferative Diabetic Retinopathy, Severe Nonproliferative Diabetic Retinopathy, and Anterior Segment Neovascularization

The only definite indication for PRP according to the DRS and ETDRS trials is high-risk PDR, which essentially entails large NVD, or any bleeding NVD or NVE. Any delay in treatment runs the risk of severe visual loss from VH or tractional complications. However, any PDR in type 2 diabetes (which constitutes about 95% of all DM) benefits from scatter photocoagulation over close observation. Therefore, high-risk characteristics are no longer included in modern grading of DR severity. Further, extensive capillary dropout areas seen on FA also constitute a valid indication for scatter photocoagulation even without the presence of new vessels. Finally, when new vessels are detected on the iris (NVI) or in the anterior chamber angle (NVA), PRP is mandatory even without any clinically obvious PDR. Other indications for PRP in early PDR/severe NPDR include a noncompliant patient, or inability to follow up at the recommended intervals; poor systemic control of DM and comorbidities; an unfavorable or fulminant course of DR in the fellow eye; and pregnancy or pending cataract surgery (conditions where DR progresses more rapidly).

Laser photocoagulation is the mainstay of treatment for PDR, and non-central DME: it reduces by half or more the chances of visual loss due to DME or PDR, eliminates the need for vitrectomy in many cases, and improves the anatomical and visual prognosis even if the lasered eyes need vitrectomy.

Nevertheless, it remains a destructive treatment. For some patients, the side effects (not to mention the complications) like scotomata, reduced dark adaptation and loss of accommodation are more troublesome than the sequelae of the disease. Convincing the patient for treatment is difficult, as the treatment is only preventive; no significant visual improvement occurs in most of the cases. Further, the treatment may have to be repeated, and in spite of repeated treatments, ETDRS reported persistent edema in a quarter of the patients at 1 year. For these reasons, a host of newer medical treatments, mainly intravitreal drugs, have replaced laser photocoagulation as the first-line treatment.

Pharmacotherapy of Diabetic Retinopathy: A Paradigm Shift

It is painful to note that despite tremendous advances in technique and instrumentation, vitrectomy has not been able to significantly improve the visual outcome in advanced PDR.[28] On the other hand, the two great clinical trials, DRS and ETDRS set a benchmark in the treatment of DR by the grading of the disease and giving guidelines for photocoagulation, which, if followed meticulously, can prevent up to 98% of blindness related to DR.[44] However, laser photocoagulation *prevents* severe visual loss; it cannot *reverse* the pre-existing visual loss. Besides, laser photocoagulation is a destructive treatment, which produces one disease (extensive chorioretinal scarring) to treat another.

With great advances in understanding the pathogenesis of DR, the last decade has seen a major paradigm shift in research on DR management, from the macro- to the molecular level. The aim of the treatments is now to treat the cause, rather than the effects of DR by drugs directed against a specific pathogenetic mechanism, injected directly into the vitreous cavity. The predominant target of pharmacotherapy is center-involving DME: mainly corticosteroids and anti-VEGF agents. For PDR, PRP vitrectomy remains the mainstay of management; anti-VEGF agents have a small niche as adjuncts, though this situation is rapidly changing. Before considering these pharmacotherapeutic agents, it is worthwhile repeating that all these treatment options target advanced stages of diabetic eye disease, and have small but significant sight-threatening complications.

Antiangiogenic Agents and Corticosteroids

Of the multitude of antiangiogenic drugs, those blocking the activity of the VEGF (anti-VEGF antibodies and their active fractions) have emerged at the forefront, after their successful use against exudative age-related macular degeneration (AMD). DR however differs from AMD in being secondary to a systemic microvascular ischemic disease, with potential implications for the long-term use of anti-VEGF agents. This concern is relevant to the treatment of DME where 12–15 injections are required in the first 3 years, despite which less than half of the treated eyes have limited visual improvement; about a fifth have residual DME, and nearly half require bailout with additional laser photocoagulation.[5] In the context of DR without DME, the benefit of anti-VEGF injections was first seen as a pleasant bonus during DME trials like RISE, RIDE, VISTA, and VIVID, where the progression of NPDR to PDR was reduced by three times (as compared to the natural course), and more than a third of the subjects actually showed regression of DR.[45] Buoyed by these findings, ranibizumab (©Lucentis; ©Accentrix)[46] and then aflibercept (©Eylea)[47] were compared against the gold standard of PRP in PDR. Though both drugs improved vision, spared visual fields, and stabilized PDR like PRP, the logistical issues like recurring costs and the need for close followup force clinicians to keep anti-VEGF injections as an adjunct treatment, preferably in PDR with concurrent DME.[48] A more viable role of anti-VEGF agents, especially bevacizumab, is as a pre-operative adjunct to complex diabetic vitrectomy. Several studies have shown that anti-VEGF injections before or during vitrectomy were likely to experience reduced intraoperative bleeding and surgical times, and improved anatomical and visual outcomes; though the cumulative evidence is not strong due to lack of large, controlled trials.[49]

Since the inflammatory aspect of diabetic vascular leakage and angiogenesis has been reported,[26] an increasing number of studies have shown the benefits of intravitreal corticosteroid (initially triamcinolone acetonide; now mainly dexamethasone depot [©Ozurdex]) in treating DME refractory to photocoagulation or anti-VEGF drugs. The main disadvantage is a rise in intraocular pressure in a large number of cases (20–80%) and cataract formation in some. A long-term drug delivery device for intravitreal fluocinolone acetonide (©Iluvien, in FAME trial) showed beneficial effects on DR progression similar to anti-VEGF molecules, but of a smaller order.[50]

Drugs Peddled by Medical Representatives

Aspirin and dipyridamole lower microaneurysm count but do not check the progression to PDR in aspirin [Microangiopathy of Diabetes (DAMAD) study]. The same is true of ticlopidine in a French study (TIMAD), promising but not definitive results.[41] Similarly, rheological agents like pentoxifylline increase RBC deformability and decrease blood viscosity, thus improving blood flow; the effect on the progression of DR remains unproven.[51] Agents to improve capillary fragility like calcium dobesilate decreases capillary leakage. The initial promise, like in the above drugs, failed to show concrete results in controlled studies.[52] High-dose vitamin E has been shown to improve blood flow and renal function in diabetic patients. However, another large study failed to show any benefit from vitamin C, E and B-carotene.[14] To cut the long story short, none of the above drugs, from aspirin to vitamins (*all of which have some pathogenetic basis for use in DR*), are at present recommended for diabetic patients till clinical trials settle the issue.

VITRECTOMY

When preventive (optimal glucose control) or early treatment (photocoagulation) strategies fail to stop the progression to advanced PDR, pars plana vitrectomy (PPV) is usually required to deal with the sequelae and complications. However, it is important to remember that visual prognosis is much better in eyes undergoing vitrectomy if prior scatter photocoagulation has been done. PRP should be done whenever possible before considering vitrectomy.

Surgical Indications

Vitreous Hemorrhage

Historically, non-clearing VH was the first indication for PPV. Surgery, however, is deferred in a fresh VH (Fig. 6.3A) if B-scan ultrasound rules out macular tractional detachment (TRD) or any rhegmatogenous retinal detachment (RRD)] for many reasons: in some eyes, VH spontaneously clears and PRP can be done; the incomplete PVD progresses toward completion (making PPV easier); the active new vessels regress (reducing risk of intraoperative bleeds); and the systemic parameters can be assessed and stabilized. It is worth remembering that DR is actually a *vitreoretinopathy*: with every resolved episode of VH, some fibrosis and vitreoretinal traction ensues; and the patient almost never reports after the very first episode of VH (perceived only as a few floaters, that subside). However, a dense VH (vision reduced to <3/60) is generally operated if persisting beyond 4 weeks.[53] Earlier surgery is recommended if the patient is young (type 1 DM), extensive fibrous proliferations or traction are present, VH is bilateral, fellow eye is blind, no PRP has been done, or a taut subhyaloid hemorrhage (which hastens fibrous proliferation at macula) is present.

Macular Tractional Detachment

Tractional retinal detachments involving or threatening the macula (Figs. 6.8A and 6.9A) are the most definitive and urgent indication for vitrectomy, as such detachment hits macular nutrition both by ischemia and detachment.[53] For the same reason, a chronic macular TRD, (lasting more than 6 months) is not likely to improve with surgery (Fig. 6.10).[54,55] As extramacular TRDs rarely advance (15% per year) into macula, they constitute a relative indication, generally in the presence of VH.

Rhegmatogenous Retinal Detachment

An RRD, alone or complicating a TRD, is a strong indication for surgery even if the macula is attached. RRD, unlike TRD, is known to progress, and therefore macular detachment is only a matter of time. The tears are typically posterior, slit-like or invisible, and close to an area of vitreous traction.[24,53]

Epimacular Membrane or Vitreomacular Traction

Epimacular or tractional membranes may form due to PRP, chronic DME, PVD, or spontaneously in florid cases. Sometimes, DME itself is caused by

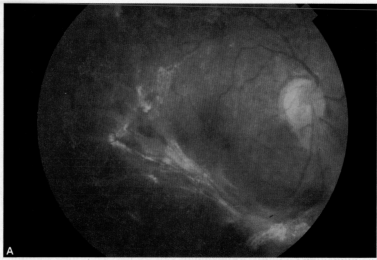

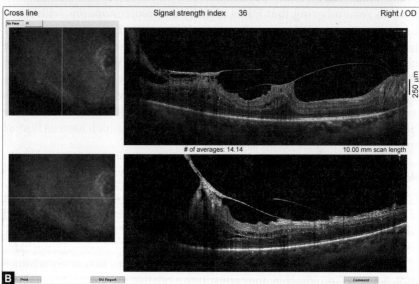

Figs. 6.8A and B: (A) This picture would be described as a macula-threatening tractional retinal detachment (TRD) in the preoptical coherence tomography (OCT) era, with a florid, massive fibrovascular membrane lifting inferior edge of macula. (B) OCT however shows that macula is already involved by the tractional membranes, and a candidate for early surgery.

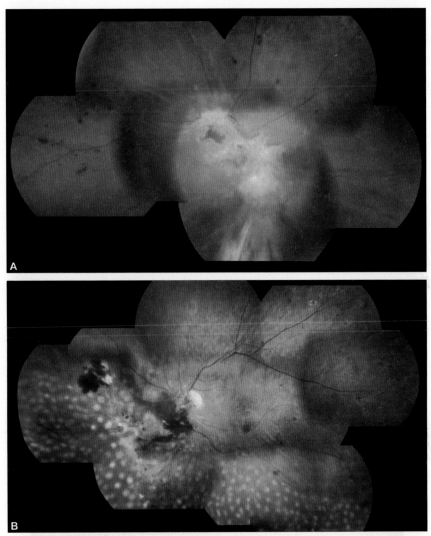

Figs. 6.9A and B: (A) This is a classic indication for early vitrectomy: macula-involving tractional retinal detachment (TRD): notice the florid new vessels on the disk and previous scatter photocoagulation (panretinal photocoagulation, PRP) marks superiorly. (B) 25-gauge vitrectomy with a 3-day prior antivascular endothelial growth factor (VEGF) injection led to a complete retinal reattachment; note the fresh PRP laser marks inferiorly.

vitreomacular traction/taut posterior hyaloid, seen clinically or on OCT (Fig. 6.8B). These patients would actually worsen with macular photocoagulation, and are candidates for PPV.[53]

Other Indications

Anterior segment rubeosis requires an urgent PRP to prevent neovascular glaucoma; therefore, any media opacities need to be removed to facilitate PRP. Eyes with very large NVD and NVE, especially when associated with fibrosis, which are refractory to scatter photocoagulation, fare better with early vitrectomy rather than with waiting for macular traction or VH.[53,54]

Surgical Objectives and Techniques

The primary aims of surgery are to remove the media (vitreous) opacities and restore normal retinal anatomy by removing anteroposterior (A-P) and tangential vitreoretinal traction; and epiretinal membrane-induced surface traction. PRP is done or added in all cases. Diathermy is used to stop bleeders and outline breaks. The surgical outcomes in DR have improved significantly after small gauge (23 G and 25 G) vitrectomy, which allows better fluidics, more control, cleaner surgery and faster recovery in simple as well as complex cases (Fig. 6.9B).[53,56]

SUMMARY AND FUTURE DIRECTIONS

Diabetic retinal disease is the most-studied microvascular complication of systemic diabetes. Several epidemiological studies and randomized clinical

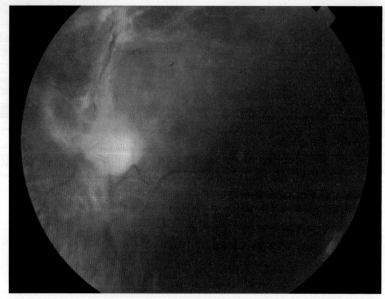

Fig. 6.10: Longstanding macular tractional retinal detachment (TRD), as shown in this figure, is not worth the effort of surgery, as the visual outcomes are bleak.

trials have described the natural history of DR and its response to therapeutic intervention. Proven beneficial treatments include improved control of hyperglycemia and hypertension, photocoagulation, vitrectomy, and more recently, antiangiogenic pharmacotherapy.

Guided by new insights in pathogenesis, pharmacotherapy promises to replace photocoagulation as the main intervention in DR. The focus of attention in future may shift from sight–threatening retinopathy to early retinopathy, from treatment to prevention. Looking at the global statistics of diabetes, such an approach is probably warranted. This approach also necessitates greater communication between ophthalmologists, diabetologists and primary-care physicians. This interdisciplinary teamwork will not only aid in identifying patients most at risk for visual loss and who are therefore urgent candidates for the existing treatments, but also those likely to benefit from new treatments on the horizon. Meanwhile, it serves us well to remember that the most effective option for pharmacotherapy remains a robust control of diabetes and associated systemic comorbidities.

REFERENCES

1. Meyer AH. World Diabetes Foundation: Annual Review 2002. Lyngby, Denmark: Videback Bogtrykken; 2002.
2. International Diabetes Federation. The Diabetes Atlas, 4th edition. Brussels, BelgiumL IDF; 2009.
3. International Diabetes Federation. The Diabetes Atlas, 7th edition. Brussels, Belgium: IDF; 2015.
4. International Diabetes Foundation. The Diabetes Atlas, 2nd edition. Brussels, Belgium: IDF; 2003.
5. Stitt AW, Curtis TM, Chen M, et al. The progress in understanding and treatment of diabetic retinopathy. Prog Retin Eye Res. 2016;51:156-86.
6. Klein R, Klein BE, Moss SE, et al. The Wisconsin Epidemiologic Study of Diabetic Retinopathy, II: prevalence and risk of diabetic retinopathy when age at diagnosis is less than 30 years. Arch Ophthalmol. 1984;102:520-6.
7. Klein R, Klein BE, Moss SE, et al. The Wisconsin Epidemiologic Study of Diabetic Retinopathy, III: prevalence and risk of diabetic retinopathy when age at diagnosis is 30 or more years. Arch Ophthalmol. 1984;102:527-32.
8. Silva PS, Cavallerano JD, Sun JK, et al. Effect of systemic medications on onset and progression of diabetic retinopathy. Nat Rev Endocrinol. 2010;6:494-508.
9. Klein R, Klein BE. Epidemiology of eye disease in diabetes. In: Flynn HW, Smiddy WE (Eds). Ophthalmology Monograph 14: Diabetes and ocular disease: past, present and future therapies. San Francisco: The Foundation of the American Academy of Ophthalmology; 2000. pp. 19-67.
10. Diabetes control and complications trial research group: the effect of intensive treatment of diabetes on the development and progression of long term complications in insulin dependent diabetes mellitus. N Engl J Med. 1993;329:977-86.
11. UK Prospective Diabetes Study Group. Intensive blood-glucose control with sulphonylureas or insulin compared with conventional treatment and risk of complications in patients with type 2 diabetes. UKPDS 33. Lancet. 1998;352:837-53.
12. Wong TY, Cruickshank KJ, Klein R, et al. HLA-DR3 and DR4 and their relation to the incidence and progression of diabetic retinopathy. Ophthalmology. 2002;109:275-81.

13. Foster DW. Diabetes Mellitus. In: Fauci AS, Braunwald E, Isselbacher KJ (Eds).. Harrison's principles of internal medicine, 14th edition. New York: McGraw-Hill Inc.; 1998. pp. 2060-81.

14. Aiello LP, Catrill MT, Wong JS. Systemic considerations in the management of diabetic retinopathy. Am J Ophthalmol. 2001;132:760-76

15. Chew EY, Klein ML, Ferris FL, et al. Association of elevated serum lipid levels with retinal hard exudates in diabetic retinopathy. Early Treatment Diabetic Retinopathy Study (ETDRS) Report 22. Arch Ophthalmol. 1996;114:1079-84.

16. Rosenblatt BJ, Benson WE. Diabetic retinopathy. In: Yanoff M, Duker JS (Eds). Ophthalmology, 2nd edition. St Louis: Mosby; 2004. p.877.

17. Dandona L, Dandona R, Naduvilath TJ, et al. Population based assessment of diabetic retinopathy in an urban population in southern India. Br J Ophthalmol. 1999;83(8):937-40.

18. Shah AS, Chen SH. Cataract surgery and diabetes. Curr Opin Ophthalmol. 2010;21(1):4-9.

19. Shukla D, Rajendran A, Singh J, et al. Atypical manifestations of diabetic retinopathy. Curr Opin Ophthalmol. 2003;14(6):371-7.

20. Gardner TW, Aiello LP. Pathogenesis of diabetic retinopathy. In: Flynn HW, Smiddy WE (Eds). Ophthalmology Monograph 14. Diabetes and ocular disease: Past, present and future therapies. San Francisco: The Foundation of the American Academy of Ophthalmology; 2000; pp. 1-17.

21. Frank RN. Etiologic mechanisms in diabetic retinopathy. In: Ryan SJ, Schachat AP, Hengst TC (Eds). Retina, 3rd edition. St Louis: Mosby; 2001; pp. 1259-94.

22. Rosenblatt BJ, Benson WE. Diabetic retinopathy. In: Yanoff M, Duker JS (Eds). Ophthalmology, 2nd edition. St Louis: Mosby; 2004. p.878.

23. Frank RN. Diabetic retinopathy New Engl J Med. 2004;350:48-58.

24. Ryan SJ, Schachat AP, Sadda SR. Retina, 5th edition. St Louis: Elsevier; 2013. pp. 907-1000.

25. Arden GB. The absence of diabetic retinopathy in patients with retinitis pigmentosa: implications for pathophysiology and possible treatment. Br J Ophthalmol. 2001;85:366-70.

26. Adamis AP. Is diabetic retinopathy an inflammatory disease? Br J Ophthalmol. 2002;86:363-5.

27. Grading diabetic retinopathy from stereoscopic color fundus photographs—an extension of the modified Airlie House classification. ETDRS report number 10. Early Treatment Diabetic Retinopathy Study Research Group. Ophthalmology. 1991;98(5 Suppl):786-806.

28. Fundus photographic risk factors for progression of diabetic retinopathy. ETDRS report number 12. Early Treatment Diabetic Retinopathy Study Research Group. Ophthalmology. 1991;98(5 Suppl):823-33.

29. Wilkinson CP, Ferris FL 3rd, Klein RE, et al. Global Diabetic Retinopathy Project Group. Proposed international clinical diabetic retinopathy and diabetic macular edema disease severity scales. Ophthalmology. 2003;110(9):1677-82.

30. Silva PS, Walia S, Cavallerano JD, et al. Comparison of low-light nonmydriatic digital imaging with 35-mm ETDRS seven-standard field stereo color fundus photographs and clinical examination. Telemed J E Health. 2012;18(7):492-9.

31. Silva PS, Cavallerano JD, Haddad NM, et al. Peripheral Lesions Identified on Ultrawide Field Imaging Predict Increased Risk of Diabetic Retinopathy Progression over 4 Years. Ophthalmology. 2015;122(5):949-56.

32. Tan CS, Chew MC, Lim LW, et al. Advances in retinal imaging for diabetic retinopathy and diabetic macular edema. Indian J Ophthalmol. 2016;64(1):76-83.

33. Shukla D, Gupta SR, Neelakantan N, et al. Type 2 idiopathic macular telangiectasia. Retina. 2012;32(2):265-74.
34. Bresnick GH. Nonproliferative diabetic retinopathy. In: Ryan SJ, Schachat AP, Murphy RB (Eds). Retina, 2nd edition. St. Louis: Mosby; 1994. pp. 1277-318.
35. Aiello LM. Perspectives on diabetic retinopathy. Am J Ophthalmol. 2003;136:122-35.
36. Shukla D, Kolluru CM, Singh J, et al. Macular ischaemia as a marker for nephropathy in diabetic retinopathy. Indian J Ophthalmol. 2004;52(3):205-10.
37. Berkon JW, Kelley JS, Orth DH. Fluorescein angiography. San Francisco, American Academy of Ophthalmology; 1984. pp. 39-74.
38. Sophie R, Lu N, Campochiaro PA. Predictors of functional and anatomic outcomes in patients with diabetic macular edema treated with ranibizumab. Ophthalmology. 2015;122:1395-401.
39. Fortune B, Schreck ME, Adams AJ. Multifocal electroretinogram delays reveal local retinal dysfunction in early diabetic retinopathy. Invest Ophthalmol Vis Sci. 1999;40:2638-51.
40. Williams GA, Scott IU, Haller JA, et al. Single field fundus photography for diabetic retinopathy screening: a report of the American Academy of Ophthalmology. Ophthalmology. 2004;111:1055-62.
41. Skyler JS. Medical management of diabetic retinopathy. In: Flynn HW, Smiddy WE (Eds). Ophthalmology Mono 14: Diabetes and ocular disease: past, present and future therapies. San Francisco: The Foundation of the American Academy of Ophthalmology; 2000. pp. 181-201.
42. American Academy of Ophthalmology. Preferred practice patterns in ophthalmology. San Francisco: American Academy of Ophthalmology;2016.
43. Folk JC, Oh KT. Photocoagulation for diabetic macular edema and diabetic retinopathy. In: Flynn HW, Smiddy WE (Eds). Oph Mono 14: Diabetes and ocular disease: past, present and future therapies. San Francisco: The Foundation of the American Academy of Ophthalmology; 2000. pp. 115-53.
44. Taylor HR. Diabetic retinopathy: a public health challenge. Am J Ophthalmol. 1996;123:543-5.
45. Wykoff CC. Impact of intravitreal pharmacotherapies including antivascular endothelial growth factor and corticosteroid agents on diabetic retinopathy. Curr Opin Ophthalmol. 2017;28(3):213-8.
46. Gross JG, Glassman AR, Jampol LM, et al. Writing Committee for the Diabetic Retinopathy Clinical Research Network. Panretinal photocoagulation vs intravitreous ranibizumab for proliferative diabetic retinopathy: a randomized clinical trial. JAMA. 2015;314:2137-46.
47. Sivaprasad S, Prevost AT, Vasconcelos JC, et al. CLARITY Study Group. Clinical efficacy of intravitreal aflibercept versus panretinal photocoagulation for best corrected visual acuity in patients with proliferative diabetic retinopathy at 52 weeks (CLARITY): a multicentre, single-blinded, randomised, controlled, phase 2b, non-inferiority trial. Lancet. 2017;389(10085):2193-203.
48. Ting DSW, Wong TY. Proliferative diabetic retinopathy: laser or eye injection? Lancet. 2017;389(10085):2165-6.
49. Martinez-Zapata MJ, Martí-Carvajal AJ, Solà I, et al. Anti-vascular endothelial growth factor for proliferative diabetic retinopathy. Cochrane Database Syst Rev. 2014;11:CD008721.
50. Wykoff CC, Chakravarthy U, Campochiaro PA, et al. Long-term Effects of Intravitreal 0.19 mg Fluocinolone Acetonide Implant on Progression and Regression of Diabetic Retinopathy. Ophthalmology. 2017;124(4):440-9.

51. Ferrai E, Fioravanti M, Patti AL, et al. Effects of long term treatment (4 years) with pentoxifylline on haemorheological changes and vascular complications in diabetic patients. Pharmatherapeutica. 1987;5:26-39.

52. Stamper RL, Smith, Aronson SB, et al. The effect of calcium dobesilate on nonproliferative diabetic retinopathy: a controlled study. Ophthalmology. 1978;85:594-606.

53. Sharma T, Fong A, Lai TY, et al. Surgical treatment for diabetic vitreoretinal diseases: a review. Clin Experiment Ophthalmol. 2016;44:340-54.

54. Davis MD, Blodi BA. Proliferative diabetic retinopathy. In: Ryan SJ, Schachat AP (Eds). Retina, 3rd edition. St. LouisL Mosby; 2001. pp. 1309-49.

55. Early vitrectomy for severe proliferative diabetic retinopathy in eyes with useful vision. Clinical application of results of a randomized trial—Diabetic Retinopathy Vitrectomy Study Report 4. The Diabetic Retinopathy Vitrectomy Study Research Group. Ophthalmology. 1988;95(10):1321-34.

56. Mikhail M, Ali-Ridha A, Chorfi S, et al. Long-term outcomes of sutureless 25-G+ pars-plana vitrectomy for the management of diabetic tractional retinal detachment. Graefes Arch Clin Exp Ophthalmol. 2017;255:255-61.

CHAPTER 7

Diabetic Macular Edema

Peter N Youssef, Suresh R Chandra

INTRODUCTION

The effects of diabetes on the eye have been well-studied and -documented. Our understanding of the epidemiology has mostly come from studies conducted in the United States and Europe. The impact of diabetes and diabetic retinopathy is now starting to become manifested and studied in other parts of the world. The World Health Organization estimates that the number of individuals living with diabetes mellitus throughout the world was 171 million in the year 2000 and will increase to 336 million by the year 2030. The three countries found to have the highest prevalence of diabetes in the year 2000 were India, China, and the United States with estimates of 32, 21, and 17 million affected individuals respectively (Fig. 7.1).

India is forecasted to have an estimated prevalence of 79.4 million people living with diabetes mellitus by 2030.[1-3] In the Andhra Pradesh Eye Disease Study (APEDS), the prevalence of diabetic retinopathy in individuals with diabetes mellitus was found to be 22.4%.[4,5] In the Chennai Urban Rural Epidemiology Study (CURES), in which an urban sample of diabetic patients was evaluated, the overall prevalence of diabetic retinopathy was found to be 17.6%.[6,7] The predicted increase in the prevalence of diabetes in conjunction with the already high prevalence of retinopathy among diabetics suggests that the diagnosis and treatment of patients with diabetic retinopathy is becoming increasingly important, both globally and specifically in India.

Studies such as the Diabetes Control and Complications Trial (DCCT) and United Kingdom Prospective Diabetes Study (UKPDS) have demonstrated that patients with diabetes mellitus and poor glycemic control are more likely to experience worsening retinopathy and vision loss. Causes for vision loss in patients with diabetic retinopathy include lenticular changes, macular ischemia, vitreous hemorrhage, traction retinal detachment secondary to proliferative diabetic retinopathy, and macular edema.

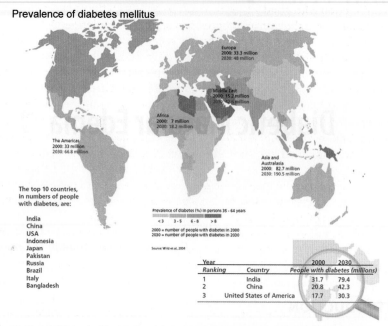

Fig. 7.1: World Map depicting the World Health Organization's estimate of the prevalence of diabetes mellitus in the year 2000 and forecasted prevalence for the year 2030.
Source: Wild S. Diabetes action now: an initiative of the World Health Organization and the International Diabetes Federation. Geneva: World Health Organization.

The onset of visual change associated with diabetes mellitus usually lags several years behind the onset of the disease itself. Retinal changes in patients with type 1 diabetes generally do not occur for at least 3–5 years after the onset of the systemic disease. While it is more difficult to determine the onset of diabetes in patients with type 2 diabetes due to the frequent presence of subclinical systemic disease prior to diagnosis, patients with type 2 diabetes mellitus are also thought to develop ocular disease and vision loss several years after disease onset.[8–12]

The most important risk factor for the development and progression of diabetic retinopathy is poor chronic blood sugar control. The advent of home glucose monitors to rapidly and accurately assess blood sugar levels along with the development of the hemoglobin A1c serum test have made it possible to study the control of blood sugar and the effect of long-term control on diabetic retinopathy. Through studies such as the UKPDS and DCCT, it has been definitively determined that the maintenance of well-controlled blood sugar decreases the likelihood of the progression of diabetic retinopathy at all stages of the disease.[8,12]

Additionally, several studies support the contention that the control of systemic comorbidities also plays a role in the development and progression of diabetic retinopathy. The UKPDS demonstrated that both increased blood sugar levels and increased blood pressure levels present an increased risk for the development and progression of retinopathy.[11,12] Several studies have also suggested that the control of hypercholesterolemia and hyperlipidemia in conjunction with good glycemic control can lessen the effects of exudative maculopathy and the overall progression of diabetic retinopathy.[11,13-17]

Macular edema remains by far the most common cause of vision loss from diabetes. While vision loss is often measured in terms of letters lost on a visual acuity chart, the true impact of this vision loss from diabetic macular edema often extends beyond the clinic into daily life. Patients can experience functional vision loss, which negatively impacts social interactions and emotional health. Studies using the 25-item Visual Function Questionnaire (VFQ-25), created by the National Eye Institute (NEI) to assess the impact of vision loss on quality of life, have suggested that vision loss from diabetic macular edema can have effects greater than those seen in patients with glaucoma and cataracts, and can even approach the magnitude of effect of vision loss in patients with age-related macular degeneration. Such data necessitates addressing the diagnosis and treatment of macular edema as a public health concern.[18,19]

While it has been assumed that macular edema is more common in older individuals with type 2 diabetes than in younger individuals with type 1 diabetes, recent epidemiological studies have suggested that the prevalence of macular edema as a function of duration of diabetes was virtually identical in persons with type 1 and type 2 diabetes. A more recent follow-up to the Wisconsin Epidemiologic Study of Diabetic Retinopathy reported that the 10-year incidence of diabetic macular edema was 20.1% in type 1 diabetics, 25.4% in type 2 diabetics requiring insulin, and 13.9% in type 2 diabetics not requiring insulin.[20-23]

The diagnosis of diabetic macular edema has classically been defined by findings of retinal thickening on dilated ophthalmoscopic examination. The Early Treatment of Diabetic Retinopathy Study (ETDRS) defined DME as retinal thickening or hard exudates within 1 disc diameter of the central macula. DME is generally further classified as clinically significant macular edema (CSME) if at least one of the following conditions is present: retinal thickening at or within 500 μm of the center of the macula, hard exudates within 500 μm of the central

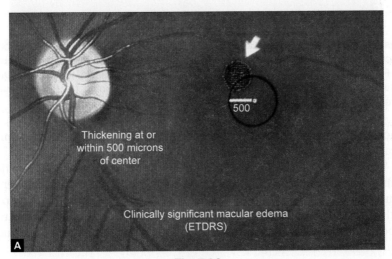

Fig. 7.2A

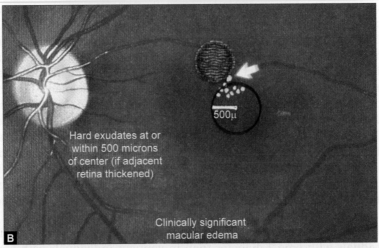

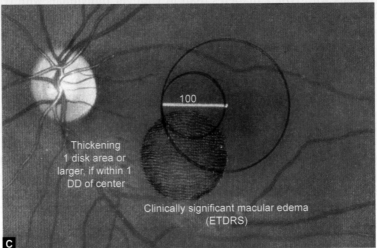

Figs. 7.2B and C

Figs. 7.2A to C: Color schematics showing the definition of clinically significant diabetic macular edema as defined by the Early Treatment of Diabetic Retinopathy Study. (A) Retinal thickening at or within 500 μm of the center of the macula. (B) Hard exudates within 500 μm of the central macula with adjacent retinal thickening. (C) 1 disk diameter of retinal thickening located at or within 1 disk diameter of the central macula.

macula with adjacent retinal thickening, or 1 disc diameter of retinal thickening located at or within 1 disc diameter of the central macula (Figs. 7.2A to C).[24-28]

While the diagnosis of macular edema is classically made on examination with slit lamp biomicroscopy, fluorescein angiography and optical coherence tomography can both be useful ancillary studies to assist in the diagnosis and management of the DME. CSME is generally further subdivided into two subcategories, focal edema and diffuse edema, based on patterns of leakage seen on fluorescein angiography.

PATHOGENESIS

Normal retinal function depends on a homeostatic balance between the potential of fluid to leak from retinal vessels and the ability of the retina to absorb any excess fluid. As evidenced by epidemiological studies, poorly-controlled longstanding diabetes is highly correlated with the development of systemic and ocular morbidity. Prolonged and chronic hyperglycemia undoubtedly plays a major role in the development of both systemic and ocular microvasculature pathology in patients with diabetes. While the pathogenesis of diabetic macular edema on a cellular level is undoubtedly complex and multifactorial, there are several known contributors to the disruption of this balance, including alterations in the vascular permeability via the formation of microaneurysms and blood-retinal barrier (BRB) dysfunction, changes in vascular permeability caused by alterations in vasoactive substances, and changes in permeability secondary to complex interactions along the vitreoretinal interface.[29-33]

Blood-retinal Barrier

The blood-retinal barrier is comprised of the inner blood-retinal barrier at the level of the neurosensory retina and the outer blood-retinal barrier at the level of the retina pigment epithelium. Both the inner and outer blood-retinal barriers rely on the integrity of tight junctions that form between the retinal vascular endothelial cells and retinal pigment epithelial cells, respectively. The dysfunction of both of the inner and outer components of the blood-retinal barrier has been implicated in the pathogenesis of diabetic macular edema. Additionally, it has been demonstrated that diabetes can induce pathologic changes in and alter the permeability of both barriers.[29,34-40]

Alterations in the integrity of either the outer or the inner blood-retinal barrier can cause the inflow of fluid into the neurosensory retina to exceed the egress of fluid and result in an accumulation of fluid or diabetic macular edema. Anatomic changes to the blood-retinal barrier include changes inherent to the vascular endothelial cells and changes in the supporting matrix of the neurosensory retina.[29,34-40]

Vascular Endothelial Cells

The retinal capillary microaneurysm is usually the first recognizable sign of diabetic retinopathy on clinical examination. Histologically, microaneurysms are hypercellular outpouchings of capillary walls. Microaneurysms are thought to form in conjunction with the depletion of capillary pericytes, another change seen early in diabetes on histological examination. In addition to contributing to the BRB, pericytes are also thought to help provide structure and support to the retinal vasculature. Ultrastructural analyses of retinal microaneurysms reveal a consistent absence of pericytes, suggesting that the loss of vessel integrity due to the absence of pericytes may render vessels vulnerable to forming aneurysms. In fact, mice that are genetically selected to have a relative absence of pericytes form early signs of retinopathy similar to those seen in nonproliferative diabetic retinopathy. It is thought that the tight junctions in microaneurysms are somewhat compromised in diabetic retinopathy and, hence, demonstrate an increase in permeability that results in fluid and lipoprotein leakage and subsequent macular edema.[10,29,33-35,37-39,41-44]

In addition to the loss of pericytes and the formation of microaneurysms, patients with diabetic retinopathy exhibit characteristic changes of endothelial cell death, basement membrane thinning, and increased leukocyte adhesion, as demonstrated in various animal studies. While the cause of these changes is not fully understood, they are thought to contribute to the disruption of the blood-retinal barrier and macular ischemia seen in patients with diabetic retinopathy.[29,32,37,39,45-47]

Vasoactive Substances

Changes in vascular permeability are also likely affected by the alteration of the local milieu of so-called vasoactive agents such as protein kinase C (PKC), vascular endothelial growth factor (VEGF), pigment epithelial derived factor (PEDF), and angiotensin II, among others. Hyperglycemia and relative ischemia may affect the levels of these substances, and these changes may be interrelated to one another.[48-60]

Of particular recent interest is the role of VEGF in altering vascular permeability; anti-VEGF pharmacotherapy is gaining wider acceptance for the treatment of various chorioretinal disorders including age-related macular degeneration, retinal vein occlusion, proliferative diabetic retinopathy and diabetic macular edema. While many cells in the retina are capable of producing VEGF, perhaps the most important of these cells are the Müller cells, which demonstrate particularly high rates of glycolysis. VEGF expression is increased in the tissue by a variety of factors, including substantial upregulation in response to hypoxia. The hypoxia-driven upregulation seen in diabetic retinopathy leads to an increase in vascular permeability. One possible mechanism for the effect of VEGF on vascular permeability is the ability of VEGF to cause structural changes in the tight junctions of vascular endothelial cells. VEGF is thought to cause the phosphorylation of tight junction proteins, thereby leading to conformational changes that alter the fenestrations in endothelial cell membranes. Additionally, VEGF may also be associated with early inflammatory changes seen in diabetic retinopathy through the upregulation of the endothelial cell proteins responsible for leukocyte adhesion and consequent increases in vascular permeability. *In vivo* studies have demonstrated increased aqueous levels of VEGF in patients with macular edema versus those without. More recent studies have corroborated these findings, demonstrating increased levels of VEGF among other vasoactive markers in the vitreous cavity of patients with macular edema.[33,50,53-61]

Vitreoretinal Interface

It has long been recognized that diabetic patients demonstrate abnormalities of the vitreoretinal interface. In particular, subsets of patients with diabetic macular edema have a persistently taut, thickened posterior hyaloid which remains attached to the retina and can cause vitreomacular traction and subsequent macular edema. In fact, diabetic patients without a history of posterior vitreous detachment are more likely to have diabetic macular edema than those patients with a history of posterior vitreous detachment. Additionally, it has been reported that the formation of a posterior vitreous detachment, whether surgical or spontaneous, has led to the resolution or improvement of diabetic macular edema in certain cases.[29,32,62-66]

Patients with diabetes have been noted to possess particularly adherent vitreoretinal adhesions that may be mediated by an increase in collagen cross-linkages between the cortical vitreous and internal limiting membrane (ILM). These firmly-adherent adhesions are thought to contribute to the propensity for diabetic patients to develop macular traction and edema. The hyaloid itself may become thickened due to infiltration with glial and inflammatory cells. This thickening can result in tangential traction on the macula independent of vitreomacular traction and potentially contribute to DME[63-68] (Figs. 7.3A and B).

TREATMENT

The most important treatment measure in a patient with any form of diabetic retinopathy is to prevent further progression of disease by improving blood sugar control and other associated risk factors such as hypertension and hyperlipidemia as demonstrated by the DCCT and UKPDS. The ophthalmologist can have a meaningful impact on improving these metabolic indices by encouraging patients to work with their primary care physicians to improve their risk factors for disease progression. Several studies reinforce the positive effect of patient education.[13,69,70]

The long-established gold standards for the treatment of macular edema have been focal and grid laser. With the advent of new surgical techniques and new pharmacotherapy, there has been an effort to improve prior treatment strategies. In the section below, we will discuss the various treatment modalities and the rationale for their use.

Laser

Strong evidence from many clinical trials indicates that laser photocoagulation preserves vision in patients with diabetic macular edema. Currently, argon laser photocoagulation is the most common form of treatment for eyes with clinically significant macular edema. The ETDRS demonstrated the beneficial effect of laser treatment; there was a 50% reduction in moderate vision loss in the laser treatment group compared with the observation group. Patients in the ETDRS with mild or moderate nonproliferative diabetic retinopathy and

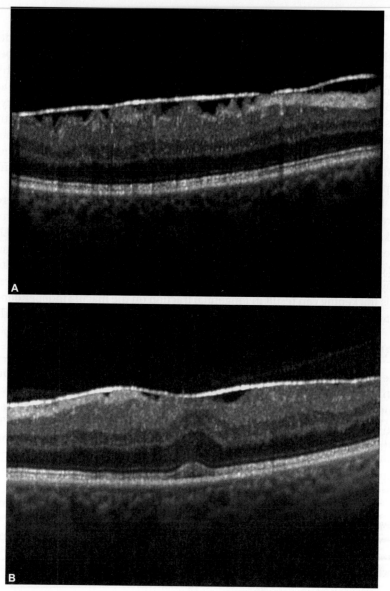

Figs. 7.3A and B: High resolution optical coherence tomography showing an abnormal vitreoretinal interface with a taut hyaloid membrane—(A) Right eye; (B) Left eye in the same patient.

macular edema were randomized to either focal/grid laser vs observation. After 3 years, 24% of the patients in the observation group experienced a loss of greater than or equal to 15 letters, which is equivalent to a doubling of the visual angle. Only 12% of treated eyes experienced similar vision loss.[24-27]

Laser was applied using either a focal or grid technique or a combination of the two in the ETDRS study. Focal laser refers to the application of laser to individual microaneurysms located between 500 μm to 3,000 μm from the foveal center. Individual microaneurysms are generally treated to attain either the whitening or darkening of the microaneurysm in an attempt to minimize the amount of energy delivered to attain these treatment endpoints. The laser is generally set to a 50–100 micron spot size with an exposure time of 0.1 seconds. The laser power settings are typically started low, between 50 mW and 60 mW for a standard 532 nm laser and titrated upward to achieve the desired treatment effect. The treating physician may need to adjust the laser settings when lasering through a particularly dense cataract or a particularly thickened retina. A grid laser is often used to treat more diffuse macular edema. The grid is composed of light-intensity burns ranging between 50 μm and 100 μm in diameter, spaced more than one burn-width apart over the area of the diffuse edema (Figs. 7.4A to D).[24-27] Adverse effects reported after the treatment of diabetic macular edema with either the focal or the grid laser include scotoma formation, the development of subretinal fibrosis, the development of choroidal neovascular membranes, and the expansion of laser scars over time (Fig. 7.5). These adverse effects can be minimized by the uptitrating the intensity of the laser delivered to the desired treatment effect.[19,26,71-81]

Patients may require multiple treatments in order to maximize treatment outcomes. Retreatments are generally performed at least three months after previous treatments, as the response of macular edema usually lags behind laser treatment. Recent randomized prospective trials, including the most recent Diabetic Retinopathy Clinical Research Network (DRCR.net) trials, have supported the use of focal and grid laser over the use intravitreal steroids for the treatment of diabetic macular edema.[82,83] Randomized prospective trials examining the use of anti-VEGF agents versus focal/grid laser in diabetic macular edema are currently underway.

Corticosteroids

As the pathogenesis for diabetic macular edema has in part been described as an inflammatory process, corticosteroids have been employed as a method of treatment. Corticosteroids have both potent antiangiogenic and anti-inflammatory effects. The ability of corticosteroids to suppress the expression of the VEGF as well as mitigate inflammatory pathways contributing to macular edema has led to the injection of these agents, triamcinolone in particular, for the treatment of diabetic macular edema.[84-96] While early reports of reduced retinal thickness and improved visual acuity seemed to indicate a potential role for the treatment of diabetic macular edema with intravitreal triamcinolone, a randomized controlled prospective study by the DRCR.net did not demonstrate the superiority of intravitreal triamcinolone over focal/grid laser.[82,83] Due to the morbidity profile of intravitreal corticosteroids, such as the potential for the development of glaucoma and significantly higher rate of cataract formation, most physicians continue to advocate the usage of focal and grid laser over the use of triamcinolone for the treatment of DME.[97,98]

While focal and grid laser remain the gold standard for the treatment of diabetic macular edema, some physicians have used corticosteroids for the treatment of diffuse, refractory edema. While there has been some suggestion of improvement in visual acuity and decreased central macular thickness after the injection of intravitreal triamcinolone, there exists conflicting data as to the long-term efficacy of steroid injections for the treatment of refractory macular edema. A recent systematic meta-analysis suggests that while corticosteroids may produce short-term improvements in vision and retinal thickness, treatment with corticosteroids confers no advantage over a placebo 6 months post-treatment.[99] With the development of more long-term corticosteroid delivery devices such as Retisert or Osurdex, it is possible that corticosteroids may become a long-term option for the treatment of refractory edema. Still other investigators have sought to combine the injection of intravitreal steroids with other modalities of treatment such as laser photocoagulation or the so-called triple therapy where the intravitreal injection of corticosteroids is combined with anti-VEGF therapy and laser photocoagulation.[100,101]

Anti-VEGF

As anti-VEGF agents have become the standard of care for the treatment of age-related macular degeneration, they have gained more widespread acceptance for the treatment of other ocular conditions. Several studies have suggested the potential for anti-VEGF agents to both improve visual acuity and decrease central macular thickness in patients with diabetic macular edema.[102-111] Currently, a prospective randomized control trial, Ranibizumab for Edema

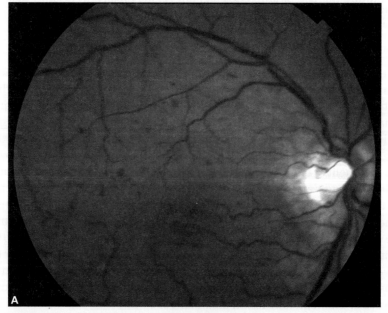

Fig. 7.4A

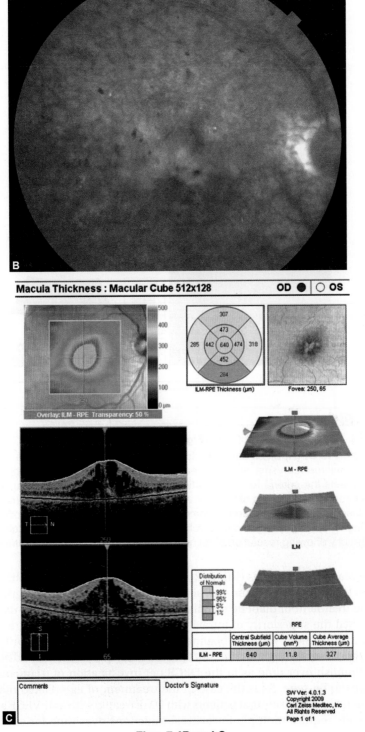

Figs. 7.4B and C

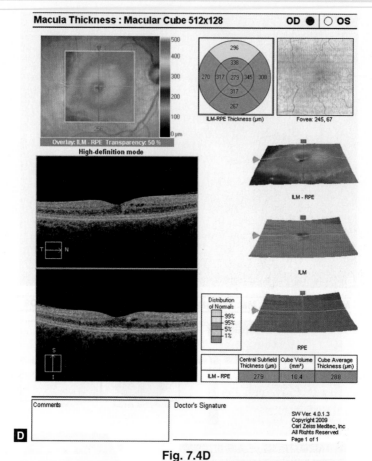

Fig. 7.4D

Figs. 7.4A to D: (A) Black and white fundus photograph of the right eye showing macular microaneurysms and an area of associated inferior retinal thickening which meets the criteria for classification of clinically significant macular edema. (B) Fluorescein angiogram of the right eye showing leakage prior to treatment with focal laser. (C) Optical coherence tomography prior to treatment with focal laser showing retinal thickening and cystic changes of the retina. (D) Optical coherence tomography showing resolution of retinal thickening after focal laser treatment.

of the Macula in Diabetes (READ-2), is investigating the use of ranibizumab versus focal/grid laser vs the combination ranibizumab and focal/grid laser for the treatment of diabetic macular edema.[112] Thus far, 6-month data has suggested the superiority of intravitreal ranibizumab over focal/grid laser. Whether treatment with ranibizumab continues to confer superiority over focal/grid laser throughout the course of the study or whether this advantage will diminish over time as in the DRCR.net investigation of triamcinolone remains to be seen. As is the case in the treatment of age-related macular degeneration, it is likely that patients with DME treated with anti-VEGF agents will likely require multiple intravitreal injections over time for sustained

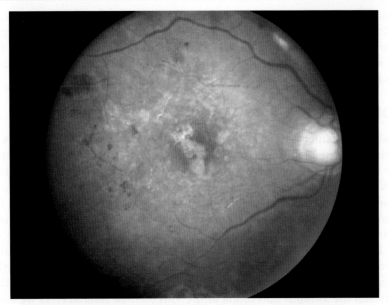

Fig. 7.5: Color fundus photograph showing atrophic macular changes secondary to scar creep from an area previously treated with focal laser.

treatment effect. Several other studies are currently underway to investigate the usage of both ranibizumab and bevacizumab in the treatment of clinically significant diabetic macular edema.

Surgical

Pars plana vitrectomy has been used for the treatment of refractory diabetic macular edema. As previously discussed, vitreomacular traction, the presence of a taught hyaloid, or diabetes-associated changes to the vitreoretinal interface and internal limiting membrane are all potential contributors to the development of diabetic macular edema. With the advent of optical coherence tomography and the ability to better image and assess the vitreoretinal interface, there exists increased rationale for the use of vitrectomy surgery in order to induce a posterior vitreous detachment and alter the pathologic vitreoretinal interface. Lewis et al. were the first to report the improvement of macular edema in patients with a thickened or taut hyaloid following a vitrectomy.[113] Since that time, many retrospective studies have indicated the potential for improvement in DME and visual acuity following pars plana vitrectomy. While some investigators have reported the improvement of macular edema and visual improvement after vitrectomy without detachment of the posterior hyaloid, most advocate the detachment of the posterior hyaloid with or without peeling the internal limiting membrane.[66,68,100,101,113-124]

The necessity of peeling the internal limiting membrane remains unclear. While many studies have been conducted to determine the effect of peeling the ILM on the resolution of macular edema and improvement of visual acuity, the results of these studies remain mixed. In 2000, Gandorfer reported a 92% success rate of both decreased retinal thickening and improvement in visual acuity after peeling the ILM.[125-127] These findings, however, were not corroborated by Kumagai et al., Kralinger et al., or Hartley et al., and as such, the benefit of peeling the ILM remains controversial.[67,128,129]

CONCLUSION

Diabetic macular edema is the leading cause of significant vision loss in patients with diabetic retinopathy. With the increased prevalence of diabetes, the treatment of diabetic retinopathy has become an increasingly important public health concern. The propensity for poorly-controlled diabetes to incur visual changes through the development of macular edema has made the treatment of diabetic macular edema one of the more pressing challenges facing ophthalmologists at this time.

It is clear that the pathogenesis of diabetic macular edema remains a complex interaction between the maintenance of blood-retinal barrier integrity, the development of vasoactive substances, and the unique interaction between the vitreous and retina at the vitreoretinal interface. As we learn more about these interactions through continued scientific exploration and experimentation, it is likely that we will develop a more sophisticated understanding of the factors that contribute to both the progression of retinopathy and diabetic macular edema.

While improving glycemic control and the control of other systemic risk factors remains the most important prognostic factors for the progression of retinopathy, increased understanding of the pathophysiology of diabetic macular edema will allow us to continue to develop new and improved modalities of treatment. While focal and grid laser remain the gold standard for the treatment of diabetic macular edema, the use of intravitreal corticosteroids, anti-VEGF therapy, and vitrectomy remain alternatives to photocoagulation. Continued investigation into these and other alternative modalities used individually or in conjunction with laser will help provide answers regarding which treatment strategies will be employed in the future for the treatment of diabetic macular edema.

REFERENCES

1. Rathmann W, Giani G. Global prevalence of diabetes: estimates for the year 2000 and projections for 2030. Diabetes Care. 2004;27(10):2568-9.
2. Shaw JE, Sicree RA, Zimmet PZ. Global estimates of the prevalence of diabetes for 2010 and 2030. Diabetes Res Clin Pract. 2009;87(1):4-14.
3. Wild S, Roglic G, Green A, et al. Global prevalence of diabetes: estimates for the year 2000 and projections for 2030. Diabetes Care. 2004;27(5):1047-53.
4. Dandona L, Dandona R, Naduvilath TJ, et al. Population based assessment of diabetic retinopathy in an urban population in southern India. Br J Ophthalmol. 1999;83(8):937-40.

5. Krishnaiah S, Das T, Nirmalan PK, et al. Risk factors for diabetic retinopathy: findings from The Andhra Pradesh eye disease study. Clin Ophthalmol. 2007;1(4):475-82.
6. Pradeepa R, Anitha B, Mohan V, et al. Risk factors for diabetic retinopathy in a South Indian Type 2 diabetic population—the Chennai Urban Rural Epidemiology Study (CURES) eye study 4. Diabet Med. 2008;25(5):536-42.
7. Rema M, Premkumar S, Anitha B, et al. Prevalence of diabetic retinopathy in urban India: the Chennai Urban Rural Epidemiology Study (CURES) eye study, I. Invest Ophthalmol Vis Sci. 2005;46(7):2328-33.
8. The effect of intensive treatment of diabetes on the development and progression of long-term complications in insulin-dependent diabetes mellitus. The Diabetes Control and Complications Trial Research Group. N Engl J Med. 1993;329(14):977-86.
9. Kohner EM, Stratton IM, Aldington SJ, et al. Relationship between the severity of retinopathy and progression to photocoagulation in patients with Type 2 diabetes mellitus in the UKPDS (UKPDS 52). Diabet Med. 2001;18(3):178-84.
10. Kohner EM, Stratton IM, Aldington SJ, et al. Microaneurysms in the development of diabetic retinopathy (UKPDS 42). UK Prospective Diabetes Study Group. Diabetologia. 1999;42(9):1107-12.
11. Matthews DR, Stratton IM, Aldington SJ, et al. Risks of progression of retinopathy and vision loss related to tight blood pressure control in type 2 diabetes mellitus: UKPDS 69. Arch Ophthalmol. 2004;122(11):1631-40.
12. Stratton IM, Kohner EM, Aldington SJ, et al. UKPDS 50: risk factors for incidence and progression of retinopathy in Type II diabetes over 6 years from diagnosis. Diabetologia. 2001;44(2):156-63.
13. Dodson PM, Gibson JM. Long-term follow-up of and underlying medical conditions in patients with diabetic exudative maculopathy. Eye. 1991;5(Pt 6):699-703.
14. Gallego PH, Craig ME, Hing S, Donaghue KC. Role of blood pressure in development of early retinopathy in adolescents with type 1 diabetes: prospective cohort study. Br Med J. 2008;337:a918.
15. Janka HU, Ziegler AG, Valsania P, et al. Impact of blood pressure on diabetic retinopathy. Diabete Metab. 1989;15(5 Pt 2):333-7.
16. Parving HH. Impact of blood pressure and antihypertensive treatment on incipient and overt nephropathy, retinopathy, and endothelial permeability in diabetes mellitus. Diabetes Care. 1991;14(3):260-9.
17. Sen K, Misra A, Kumar A, Pandey RM. Simvastatin retards progression of retinopathy in diabetic patients with hypercholesterolemia. Diabetes Res Clin Pract. 2002;56(1):1-11.
18. Hariprasad SM, Mieler WF, Grassi M, et al. Vision-related quality of life in patients with diabetic macular oedema. Br J Ophthalmol. 2008;92(1):89-92.
19. Tranos PG, Topouzis F, Stangos NT, et al. Effect of laser photocoagulation treatment for diabetic macular oedema on patient's vision-related quality of life. Curr Eye Res. 2004;29(1):41-9.
20. Giuffre G, Lodato G, Dardanoni G. Prevalence and risk factors of diabetic retinopathy in adult and elderly subjects: the Casteldaccia eye study. Graefes Arch Clin Exp Ophthalmol. 2004;242(7):535-40.
21. Klein R, Klein BE, Moss SE, et al. The Wisconsin epidemiologic study of diabetic retinopathy. III. Prevalence and risk of diabetic retinopathy when age at diagnosis is 30 or more years. Arch Ophthalmol. 1984;102(4):527-32.

22. Klein R, Klein BE, Moss SE, et al. The Wisconsin epidemiologic study of diabetic retinopathy. II. Prevalence and risk of diabetic retinopathy when age at diagnosis is less than 30 years. Arch Ophthalmol. 1984;102(4):520-6.

23. Klein R, Klein BE, Moss SE, et al. The Wisconsin epidemiologic study of diabetic retinopathy. IV. Diabetic macular edema. Ophthalmology. 1984;91(12):1464-74.

24. Photocoagulation for diabetic macular edema. Early Treatment Diabetic Retinopathy Study report number 1. Early Treatment Diabetic Retinopathy Study research group. Arch Ophthalmol. 1985;103(12):1796-806.

25. Treatment techniques and clinical guidelines for photocoagulation of diabetic macular edema. Early Treatment Diabetic Retinopathy Study Report Number 2. Early Treatment Diabetic Retinopathy Study Research Group. Ophthalmology. 1987;94(7):761-74.

26. Photocoagulation for diabetic macular edema: Early Treatment Diabetic Retinopathy Study Report no. 4. The Early Treatment Diabetic Retinopathy Study Research Group. Int Ophthalmol Clin. 1987;27(4):265-72.

27. Focal photocoagulation treatment of diabetic macular edema. Relationship of treatment effect to fluorescein angiographic and other retinal characteristics at baseline: ETDRS report no. 19. Early Treatment Diabetic Retinopathy Study Research Group. Arch Ophthalmol. 1995;113(9):1144-55.

28. Kinyoun J, Barton F, Fisher M, et al. Detection of diabetic macular edema. Ophthalmoscopy versus photography—Early Treatment Diabetic Retinopathy Study Report Number 5. The ETDRS Research Group. Ophthalmology. 1989;96(6):746-50; discussion 50-1.

29. Bhagat N, Grigorian RA, Tutela A, et al. Diabetic macular edema: pathogenesis and treatment. Surv Ophthalmol. 2009;54(1):1-32.

30. Chmielewska K, Robaszkiewicz J, Kosatka M. [Role of the retinal pigment epithelium (RPE) in the pathogenesis and treatment of diabetic macular edema (DME)]. Klin Oczna. 2008;110(7-9):318-20.

31. Ciulla TA, Amador AG, Zinman B. Diabetic retinopathy and diabetic macular edema: pathophysiology, screening, and novel therapies. Diabetes Care. 2003;26(9):2653-64.

32. Joussen AM, Smyth N, Niessen C. Pathophysiology of diabetic macular edema. Dev Ophthalmol. 2007;39:1-12.

33. Singh A, Stewart JM. Pathophysiology of diabetic macular edema. Int Ophthalmol Clin. 2009;49(2):1-11.

34. Cunha-Vaz J, Faria de Abreu JR, Campos AJ. Early breakdown of the blood-retinal barrier in diabetes. Br J Ophthalmol. 1975;59(11):649-56.

35. Cunha-Vaz J, Leite E, Sousa JC, et al. Blood-retinal barrier permeability and its relation to progression of retinopathy in patients with type 2 diabetes. A four-year follow-up study. Graefes Arch Clin Exp Ophthalmol. 1993;231(3):141-5.

36. Cunha-Vaz J, Lobo C, Sousa JC, et al. Progression of retinopathy and alteration of the blood-retinal barrier in patients with type 2 diabetes: a 7-year prospective follow-up study. Graefes Arch Clin Exp Ophthalmol. 1998;236(4):264-8.

37. Cunha-Vaz JG. Studies on the pathophysiology of diabetic retinopathy. The blood-retinal barrier in diabetes. Diabetes. 1983;32 Suppl 2:20-7.

38. Dorchy H. Characterization of early stages of diabetic retinopathy. Importance of the breakdown of the blood-retinal barrier. Diabetes Care. 1993;16(8):1212-4.

39. Frank RN. The mechanism of blood-retinal barrier breakdown in diabetes. Arch Ophthalmol. 1985;103(9):1303-4.

40. Krogsaa B, Lund-Andersen H, Mehlsen J, Sestoft L. Blood-retinal barrier permeability versus diabetes duration and retinal morphology in insulin dependent diabetic patients. Acta Ophthalmol. 1987;65(6):686-92.
41. Chazan BI. Microaneurysms in diabetes mellitus. Acta Diabetol Lat. 1972;9(3):337-49.
42. Klein R, Meuer SM, Moss SE, Klein BE. The relationship of retinal microaneurysm counts to the 4-year progression of diabetic retinopathy. Arch Ophthalmol. 1989;107(12):1780-5.
43. Klein R, Meuer SM, Moss SE, Klein BE. Retinal microaneurysm counts and 10-year progression of diabetic retinopathy. Arch Ophthalmol. 1995;113(11):1386-91.
44. Stitt AW, Gardiner TA, Archer DB. Histological and ultrastructural investigation of retinal microaneurysm development in diabetic patients. Br J Ophthalmol. 1995;79(4):362-7.
45. Lobo CL, Bernardes RC, Cunha-Vaz JG. Alterations of the blood-retinal barrier and retinal thickness in preclinical retinopathy in subjects with type 2 diabetes. Arch Ophthalmol. 2000;118(10):1364-9.
46. Lobo CL, Bernardes RC, de Abreu JR, et al. One-year follow-up of blood-retinal barrier and retinal thickness alterations in patients with type 2 diabetes mellitus and mild nonproliferative retinopathy. Arch Ophthalmol. 2001;119(10):1469-74.
47. Lobo CL, Bernardes RC, Figueira JP, et al. Three-year follow-up study of blood-retinal barrier and retinal thickness alterations in patients with type 2 diabetes mellitus and mild nonproliferative diabetic retinopathy. Arch Ophthalmol. 2004;122(2):211-7.
48. Aiello LP. The potential role of PKC beta in diabetic retinopathy and macular edema. Surv Ophthalmol. 2002;47 Suppl 2:S263-9.
49. Benitez del Castillo JM, Castillo A, Fernandez PC, Garcia Sanchez J. Clinical and metabolic factors associated with the blood retinal barrier permeability in insulin dependent diabetes mellitus without retinopathy. Doc Ophthalmol. 1993;84(2):127-33.
50. Churchill AJ, Carter JG, Ramsden C, et al. VEGF polymorphisms are associated with severity of diabetic retinopathy. Invest Ophthalmol Vis Sci. 2008;49(8):3611-6.
51. Galvez MI. Rubosixtaurin and other PKC inhibitors in diabetic retinopathy and macular edema. Review. Curr Diabetes Rev. 2009;5(1):14-7.
52. Kaji Y, Oshika T. Role of advanced glycation end products and activation of PKC in diabetic retinopathy. Nippon Rinsho. 2005;63(Suppl 6):188-93.
53. Kim JH, Yu YS, Cho CS, et al. Blockade of angiotensin II attenuates VEGF-mediated blood-retinal barrier breakdown in diabetic retinopathy. J Cereb Blood Flow Metab. 2009;29(3):621-8.
54. Malik RA, Li C, Aziz W, et al. Elevated plasma CD105 and vitreous VEGF levels in diabetic retinopathy. J Cell Mol Med. 2005;9(3):692-7.
55. Nakamura S, Iwasaki N, Funatsu H, et al. Impact of variants in the VEGF gene on progression of proliferative diabetic retinopathy. Graefes Arch Clin Exp Ophthalmol. 2009;247(1):21-6.
56. Qaum T, Xu Q, Joussen AM, et al. VEGF-initiated blood-retinal barrier breakdown in early diabetes. Invest Ophthalmol Vis Sci. 2001;42(10):2408-13.
57. Song E, Dong Y, Han LN, et al. Diabetic retinopathy: VEGF, bFGF and retinal vascular pathology. Chin Med J. 2004;117(2):247-51.
58. Stoschitzky K. Angiotensin II, VEGF, and diabetic retinopathy. Lancet. 1998;351(9105):836-7.
59. Williams B. Angiotensin II, VEGF, and diabetic retinopathy. Lancet. 1998;351(9105):837-8.

60. Zhang SX, Wang JJ, Gao G, et al. Pigment epithelium-derived factor downregulates vascular endothelial growth factor (VEGF) expression and inhibits VEGF-VEGF receptor 2 binding in diabetic retinopathy. J Mol Endocrinol. 2006;37(1):1-12.

61. Skondra D, Noda K, Almulki L, et al. Characterization of azurocidin as a permeability factor in the retina: involvement in VEGF-induced and early diabetic blood-retinal barrier breakdown. Invest Ophthalmol Vis Sci. 2008;49(2):726-31.

62. Hatano N, Mizota A, Tanaka M. Vitreous surgery for diabetic macular edema—its prognosis and correlation between preoperative systemic and ocular conditions and visual outcome. Ann Ophthalmol. 2007;39(3):222-7.

63. Mackay CJ. Tomographic assessment of vitreous surgery for diabetic macular edema. Am J Ophthalmol. 2002;133(1):166.

64. Nasrallah FP, Jalkh AE, Van Coppenolle F, et al. The role of the vitreous in diabetic macular edema. Ophthalmology. 1988;95(10):1335-9.

65. Otani T, Kishi S. Tomographic assessment of vitreous surgery for diabetic macular edema. Am J Ophthalmol. 2000;129(4):487-94.

66. Yamamoto S, Yamamoto T, Ogata K, et al. Morphological and functional changes of the macula after vitrectomy and creation of posterior vitreous detachment in eyes with diabetic macular edema. Doc Ophthalmol. 2004;109(3):249-53.

67. Kumagai K, Ogino N, Furukawa M, et al. Internal limiting membrane peeling in vitreous surgery for diabetic macular edema. Nippon Ganka Gakkai Zasshi. 2002;106(9):590-4.

68. Yamamoto T, Akabane N, Takeuchi S. Vitrectomy for diabetic macular edema: the role of posterior vitreous detachment and epimacular membrane. Am J Ophthalmol. 2001;132(3):369-77.

69. Fritsche A, Stumvoll M, Goebbel S, et al. Long term effect of a structured inpatient diabetes teaching and treatment programme in type 2 diabetic patients: influence of mode of follow-up. Diabetes Res Clin Pract. 1999;46(2):135-41.

70. Rachmani R, Slavachevski I, Berla M, et al. Teaching and motivating patients to control their risk factors retards progression of cardiovascular as well as microvascular sequelae of Type 2 diabetes mellitus-a randomized prospective 8 years follow-up study. Diabet Med. 2005;22(4):410-4.

71. The Diabetic Retinopathy Clinical Research Network. The course of response to focal/grid photocoagulation for diabetic macular edema. Retina. 2009;29(10):1436-43.

72. Berger AR, Boniuk I. Bilateral subretinal neovascularization after focal argon laser photocoagulation for diabetic macular edema. Am J Ophthalmol. 1989;108(1):88-90.

73. Friberg TR. Subthreshold (invisible) modified grid diode laser photocoagulation and diffuse diabetic macular edema (DDME). Ophthalmic Surg Lasers. 1999;30(9):705.

74. Guyer DR, D'Amico DJ, Smith CW. Subretinal fibrosis after laser photocoagulation for diabetic macular edema. Am J Ophthalmol. 1992;113(6):652-6.

75. Han DP, Mieler WF, Burton TC. Submacular fibrosis after photocoagulation for diabetic macular edema. Am J Ophthalmol. 1992;113(5):513-21.

76. Haut J, Monin C, Ancel JM, et al. Limitations of photocoagulation in the treatment of diabetic maculo-foveolar edema: macular neuro-epithelium detachment. Bull Soc Ophtalmol Fr. 1990;90(8-9):745-6.

77. Kojima K, Yamagishi Z, Shimizu Y, et al. Effects of photocoagulation on diabetic macular edema. Nippon Ganka Gakkai Zasshi. 1990;94(1):54-60.

78. Lai Y, Gao R, Wu D. The study on changes of macular light sensitivity before and after photocoagulation for diabetic macular edema. Zhonghua Yan Ke Za Zhi. 1996;32(5):362-5.

79. Rutledge BK, Wallow IH, Poulsen GL. Sub-pigment epithelial membranes after photocoagulation for diabetic macular edema. Arch Ophthalmol. 1993;111(5):608-13.

80. Schatz H, Madeira D, McDonald HR, et al. Progressive enlargement of laser scars following grid laser photocoagulation for diffuse diabetic macular edema. Arch Ophthalmol. 1991;109(11):1549-51.

81. Sims LM, Stoessel K, Thompson JT, et al. Assessment of visual-field changes before and after focal photocoagulation for clinically significant diabetic macular edema. Ophthalmologica. 1990;200(3):133-41.

82. Beck RW, Edwards AR, Aiello LP, et al. Three-year follow-up of a randomized trial comparing focal/grid photocoagulation and intravitreal triamcinolone for diabetic macular edema. Arch Ophthalmol. 2009;127(3):245-51.

83. Ip MS, Bressler SB, Antoszyk AN, et al. A randomized trial comparing intravitreal triamcinolone and focal/grid photocoagulation for diabetic macular edema: baseline features. Retina. 2008;28(7):919-30.

84. Bae JS, Park SJ, Ham IR, et al. Dose dependent effects of intravitreal triamcinolone acetonide on diffuse diabetic macular edema. Korean J Ophthalmol. 2009;23(2):80-5.

85. Bakri SJ, Beer PM. Intravitreal triamcinolone injection for diabetic macular edema: a clinical and fluorescein angiographic case series. Can J Ophthalmol. 2004;39(7):755-60.

86. Bonini-Filho MA, Jorge R, Barbosa JC, et al. Intravitreal injection versus sub-Tenon's infusion of triamcinolone acetonide for refractory diabetic macular edema: a randomized clinical trial. Invest Ophthalmol Vis Sci. 2005;46(10):3845-9.

87. Chan CK, Chan WM, Cheung BT, et al. Intravitreal injection of triamcinolone for diffuse diabetic macular edema. Arch Ophthalmol. 2004;122(7):1083-5; author reply 6-8.

88. Chieh JJ, Roth DB, Liu M, et al. Intravitreal triamcinolone acetonide for diabetic macular edema. Retina. 2005;25(7):828-34.

89. Dubey AK. Intravitreal injection of triamcinolone acetonide for diabetic macular edema: principles and practice. Indian J Ophthalmol. 2006;54(4):290.

90. Hauser D, Bukelman A, Pokroy R, et al. Intravitreal triamcinolone for diabetic macular edema: comparison of 1, 2, and 4 mg. Retina. 2008;28(6):825-30.

91. Jonas JB, Degenring RF, Kamppeter BA, et al. Duration of the effect of intravitreal triamcinolone acetonide as treatment for diffuse diabetic macular edema. Am J Ophthalmol. 2004;138(1):158-60.

92. Kuhn F, Barker D. Intravitreal injection of triamcinolone acetonide for diabetic macular edema. Arch Ophthalmol. 2004;122(7):1082-3.

93. Martidis A, Duker JS, Greenberg PB, et al. Intravitreal triamcinolone for refractory diabetic macular edema. Ophthalmology. 2002;109(5):920-7.

94. Ozkiris A, Evereklioglu C, Erkilic K, et al. Intravitreal triamcinolone acetonide injection as primary treatment for diabetic macular edema. Eur J Ophthalmol. 2004;14(6):543-9.

95. Vedantham V, Kim R. Intravitreal injection of triamcinolone acetonide for diabetic macular edema: principles and practice. Indian J Ophthalmol. 2006;54(2):133-7.

96. Zhang X, Bao S, Lai D, et al. Intravitreal triamcinolone acetonide inhibits breakdown of the blood-retinal barrier through differential regulation of VEGF-A and its receptors in early diabetic rat retinas. Diabetes. 2008;57(4):1026-33.

97. Kreissig I, Degenring RF, Jonas JB. Diffuse diabetic macular edema. Intraocular pressure after intravitreal triamcinolone acetonide. Ophthalmologe. 2005;102(2):153-7.

98. Lopez-Galvez MI, Pastor-Jimeno JC. Efficacy and safety of intravitreal injection of triamcinolone acetonide as treatment for diffuse diabetic macular edema. Arch Soc Esp Oftalmol. 2009;84(11):547-8.

99. Grover D, Li TJ, Chong CC. Intravitreal steroids for macular edema in diabetes. Cochrane Database Syst Rev. 2008(1):CD005656.

100. Er H. Triple therapy of vitrectomy, intravitreal triamcinolone, and macular laser photocoagulation for intractable diabetic macular edema. Am J Ophthalmol. 2008;146(2):332-3; author reply 3.

101. Kang SW, Park SC, Cho HY, et al. Triple therapy of vitrectomy, intravitreal triamcinolone, and macular laser photocoagulation for intractable diabetic macular edema. Am J Ophthalmol. 2007;144(6):878-85.

102. Arevalo JF, Fromow-Guerra J, Quiroz-Mercado H, et al. Primary intravitreal bevacizumab (Avastin) for diabetic macular edema: results from the Pan-American Collaborative Retina Study Group at 6-month follow-up. Ophthalmology. 2007;114(4):743-50.

103. Arevalo JF, Sanchez JG, Fromow-Guerra J, et al. Comparison of two doses of primary intravitreal bevacizumab (Avastin) for diffuse diabetic macular edema: results from the Pan-American Collaborative Retina Study Group (PACORES) at 12-month follow-up. Graefes Arch Clin Exp Ophthalmol. 2009;247(6):735-43.

104. Chun DW, Heier JS, Topping TM, et al. A pilot study of multiple intravitreal injections of ranibizumab in patients with center-involving clinically significant diabetic macular edema. Ophthalmology. 2006;113(10):1706-12.

105. Haritoglou C, Kook D, Neubauer A, et al. Intravitreal bevacizumab (Avastin) therapy for persistent diffuse diabetic macular edema. Retina. 2006;26(9):999-1005.

106. Khurana RN, Do DV, Nguyen QD. Anti-VEGF therapeutic approaches for diabetic macular edema. Int Ophthalmol Clin. 2009;49(2):109-19.

107. Kook D, Wolf A, Kreutzer T, et al. Long-term effect of intravitreal bevacizumab (avastin) in patients with chronic diffuse diabetic macular edema. Retina. 2008;28(8):1053-60.

108. Kumar A, Sinha S. Intravitreal bevacizumab (Avastin) treatment of diffuse diabetic macular edema in an Indian population. Indian J Ophthalmol. 2007;55(6):451-5.

109. Nagasawa T, Naito T, Matsushita S, et al. Efficacy of intravitreal bevacizumab (Avastin) for short-term treatment of diabetic macular edema. J Med Invest. 2009;56(3-4):111-5.

110. Velez-Montoya R, Fromow-Guerra J, Burgos O, et al. The effect of unilateral intravitreal bevacizumab (avastin), in the treatment of diffuse bilateral diabetic macular edema: a pilot study. Retina. 2009;29(1):20-6.

111. Yanyali A, Aytug B, Horozoglu F, et al. Bevacizumab (Avastin) for diabetic macular edema in previously vitrectomized eyes. Am J Ophthalmol. 2007;144(1):124-6.

112. Nguyen QD, Shah SM, Heier JS, et al. Primary End Point (Six Months) Results of the Ranibizumab for Edema of the mAcula in diabetes (READ-2) study. Ophthalmology. 2009;116(11):2175-81 e1.

113. Lewis H. The role of vitrectomy in the treatment of diabetic macular edema. Am J Ophthalmol. 2001;131(1):123-5.

114. Bahadir M, Ertan A, Mertoglu O. Visual acuity comparison of vitrectomy with and without internal limiting membrane removal in the treatment of diabetic macular edema. Int Ophthalmol. 2005;26(1-2):3-8.

115. Diaz-Llopis M, Udaondo P, Arevalo F, et al. Intravitreal plasmin without associated vitrectomy as a treatment for refractory diabetic macular edema. J Ocul Pharmacol Ther. 2009;25(4):379-84.

116. Diaz-Llopis M, Udaondo P, Garcia-Delpech S, et al. Enzymatic vitrectomy by intravitreal autologous plasmin injection, as initial treatment for diffuse diabetic macular edema. Arch Soc Esp Oftalmol. 2008;83(2):77-84.

117. Hernandez-Da Mota SE, Chacon-Lara A, Hernández-Vázquez E. Use of triamcinolone and bevacizumab in 25G phaco-vitrectomy surgery for the treatment of cataract and diabetic macular edema. Arch Soc Esp Oftalmol. 2008;83(5):293-300.

118. Higuchi A, Ogata N, Jo N, et al. Pars plana vitrectomy with removal of posterior hyaloid face in treatment of refractory diabetic macular edema resistant to triamcinolone acetonide. Jpn J Ophthalmol. 2006;50(6):529-31.

119. Jahn CE, Schopfer DC, Heinzle T, et al. Lasting resolution of diabetic macular edema and stable improvement of visual acuity after treatment with pars plana vitrectomy. Ophthalmologica. 2009;223(3):219-20.

120. Jahn CE, Topfner von Schutz K, Richter J, et al. Improvement of visual acuity in eyes with diabetic macular edema after treatment with pars plana vitrectomy. Ophthalmologica. 2004;218(6):378-84.

121. Kim YM, Chung EJ, Byeon SH, et al. Pars plana vitrectomy with internal limiting membrane peeling compared with intravitreal triamcinolone injection in the treatment of diabetic macular edema. Ophthalmologica. 2009;223(1):17-23.

122. Lai WW, Mohamed S, Lam DS. Improvement of visual acuity in eyes with diabetic macular edema after treatment with pars plana vitrectomy. Ophthalmologica. 2005;219(3):189.

123. Parolini B, Panozzo G, Gusson E, et al. Diode laser, vitrectomy and intravitreal triamcinolone. A comparative study for the treatment of diffuse non tractional diabetic macular edema. Semin Ophthalmol. 2004;19(1-2):1-12.

124. Recchia FM, Ruby AJ, Carvalho Recchia CA. Pars plana vitrectomy with removal of the internal limiting membrane in the treatment of persistent diabetic macular edema. Am J Ophthalmol. 2005;139(3):447-54.

125. Gandorfer A, Kampik A. Role of vitreoretinal interface in the pathogenesis and therapy of macular disease associated with optic pits. Ophthalmology. 2000;97(4):276-9.

126. Gandorfer A, Kampik A. Pars plana vitrectomy with and without peeling of the inner limiting membrane (ILM) for diabetic macular edema. Retina. 2008;28(1):187-8.

127. Gandorfer A, Messmer EM, Ulbig MW, et al. Resolution of diabetic macular edema after surgical removal of the posterior hyaloid and the inner limiting membrane. Retina. 2000;20(2):126-33.

128. Hartley KL, Smiddy WE, Flynn HW Jr, et al. Pars plana vitrectomy with internal limiting membrane peeling for diabetic macular edema. Retina. 2008;28(3):410-9.

129. Kralinger MT, Pedri M, Kralinger F, et al. Long-term outcome after vitrectomy for diabetic macular edema. Ophthalmologica. 2006;220(3):147-52.

CHAPTER 8

Diabetic Papillopathy

Michael M Altaweel, Richard E Appen, Suresh R Chandra

INTRODUCTION

Diabetic papillopathy is classically described as a disorder in which young juvenile diabetics develop transient edema of the optic disks with minimal impairment of the function of the optic nerve. A mild-to-moderate visual disturbance with mild visual field abnormality is often the presenting symptom. Accompanying diabetic retinopathy is usually not severe. This disorder was first described in 1971 by Lubow and Makley as *pseudopapilledema of juvenile diabetes mellitus*[1] and was further characterized in three case series published in 1980.[2-4]

CASE PRESENTATION

A 20-year-old man with a 17-year-history of diabetes mellitus experienced brief intermittent blurring of vision of both eyes. Visual acuity was 20/20 in the right eye and 20/25 in the left eye. Color vision tested with the Munsell D15 test was normal in both eyes (OU). Pupillary reactions and extraocular movements were normal. The anterior segments of the eyes were unremarkable. The intraocular pressure was 24 mm Hg in each eye. Posterior segment examination revealed 1–2 diopters of disk swelling OU with peripapillary hemorrhages and dilated retinal vessels (Figs. 8.1A and B). The retinas were otherwise normal. Visual field testing revealed enlarged blind spots. The blood pressure was 112/78 mm Hg.

A fluorescein angiogram revealed telangiectatic vessels OU with a staining of the disk (Figs. 8.2A and B). Within 1 month, without treatment, the swelling of the right optic nerve head resolved. Within 3 months of presentation, both optic nerves had regained a normal appearance (Figs. 8.3 and 8.4). Visual

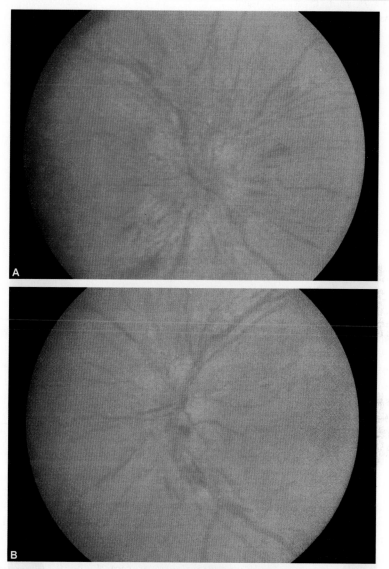

Figs. 8.1A and B: Bilateral optic nerve swelling with peripapillary hemorrhages and telangiectatic superficial vessels. Minimal diabetic retinopathy is evident.

acuity remained stable at 20/20 in the right eye and 20/40 in the left eye. The blind spot had returned to its normal size.

Three years later, the patient developed proliferative diabetic retinopathy bilaterally (Figs. 8.5 and 8.6) and required panretinal photocoagulation.

A 13-year-old female with 10-year-history of Type I diabetes had asymptomatic bilateral optic nerve swelling (Figs. 8.7A and B).

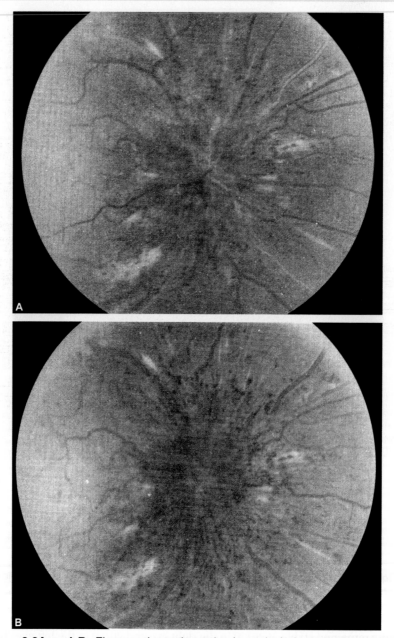

Figs. 8.2A and B: Fluorescein angiography (negative) demonstrates radially oriented dilated superficial vessels with leakage into substance of optic nerve (13 and 23 seconds).

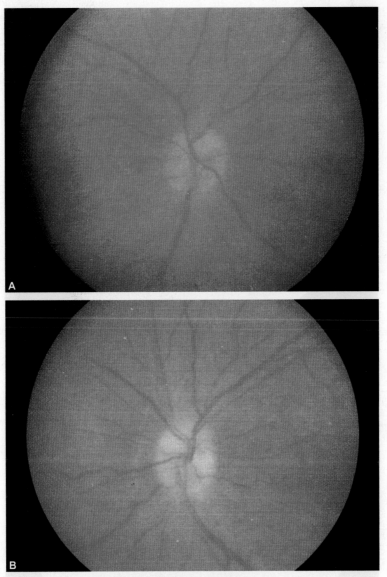

Figs. 8.3A and B: Complete resolution of optic nerve swelling and vascular changes in both eyes within 6 months.

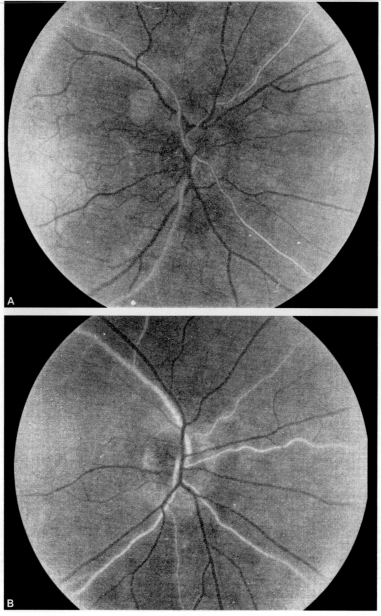

Figs. 8.4A and B: Fluorescein angiography confirms resolution of vascular abnormality.

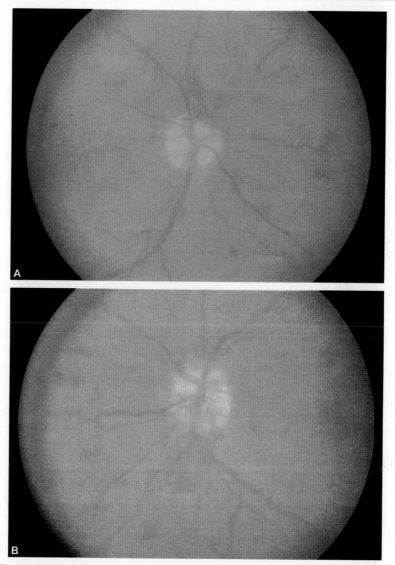

Figs. 8.5A and B: Neovascularization at the disk has developed in both eyes after 3 years requiring panretinal photocoagulation.

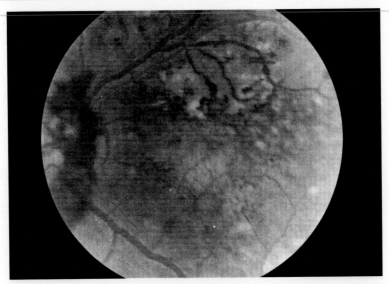

Fig. 8.6: Disk neovascularization with leakage and a large area of ischemia demonstrated on fundus fluorescein angiography.

An fundus fluorescein angiography (FFA) demonstrated the leakage of dye into the substance of optic nerve heads (Figs. 8.8A and B). Visual fields showed bilateral enlargement of blind spots and a paracentral scotoma in the left field (Fig. 8.9). The 3-month follow-up examination revealed a normal appearance of both optic nerve heads (Figs. 8.10A and B). The recharting of visual fields demonstrated normal fields (Fig. 8.11) concurring with the findings of funduscopy.

DEMOGRAPHICS

In the reports of Appen et al.,[2] Pavan et al.,[3] and Barr et al.,[4] of 25 patients, all but two patients were less than 30 years of age. The mean age was 22 years in the largest series. All the patients were Type I diabetics. This age group has continued to be the most commonly described as developing diabetic papillopathy, but a recent case series described similar findings in 27 eyes of 19 patients with an age range of 19–79 and a mean age of 50 years.[5] In this series, two-thirds were Type II diabetics. The incidence of diabetic papillopathy is approximately 4/1,000 diabetics.

SYMPTOMS

The patient may be asymptomatic, but can experience mild visual blurring, which may be transient. Eye pain and headache are generally not present.

EXAMINATION

The visual acuity is commonly mildly impaired. The anterior segment of the eye is usually normal. A relative afferent pupillary defect is not present in most

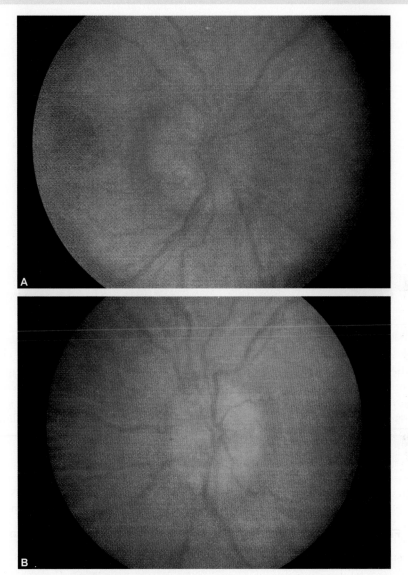

Figs. 8.7A and B: Bilateral optic nerve swelling.

cases. The color vision is generally normal. The posterior segment examination reveals unilateral or bilateral swelling of the optic disk, on the surface of which are radially oriented dilated superficial telangiectatic vessels. The degree of diabetic retinopathy accompanying this disorder is usually mild, and the systemic blood pressure is normal.

INVESTIGATION

Fluorescein angiography can be used to distinguish between telangiectatic vessels associated with the disk edema, and new vessels indicative of

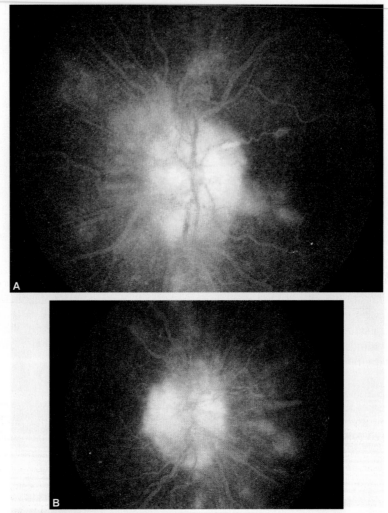

Figs. 8.8A and B: Leakage into substance of optic nerves demonstrated on fluorescein angiogram (negative).

proliferative diabetic retinopathy. With typical diabetic papillopathy, the dilated preexisting vessels lie in the plane of the disk in the retina and are radially oriented. They do not leak early but may eventually leak into the substance of the disk and retina with hyperfluorescence of the disk noted on late frames. The neovascularization of the disk (NVD) is characterized by an irregular vessel pattern in an elevated plane, with leakage of the dye into the vitreous, obscuring the underlying retinal vasculature.

The visual field in patients with diabetic papillopathy may be normal, but commonly reveals an enlarged blind spot. Cases with more severe visual field deficits such as central or paracentral scotomas have been described.[4]

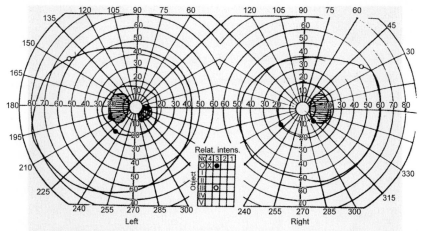

Fig. 8.9: Corresponding Goldmann visual field demonstrates enlarged blind spots OU and a paracentral scotoma OS.

Lumbar puncture was performed routinely in several case series, and in all cases the intracranial pressure was found to be normal, clarifying that the condition is not papilledema. Similarly, neuroimaging also failed to reveal evidence of elevated intracranial pressure.[5] Laboratory testing of such individuals has routinely been normal, including complete blood cell count and erythrocyte sedimentation rate.

PATHOPHYSIOLOGY

There are several theories on the pathogenesis of diabetic papillopathy. Lubow and Makley suggested that the syndrome may be a variant of anterior ischemic optic neuropathy (AION).[1] Their view was echoed by Hayreh et al. who commented that AION can vary in severity and in age of presentation.[6] However, Appen et al. concluded that the differences between diabetic papillopathy and AION are greater than their similarities. The younger age of the patients, the relative lack of symptoms of vision impairment, the bilaterality, and the absence of altitudinal visual field defects are characteristics of diabetic papillopathy that suggest it is a distinct entity different from AION. These authors suggested that a vasculopathy of the most superficial layer of disk capillaries in the optic nerve head, similar to the diffuse microvascular abnormalities of diabetic retinopathy, might cause diabetic papillopathy by producing the transient leakage of fluid into and around the optic nerve head with consequent optic disk swelling.[2]

DIFFERENTIAL DIAGNOSIS

The major differential diagnoses for diabetic papillopathy are papilledema and AION. The occurrence of the condition in a young person with Type I diabetes would raise suspicion of diabetic papillopathy. The absence of headache or

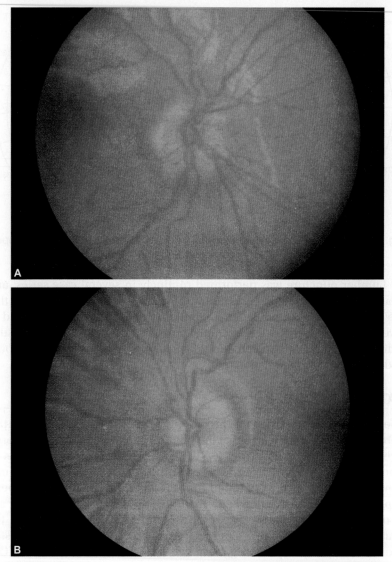

Figs. 8.10A and B: Normal optic nerve appearance in both eyes is regained within 3 months.

other neurologic symptoms, and the characteristic appearance of the radially oriented distended vessels at the optic disk in diabetic papillopathy would enable one to doubt the presence of papilledema. If there were uncertainty, demonstration of normal results of neuroimaging and normal intracranial pressure at lumbar puncture would exclude papilledema as the diagnosis.

Regarding AION, diabetic papillopathy typically presents in a much younger population without similar optic nerve function abnormalities. Altitudinal visual field defects are rare, and there is typically no relative afferent pupillary

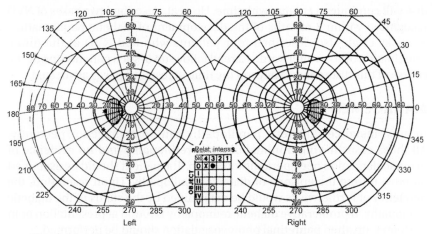

Fig. 8.11: Visual field examination concurs with findings on funduscopy.

defect, even when the disorder is unilateral. The characteristic visual acuity and visual field improvement found in diabetic papillopathy does not occur with AION.

Diabetic papillopathy is differentiated from inflammatory or demyelinating papillitis by the presence of normal pupil reactions, the absence of a central visual field defect, and the minimal impairment of visual acuity.

Papillophlebitis is more likely to be unilateral, and has more retinal hemorrhages than in diabetic papillopathy.

Malignant hypertension must be considered in the differential diagnosis. The absence of elevated brachial blood pressure and the absence of retinal arteriovenous crossing changes and localized arterial narrowing would distinguish diabetic papillopathy from malignant hypertensive retinopathy.

PROGNOSIS

A series of articles[3-5] described resolution of the optic disk edema in most eyes within 3 months. The visual acuity also returned to normal within a short period of time. In Pavan's series, 7 of 8 patients regained 20/20 visual acuity within 6 months.[3] In Barr's series, 15–21 eyes had regained better than 20/40 acuity by 3 months after presentation.[4] Regillo et al. described an older cohort of patients with diabetic papillopathy. However, the prognosis was similarly favorable, with 23 of 27 eyes attaining better than or equal to 20/50 Snellen visual acuity.[5]

Earlier reports on the diabetic papillopathy found that in most cases the degree of diabetic retinopathy was mild or moderate. It was felt that diabetic papillopathy was not a harbinger of proliferative disease. However, several recent articles described the concurrent or immediately subsequent development of NVD associated with diabetic papillopathy.[7-9] While the telangiectatic vessels found with classic diabetic papillopathy will appear normal upon resolution of the disk edema, the neovascularization at the optic disk will continue to enlarge with time. Ho et al. described two cases of NVD recognized within 3 months of the development of diabetic papillopathy.[8] Stransky et al. also described four patients who had NVD at the initial examination or soon afterward.[7] Careful follow-up of such patients during the course of this disorder and beyond the time of resolution was advocated.

MANAGEMENT

In most instances, diabetic papillopathy can be managed expectantly. All those cases having minimal diabetic retinopathy and no evidence of neovascularization need periodic follow-up. The patient should be examined monthly during the episode of diabetic papillopathy. Upon resolution, the frequency of further visits would be determined by the status of the diabetic retinopathy. If proliferative diabetic retinopathy is found at presentation or in the follow-up, then panretinal photocoagulation should be performed.

Of the 27 eyes described by Regillo et al., 19 (70%) had clinically significant macular edema. Six of the 19 required focal laser treatment.[5] Younger patients with diabetic papillopathy are less likely to require this management.

Systemically-administered corticosteroids have been used for one patient with diabetic papillopathy with no significant improvement.[3] As the prognosis is generally favorable for this disorder and corticosteroids cause difficulty with diabetic control among other side effects, they are not recommended as treatment.

SUMMARY

Diabetic papillopathy is a disorder in which diabetics develop transient swelling of one or both optic disks with no evidence of elevated intracranial pressure. Symptoms of visual blurring and mild visual field defects typically resolve within several months without treatment. Although initially described in juvenile Type I diabetics, the disorder has more recently been reported in an older population with Type II diabetes. Proliferative diabetic retinopathy occasionally may be associated with diabetic papillopathy or may develop subsequently. Most cases of diabetic papillopathy do not need any treatment unless associated with proliferative changes.

REFERENCES

1. Lubow M, Makley TA Jr. Pseudopapilledema of juvenile diabetes mellitus. Arch Ophthalmol. 1971;85:417-22.
2. Appen RE, Chandra SR, Klein R, et al. Diabetic papillopathy. Am J Ophthalmol. 1980;90:203-9.
3. Pavan PR, Aiello LM, Wafai ZW. Optic disc oedema in juvenile-onset diabetes. Arch Ophthalmol. 1980;98:2193-5.
4. Barr CC, Glaser JS, Blakenship G. Acute disc swelling in juvenile diabetes: clinical profile and natural history of 12 cases. Arch Ophthalmol. 1980;98:2185-92.
5. Regillo CD, Brown GC, Savino PJ, et al. Diabetic retinopathy: patient characteristics and fundus findings. Arch Ophthalmol. 1995;113:889-95.

6. Hayreh SS, Zahoruk RM. Anterior ischemic optic neuropathy VI in juvenile diabetics. Ophthalmologica. 1981;182(1):13-28.
7. Stransky T. Diabetic papillopathy and proliferative retinopathy. Graefes Arch Clin Exp Ophthalmol. 1986;224:46-50.
8. Ho AC, Maguire AM, Yannuzzi LA, et al. Rapidly progressive optic disk neovascularization after diabetic papillopathy. Am J Ophthalmol 1995;120:673-5.
9. DeUngria JM, DelPriore LV, Hart W. Abnormal disc vessels after diabetic papillopathy. Arch Ophthalmol. 1995;113:245-6.

CHAPTER 9

Hypertensive Retinopathy

Shreyas Temkar, Bhavya G, Pradeep Venkatesh

INTRODUCTION

Hypertension is one of the most prevalent systemic illnesses in patients encountered by an ophthalmologist during his/her practice. This clinical condition is a significant modifiable risk factor for cardiovascular catastrophes, such as myocardial infarction, stroke, aortic dissection and others. Though essential hypertension remains the most important type of hypertension, secondary causes, such as renal disease, pheochromocytoma, Cushing's syndrome, steroid therapy, etc. need to be ruled out. Despite hypertension being a common factor in the pathogenesis of multiple end-organ diseases, many patients with hypertension remain undiagnosed or undertreated.[1]

The Joint National Committee 8 (JNC 8, 2014) recommends that in a general population aged more than 60 years, pharmacological treatment should be started on anti-hypertensive drugs when systolic blood pressure is more than 150 mm Hg and diastolic blood pressure is more than 90 mm Hg. This recommendation is based on the evidence that lowering blood pressure to aforementioned limits reduces the risk of heart failure, stroke and coronary heart disease. However, the optimal management of hypertension depends on the timely diagnosis of this illness.[2]

OCULAR MANIFESTATIONS

Systemic hypertension causes series of pathological changes in retinal, choroidal and optic nerve circulations. The changes seen in these vessels depend on the onset of hypertension (acute or chronic), severity and duration. Apart from the direct effects on retinal, choroidal and optic nerve head circulation, hypertension is known to be an important risk factor in the pathogenesis of disorders, such as venous and arterial occlusions, ischemic optic neuropathy, worsening of diabetic retinopathy and retinal artery macroaneurysm.

Hypertensive Retinopathy

Retinal microvascular changes in hypertensive retinopathy include both arteriosclerotic changes and those due to vasoconstriction. Retinal vasculature changes in patients with hypertension are considered to be useful indicators of target organ damage. Tso et al. described sequential phases of retinal vascular changes in patients with hypertension. Although the changes occur serially there can be overlapping phases as well.[3]

Vasoconstrictive Phase

This is the initial response of an arteriole to an acute rise in blood pressure (autoregulatory phenomenon). This is seen clinically as generalized arteriolar narrowing. With chronicity, the vessels lose the capacity to autoregulate and the arterioles dilate instead. This is clinically seen as focal or generalized arteriolar dilatation. In younger individuals with healthy vascular system, the initial response to acute hypertension is a generalized narrowing whereas in older individuals with age-related arteriolosclerosis, both patchy dilatation and narrowing of arterioles are seen.

Sclerotic Phase

These changes are seen in individuals with chronic and persistent raise in blood pressure and are due to adaptive changes in vessel wall. Clinically, it appears as widening of arteriolar reflex and arteriovenous crossing changes.

Exudative Phase

These changes occur due to the break in the blood retinal barrier caused due to chronic vessel wall changes. Retinal hemorrhages, cotton wool spots, and hard exudates are the clinical manifestations of this stage.

Since the assessment of retinal vasculature is noninvasive and easily accessible, various classification systems for hypertensive retinopathy have been proposed and some of these systems have tried to correlate the severity of hypertensive changes in the retinal vessels with systemic comorbidities. Most of these signs can be easily picked by direct ophthalmoscopy and hence the physicians too in their clinical practice can use these systems. Keith, Wagener and Barker proposed the first classification of hypertensive retinopathy in 1939 (Table 9.1).

The Scheie classification was proposed in 1953. It divides hypertensive retinopathy into stages of arteriosclerotic changes and grades light reflex changes (Table 9.2).

The classification proposed by Wong and Mitchell in 2004 correlates the changes of hypertensive retinopathy with cardiovascular morbidity and mortality (Table 9.3).[4]

TABLE 9.1: Keith, Wagener and Barker classification of hypertensive retinopathy.

Grade	Stage	Description
1	Mild hypertension	Mild generalized arteriolar narrowing or sclerosis, broadening of arteriolar light reflex, concealment of veins
2	More marked hypertension	Marked generalized narrowing, definite focal narrowing and arteriovenous crossing changes. Moderate to marked sclerosis of the retinal arterioles. Exaggerated arterial light reflex
3	Mild angiospastic hypertensive retinopathy	Retinal hemorrhages, exudates and cotton wool spots (Figs. 9.1A and B)
4	Severe hypertensive retinopathy	Severe Grade III signs and papilledema

TABLE 9.2: Scheie classification of hypertensive retinopathy.

Stage	
0	Diagnosis of hypertension but no visible retinal abnormalities
1	Diffuse arteriolar narrowing; no focal constriction
2	More pronounced arteriolar narrowing with focal constriction
3	Focal and diffuse narrowing, retinal hemorrhages
4	Retinal edema, hard exudates and disk edema

Grade	
0	Normal
1	Broadening of light reflex with minimal arteriolovenous compression
2	Light reflex changes and crossing changes more prominent
3	Copper-wire appearance; more prominent arteriolovenous compression
4	Silver-wire appearance; severe arteriolovenous crossing changes

TABLE 9.3: Wong and Mitchell classification of hypertensive retinopathy with cardiovascular morbidity and mortality.

Grades	Description	Systemic association
No	No detectable retinal signs	None
Mild	Generalized or focal arteriolar narrowing, arteriovenous nicking, arteriolar wall opacity (silver wiring)	Modest association with risk of clinical and subclinical stroke, coronary artery disease, and mortality
Moderate	Hemorrhages, microaneurysms, cotton wool spots, hard exudates	Strong association with risk of clinical and subclinical stroke, cognitive decline, and cardiovascular mortality
Malignant	Moderate retinopathy with optic disk swelling	Strong association with risk of clinical and subclinical stroke, cognitive decline, and cardiovascular mortality

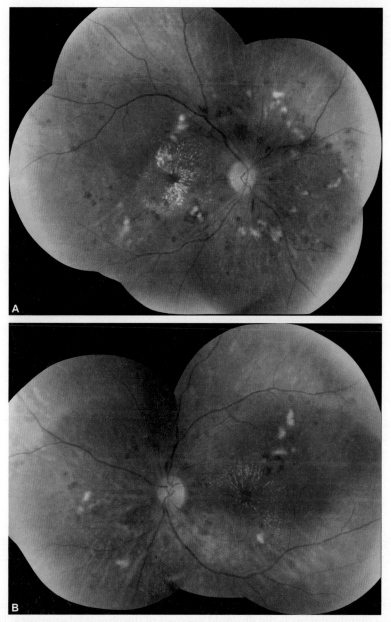

Figs 9.1A and B: Fundus pictures of both eyes suggestive of grade 3 hypertensive retinopathy (multiple retinal hemorrhages, cotton wool spots and hard exudates)

Hypertensive Choroidopathy

Hypertensive changes in choroid are typically seen in younger individuals with pliable vessels and are often seen in accelerated forms of hypertension (renal disease, pregnancy-induced hypertension, pheochromocytoma) rather

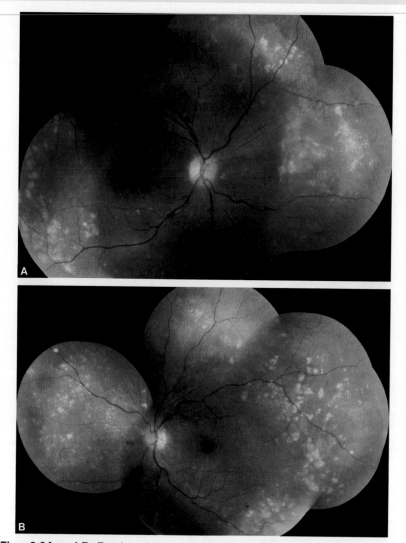

Figs. 9.2A and B: Fundus pictures of both eyes showing deep yellowish-white small patches (Elschnig spots) suggestive of hypertensive choroidopathy.

than chronic forms (e.g. essential hypertension). The main pathology behind these manifestations is the fibrinoid necrosis of the choroidal arterioles. Two distinct forms of hypertensive choroidopathy are described and include Elschnig spots (Figs. 9.2A and B) and Siegrist streaks. Elschnig spots are deep, yellow patches at the level of the retinal pigment epithelium which later become irregularly pigmented with hypopigmented halo. Siegrist streaks are linear hyperpigmented streaks of retinal pigment epithelium hyperplasia and hypertrophy. Severe uncontrolled hypertension can also lead to exudative detachment, which is often bilateral.

Hypertensive Optic Neuropathy

Bilateral optic disk involvement (papilledema) is a feature of malignant hypertension (stage 4). This is suggestive of an ongoing hypertensive crisis and requires urgent medical attention to reduce the blood pressure.

REFERENCES

1. Albert DM, Jakobiec FA, Azar D, et al. Hypertension and its ocular manifestations. In: Principles and Practice of Ophthalmology, 3rd edition. Philadelphia: Saunders; 2008. pp. 4367-84.
2. JNC 8 Guidelines for the management of hypertension in adults. Am Fam Physician. 2014;90(7):503-4.
3. Tso MO, Jampol LM. Pathophysiology of hypertensive retinopathy. Ophthalmology. 1982;89(10):1132-45.
4. Wong TY, Mitchell P. Hypertensive retinopathy. N Engl J Med. 2004;351(22):2310-7.

Recent Advances in the Management of Retinal Vein Occlusions

Deependra Vikram Singh, Yog Raj Sharma

INTRODUCTION

Retinal vein occlusion (RVO) is one of the most common causes of acquired retinal vascular abnormality in adults and a frequent cause of visual loss. There are few data on the prevalence of RVO in the general population, with current estimates derived largely from studies in white populations.[1-3] However, a recently published pooled analysis of 11 major studies from the United States, Europe, Asia, and Australia has found the incidence of branch retinal vascular occlusion (BRVO) to be 4.4/1,000 persons and 0.8/1,000 persons for central retinal vein occlusion (CRVO) in the general population.[4] The prevalence of RVO was similar for men and women, and increased with age. The prevalence of BRVO was highest in Asians and Hispanics and lowest in whites.

This chapter will focus on recent advances in the management of RVO observed over the last decade. Such discussion can be initiated only after understanding pathogenesis of RVO and a brief reference to two major studies (Table 10.1) for BRVO and CRVO. [5-9]

PATHOGENESIS

Despite being grouped together, BRVO and CRVO differ significantly in the etiology, pathogenesis, natural course and management.

Branch Retinal Vein Occlusion

The BRVO is considered to be the result of age-related arteriosclerosis of the retinal arteriole compressing the retinal venule at the A-V crossing, where they share a common sheath. Once the occlusion occurs, increased vascular pressure behind the occlusion may lead to leakage of fluid and small molecules

TABLE 10.1: Objectives, eligibility, and visual results of BVOS and CVOS.	
BVOS study[5,6]	CVOS study[7-9]
Evaluated argon laser photocoagulation for treatment of BRVO patients having BCVA from 20/40 to 20/200. 139 eyes studied. • To determine whether scatter argon laser photocoagulation can prevent the development of neovascularization • To determine whether peripheral scatter argon laser photocoagulation can prevent vitreous hemorrhage • To determine whether macular argon laser photocoagulation can improve visual acuity in eyes with macular edema reducing vision to 20/40 or worse	Multicenter, randomized, controlled clinical trial designed to answer the following three questions: • To determine whether photocoagulation therapy can help prevent iris neovascularization in eyes with CVO and evidence of ischemic retina • To assess whether grid-pattern photocoagulation therapy will reduce loss of central visual acuity due to macular edema secondary to CVO • To develop new data base describing the course and prognosis for eyes with CVO

(BVOS: Branch Vein Occlusion Study; CVOS: Central Vein Occlusion Study; BRVO: branch retinal vascular occlusion; BCVA: best corrected visual acuity; CVO: central vein occlusion)

across the vascular wall and into the surrounding retinal tissue, resulting in local edema. Vitreous traction may facilitate the development of cystoid macular edema (CME). In addition, vascular endothelial damage to the affected vein may induce low-grade, chronic inflammation of the retinal microvasculature and upregulation of inflammatory mediators. These mediators include prostaglandins, leukotrienes, intercellular adhesion molecule-1 (ICAM-1), integrins, tumor necrosis factor-α, and vascular endothelial growth factor (VEGF).[10] Many of these cytokines weaken the blood-retina barrier and perpetuate CME. Late onset retinal ischemia leads to neovascularization, recurrent vitreous hemorrhages, and tractional retinal detachments. Long-standing macular edema from BRVO can also lead to the formation of large cysts and inner lamellar or full-thickness macular hole.

Central Retinal Vein Occlusion

The pathogenesis of CRVO is poorly understood and is believed to be multifactorial. Most hypotheses revolve around the combination of factors causing external compression on the optic nerve and/or the central retinal vein, along with hematological factors promoting venous stasis and increased coagulability resulting in obstruction of central retinal vein posterior to lamina cribrosa. Increased intravascular pressure proximal to the resultant central retinal venous occlusion contributes to fluid leakage into the retina, resulting in retinal edema. Vision loss from CRVO is usually due to CME, ischemic maculopathy, capillary nonperfusion, posterior segment neovascularization, vitreous hemorrhage, anterior segment neovascularization (iris or angle), and neovascular glaucoma (NVG). Chronic CME can lead to pigmentary degeneration and photoreceptor loss with a permanent central scotoma. The common site of neovascularization is the anterior segment, but it can also occur in the posterior segment (e.g. optic nerve, retina). The risk of neovascularization increases with the degree of retinal ischemia. Anterior segment neovascularization and NVG is most likely to develop during the first few months after the occlusion (100 days glaucoma).

The argon laser treatment was evaluated in Branch Vein Occlusion Study (BVOS) and Central Vein Occlusion Study (CVOS) with special reference to eligibility criteria, prevention of vascularization, and visual recovery.

RECENT ADVANCES IN THE MANAGEMENT OF RETINAL VEIN OCCLUSION

The management of RVO has witnessed a paradigm shifts after two major advancements in the field of medical retina. The first is the availability of optical coherence tomography (OCT) and the second is intravitreal injections.

EPIDEMIOLOGY

Natural Course of Central Retinal Vein Occlusion

In an evidence-based analysis, McIntosh et al. reviewed 53 studies with data from 3,271 eyes with CRVO and found that most eyes had visual acuity (VA) of less than 20/40 at the baseline.[11] Although six studies reported an improvement in VA, none of these improvements resulted in VA better than 20/40. Up to 34% of eyes with nonischemic CRVO converted to ischemic CRVO over a 3-year period. In ischemic CRVO cases, neovascular glaucoma developed in at least 23% of eyes within 15 months. In nonischemic CRVO cases, macular edema resolved in approximately 30% of eyes over time, and subsequent neovascular glaucoma was rare. The most accepted definition of ischemic CRVO was the presence of at least 10 disk areas of capillary nonperfusion on fundus fluorescein angiography (FFA). In their retrospective analysis of 66 eyes with CRVO, Harey et al. found that among the nonischemic eyes with initial visual acuity of 20/70 or worse, 59% improved, 27% showed no change, and 14% deteriorated on resolution of macular edema, whereas in ischemic CRVO, 41% improved, 41% did not change, and 18% deteriorated.[12] While the authors have highlighted the importance of differentiating ischemic from nonischemic CRVO, they have also stressed the limitation of FFA in identifying all ischemic cases. Therefore, they have suggested the use of functional tests like relative afferent pupillary defect, electroretinography, visual acuity, and peripheral visual fields to assist in the categorization of CRVO cases.

Natural Course of Branch Retinal Vein Occlusion

Although the natural course of BRVO is much more favorable than CRVO, untreated BRVO patients can develop irreversible loss of vision from vitreous hemorrhage, traction retinal detachments and persisting macular edema and traction. Also, patients with BRVO are more likely to suffer from carotid artery obstruction and atherosclerosis. A large volume of data on natural course of BRVO is still missing from the literature.

DIAGNOSIS

Optical Coherence Tomography

Availability of time-domain and spectral-domain OCTs has revolutionized the management of many retinal diseases including RVO. Because OCT imaging is a noncontact procedure and the infrared measurement beam is barely perceived by the test subject, testing is well-tolerated by patients. The rapid acquisition time of OCT permits multiple images to be acquired simultaneously with different cross-sectional image planes, providing a comprehensive assessment of the macula. Optical coherence tomography provides information that complements the information supplied by fundus photography and fluorescein angiography. By allowing the direct visualization of retinal pathology on a morphologic level, OCT can be used for initial diagnosis and providing guidelines for management decisions. The advent of new pharmacologic therapies for the treatment of retinal diseases such as macular edema and choroidal neovascularization has enhanced the utility of OCT as a means of determining a therapeutic anatomic response. Currently, most clinical trials that are evaluating retinal treatments use OCT response as a secondary outcome. Traditionally, BVOS recommended no intervention for macular edema in BRVO till best corrected visual acuity (BCVA) is better than 20/60; however, a large number of macular BRVO patients are found to have significant macular edema and cystoid changes on the OCT with BCVA greater than 20/60. Such patients are now frequently offered treatments to prevent further visual loss and restore the macular function earlier, rather than waiting for BCVA to drop below 20/60. Figures 10.1A to H show a similar case where a macular BRVO patient was treated for macular edema with BCVA of 20/40. OCT has become an excellent noninvasive tool for serial follow-up of such patients, especially when macular edema shows recurrences. OCT allows detection, evaluation and documentation of any vitreomacular traction associated with macular edema in BRVO patients. These patients can be counseled for the possibility of vitreous surgery in future and also about the chances of worsening with laser photocoagulation. Although rare, a spontaneous posterior vitreous detachment can sometimes lead to improvement in such patients. The same can be confirmed with OCT. Figures 10.2A to H show an example of such case. OCT can precisely outline the extent of involvement by macular edema. The cases showing no foveal involvement can be safely observed with serial OCTs and subjected to peripheral scatter photocoagulation on development of retinal ischemia. Figures 10.3A to F show an example of such case.

In CRVO, OCT is again very helpful in detecting and quantifying macular edema. The resolution of macular edema and its recurrence is also nicely depicted on serial macular scans. Figures 10.4A to F show OCT scans of an ischemic CRVO with macular edema before and after the anti-VEGF injections. Late cases show thinning of the retina suggestive of loss of nerve fiber layer (NFL) and photoreceptors.

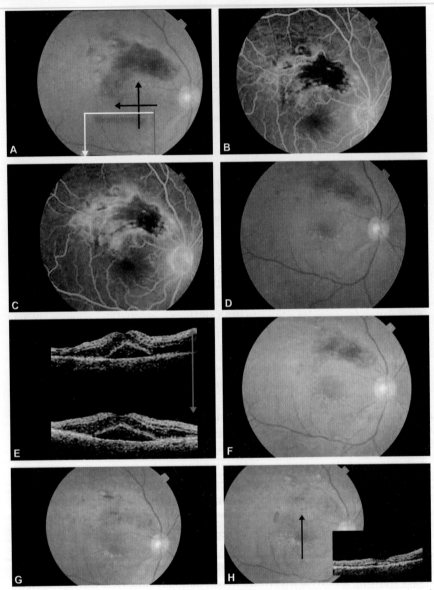

Figs. 10.1A to H: Serial fundus photographs and optical coherence tomography of a 60-year-old female with macular branch retinal vascular occlusion. (A to C) Color and fundus fluorescein angiography photographs show ischemia and retinal edema. (D) OCT scans show foveal involvement by macular edema and subretinal fluid. (E to H) Serial photographs show improvement after two intravitreal ranibizumab injections at 1, 2, 3 and 6 months, respectively.

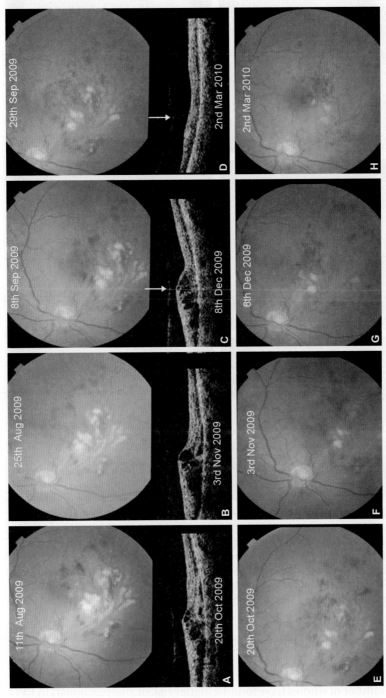

Figs. 10.2A to H: Serial fundus photographs and optical coherence tomography of a 45-year-old female with inferotemporal branch retinal vascular occlusion, and showing resolution following two bevacizumab injections and spontaneous posterior vitreous detachment (white arrow).

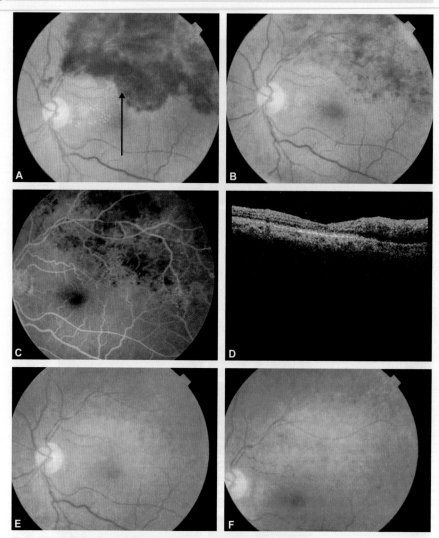

Figs. 10.3A to F: Serial fundus photographs of a 80-old-year female with superotemporal branch retinal vascular occlusion. (A and B) Fundus photographs showing retinal edema not involving macula confirmed on optical coherence tomography. (C and D) Fundus fluorescein angiography photographs done at 3 months after hemorrhages were resolved and show ischemia and collaterals. (E and F) Fundus photographs showing resolved retinal edema and laser marks. (E) At 6 months follow-up. (F) At 9 months follow-up.

SYSTEMIC WORK-UP

Role of Atherosclerosis

A large number of studies have found a higher risk of atherosclerosis in RVO patients.[3,13] In a recent meta-analysis of 21 observational studies including

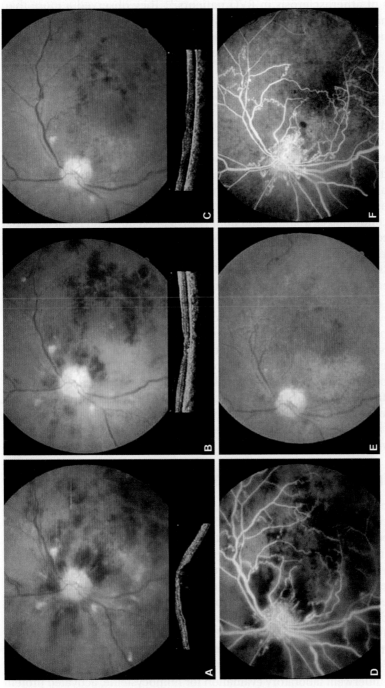

Figs. 10.4A to F: Fundus, fluorescein angiography photographs of an 85-year-old male with ischemic central retinal vein occlusion. (B to E) Serial pictures showing resolution of macular edema and hemorrhages but worsening retinal ischemia in spite of monthly bevacizumab injections. (B) At 1 month. (C) At 3 months. (E and F) At 6 months.

2915 patients with RVO, O'Mahoney et al. evaluated the role of 3 major risk factors of atherosclerosis in RVO patients.[13] They observed a more than 3.5-time higher risk of RVO in cases with systemic hypertension. About a 2.5-time higher risk of RVO was associated with hyperlipidemia, but there was only a modest correlation between RVO and the presence of diabetes mellitus.

Association with Carotid Artery Obstruction

Carotid artery changes have been regarded as an important indicator of the extent of systemic atherosclerosis.[14,15] Brown et al.[16] and Green et al.[17] have demonstrated, some association between the presence of carotid lesions and the pathogenesis of ischemic RVO, using digital subtraction angiography and histopathologic analysis, respectively. With recent advances and the wide application of ultrasonographic examinations, carotid artery evaluation is being conducted as a simple and noninvasive procedure and is encountered more commonly even in routine clinical ophthalmology. In a recent study of patients with RVO, carotid artery evaluation was done on 58 eyes of 57 patients aged between 51 years and 88 years to investigate the relationship between RVO and carotid artery lesions.[18] Thirty-nine patients (40 eyes) had CRVO, and 18 patients (18 eyes) had BRVO. It is further demonstrated that the prevalence of plaque in the carotid artery was 49% among CRVO patients older than 50 years of age; the prevalence among those older than 70 years of age was significantly higher than that among individuals of similar age who attended the examination center (controls). The clinical characteristics of CRVO patients with carotid lesions in the present study included a significantly higher frequency (79%) of the ischemic type shown by fluorescein angiography. Compared with 49% of CRVO cases, only 22% of BRVO cases had plaque in the carotid artery, showing a lower prevalence of carotid lesions in BRVO although there was no significant difference.

Role of Laboratory Investigations in Young Patients

Changes in the blood vessel wall, changes in the blood flow, and changes in blood coagulability are known as *Virchow's triad*. These inter-related factors have been known to be responsible for the formation of thrombi in blood vessels as described by Virchow in the 19th century. Increased blood viscosity, Factor V Leiden, hyperhomocysteinemia, and protein C or S deficiency have been considered to play a role in the development of CRVO.[19-22] There are certain acquired hypercoagulable states also, including elevated antiphospholipid antibodies [AP-Abs; lupus anticoagulant (LA) and anticardiolipin antibodies (ACAs)]. Lahey et al. investigated whether hypercoagulability plays a role in thrombus formation in patients with CRVO who are less than 56 years of age.[23] Fifty-five patients with CRVO less than 56 years old (mean age 44 years) underwent laboratory evaluation for homocysteine, activated protein C resistance, protein C activity, protein S activity, antithrombin III activity, antiphospholipid antibodies, and anticardiolipin antibodies. The results were compared with previously drawn age-matched control groups obtained by the same laboratory for statistical significance. Twenty-seven percent of the CRVO patients had one positive test result, suggesting hypercoagulability. Compared with the control groups, these patients less than 56 years old with CRVO had a higher incidence of coagulation abnormalities according to laboratory testing. Among the parameters tested, hyperhomocysteinemia and circulating antiphospholipid antibodies were significantly more common in the CRVO patients ($P < 0.05$) compared with age-matched controls. Another useful data comes from a meta-analysis of thrombophilic risk factors that found only elevated homocysteine and anticardiolipin antibodies to be associated with CRVO.[24] A recent large case-control study, however, found no association between CRVO and thrombophilic risk factors, including homocysteine levels and anticardiolipin antibodies.[25] Recurrent CRVO has also been reported with elevated homocysteine in one study, but associations with anticardiolipin antibodies and Factor V Leiden were not identified as risk factors in a multivariate study comparing patients with recurrent CRVO to those with one CRVO.[26] In view of contradictory results, the need for further evaluation of the role of hypercoagulability states in RVO cannot be over emphasized.

INTERVENTIONS FOR RETINAL VEIN OCCLUSION

The conventional management of RVO as outline by BVOS and CVOS has been discussed elsewhere and a brief reference is provided in Table 10.1. While grid and sectoral scatter photocoagulation has been quite rewarding for BRVO, the CRVO continues to carry very poor visual prognosis and conventional management is far from satisfactory. The high incidence of severe vision loss associated with CRVO has prompted many researchers to explore a number of new strategies for its management. The focus of these interventions is on two major issues:
1. The treatment of recurrent macular edema and the resulting photoreceptor loss
2. The reversal of retinal ischemia by either promoting collaterals, or bypassing the occluding vein, or by suppressing the overactive thrombotic mechanisms.

Intravitreal Steroids

Although the safety of intravitreal triamcinolone acetonide (IVTA) has been known since as early as 1981,[27] its wider clinical use for macular edema started only a decade back after more studies on safety and efficacy in patients with uveitis and diabetic macular edema became available.[28,29] Since TA was found to have antiangiogenic, antiproliferative, and antiedematous effects, its use for macular edema from CRVO started in 2002 with a large number of reports describing treatment benefits from intravitreal triamcinolone in terms of visual acuity and macular edema.[30-34] IVTA was used in doses of 4 mg, 2 mg and 1 mg.

However, all studies found the visual benefits to be transient and lasting for a maximum of 6 months, and a high incidence of side effects like rising intraocular pressure (IOP), cataract formation, and endophthalmitis. The need to have larger studies on steroid use in macular edema was felt.[35] Finally, to explore the role of IVTA in the management of RVO, The Standard Care versus Corticosteroid for Retinal Vein Occlusion (SCORE) study, sponsored by the National Institutes of Health, National Eye Institute, was initiated. It consisted of two multicenter, randomized, Phase III clinical trials comparing the efficacy and safety of standard care with intravitreal injection(s) of triamcinolone acetonide (hereafter referred to as intravitreal triamcinolone) in either a 1 mg or a 4 mg dose for vision loss associated with macular edema secondary to CRVO and BRVO.[36-38] Figures 10.5A to H show a CRVO patient managed with IVTA.

To summarize, while the IVTA was not found useful in patients with BRVO, it was found to improve BCVA in CRVO patients. Although the efficacy of 1 mg and 4 mg IVTA were similar, the 1 mg dose demonstrated a safety profile superior to that of the 4 mg dose. After IVTA, more steroids have been explored for their potential role in similar conditions; flucinolode implant and dexamethasone implant.[39-41]

Dexamethasone is a potent, water-soluble corticosteroid that can be delivered to the vitreous cavity by the dexamethasone intravitreal implant (DEX

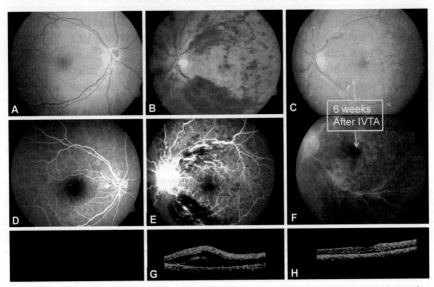

Figs. 10.5A to H: Serial fundus photographs and optical coherence tomography of a 46-year-old female with old central retinal vein occlusion (CRVO) with collaterals (OD) and acute CRVO (OS). (A and C) Fundus and fundus fluorescein angiography photographs show compensated CRVO with collaterals at disk. (B, D and E) Fundus and FFA photographs and OCT scans show acute CRVO with macular edema. (F to H) Fundus, FFA photographs and OCT scans at 6 weeks postintravitreal triamcinolone acetonide injection showing resolution of macular edema, hemorrhages and tortuosity.

implant; OZURDEX, Allergan, Inc., Irvine, CA). A DEX implant is composed of a biodegradable copolymer of lactic acid and glycolic acid containing micronized dexamethasone. The drug-copolymer complex gradually releases the total dose of dexamethasone over a series of months after insertion into the eye through a small pars plana puncture using a customized applicator system. In a recent study in eyes with persistent macular edema from several different causes (including RVO), DEX implant 0.7 mg produced improvements in visual acuity, macular thickness, and fluorescein leakage that were sustained for up to 6 months.[39] In a randomized, sham-controlled trial of dexamethasone intravitreal implant in 1,267 patients with macular edema due to retinal vein occlusion, the percentage of eyes with a greater than or equal to 15-letter improvement in BCVA was significantly higher in both DEX implant groups compared with sham at days 30–90 ($P < 0.001$). The percentage of eyes with a greater than or equal to 15-letter loss in BCVA was significantly lower in the DEX implant 0.7 mg group compared with the sham at all follow-up visits ($P \leq 0.036$).[40] Increased IOP as found in 16% of the cases at day 60 (both doses) and was not different from sham by day 180. Ozurdex received FDA approval for treatment of macular edema secondary to BRVO in 2009.

An implantable fluocinolone acetonide (Retisert, Bausch and Lomb, Rochester, NY) is also being evaluated for the treatment of BRVO and CRVO.[41] These trials help to clarify the role of corticosteroid therapy in the management of BRVO.

Intravitreal Antivascular Endothelial Growth Factor Drugs

The major stimulus for the formation of macular edema and neovascularization in patients with RVO seems to be hypoxia-induced production of VEGF, an angiogenic factor that promotes angiogenesis and increases permeability.[42] After encountering the limitations of IVTA therapy due to the high rate of side effects, such as cataract formation or increased intraocular pressure, the researchers looked upon VEGF inhibition as an alternative. Since the first report of the efficacy of intravitreal bevacizumab (a recombinant monoclonal antibody binding to all isoforms of VEGF) in a patient with macular edema secondary to CRVO in 2005,[43] several retrospective case series have shown the benefit of this treatment, with an improvement in visual acuity and a decrease of central retinal thickness (CRT) in patients with macular edema associated with both BRVO and CRVO.[44-47]

Current Role of Bevacizumab in Retinal Vein Occlusion

The initial encouraging results with intravitreal bevacizumab were followed by wide spread use in RVO patients. BRVO patients were found to have more predictable and sustained improvement in visual acuity although it required repeat injections.[47] The report on repeated bevacizumab injections demonstrated early and clinically relevant benefits from bevacizumab injections for the complications of CRVO.[46] Visual acuity improved and macular edema decreased after a single injection in the majority of treated patients as early as the 1-week visit. The data also suggested that an injection of intravitreal bevacizumab has a limited beneficial effect of approximately 2 months in most patients and that intermittent reinjection may be needed to sustain the visual benefits. Bevacizumab treatment early after the onset of CRVO was also associated with a statistically significant reduction in venous dilation, tortuosity, optic disk swelling, and macular edema in addition to the improvement of VA.[48] However, for CRVO patients the bevacizumab raised some concerns; theoretically, blocking VEGF should avert many of the complications that result from a CRVO. Alternatively, VEGF may be necessary for the formation of collaterals that would allow alternative venous drainage around the central retinal vein thrombosis. If this is the case, blocking VEGF may in fact be detrimental. The long-term role of anti-VEGF agents in the treatment of CME due to CRVO and the role of early intervention in improving outcome and potentially limiting progression to the ischemic variant still remain unanswered. Figures 10.6A to D show a case with CRVO and NVG successfully managed with bevacizumab injections and laser photocoagulation.

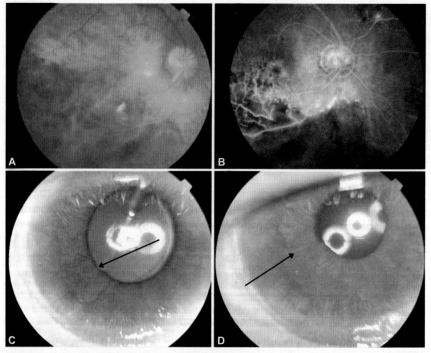

Figs. 10.6A to D: Anterior segment and fundus photographs of a 75-year-old male with ischemic hemispheric retinal vein occlusion (HRVO) leading to neovascular glaucoma. (A and B) Fundus photographs and fundus fluorescein angiography showing ischemic HRVO. (C and D) Anterior segment photographs showing regression of NVI within 48 hours of bevacizumab injection.

Role of Ranibizumab

Ranibizumab (Lucentis; Genentech Inc.) has been proposed to have potentially increased retinal penetration because of a smaller molecular size and a higher binding affinity for VEGF than bevacizumab.[49] Spaide et al. in a prospective study, evaluated intravitreal injection of ranibizumab as a potential treatment for decreased visual acuity (VA) secondary to CRVO.[50] A total of 20 eyes of 20 patients with a mean age of 72.1 years, a mean VA of 45.8 ETDRS letters, and a mean central macular thickness of 574.6 µm received 3 monthly intravitreal ranibizumab injections. The patients were given additional ranibizumab if they had macular edema as determined by optical coherence tomography or any new intraretinal hemorrhage. At 12 months of follow-up, the mean VA improved to 64.3 letters and the central macular thickness decreased to 186 µm (both different than baseline values; $P < 0.001$) using a mean of 8.5 injections. The change in macular thickness was not correlated with the change in VA. At 12 months 56.3% eyes had improvement of three lines or more and 12.5% had an improvement of more than six lines of VA. In one patient with a history of transient ischemic attack, an ischemic stroke developed but no sequel resulted. In another patient, vitreomacular traction developed, but the patient had improved acuity as compared with baseline. There were no infections, retinal tears, or detachments. Interestingly, the prolonged arm-to-early arterial filling time (measured on angiograms) at baseline showed no change at 1 year follow-up. This was despite near normalization of the retinal thickness, retinal appearance, and improvement in VA. This observation led them to hypothesis that the arterial supply into these eyes was compromised. The hypothesis is also supported by an old experiment where reduction of venous outflow with a simple ligation of the vein in primates did not produce a picture consistent with severe CRVO;[51] to produce severe CRVO, simultaneous compromise in the arterial flow was required.[38]

Pegaptanib Sodium

Pegaptanib, a 40-kDa RNA aptamer, binds to VEGF165, the predominant pathological isoform in ischemia-mediated ocular neovascularization and in diseases such as diabetic macular edema.[52-54] Clinical trials have suggested that the intravitreous injection of pegaptanib sodium can be effective in the treatment of diabetic macular edema,[55] proliferative diabetic retinopathy,[56] and neovascular age-related macular degeneration.[57,58] A recently published dose-ranging, double-masked, multicenter, phase 2 trial included subjects with CRVO for 6 months' or less duration randomly assigned (1:1:1) to receive pegaptanib sodium or sham injections every 6 weeks for 24 weeks (0.3 mg and 1 mg, n = 33; sham, n = 32).[59] At week 30, 36% subjects treated with 0.3 mg of pegaptanib sodium and 39% treated with 1 mg gained 15 or more letters from the baseline as against 28% sham treated subjects. Also subjects treated with pegaptanib sodium were less likely to lose 15 or more letters (9% and 6%; 0.3 mg and 1 mg pegaptanib sodium groups, respectively) compared with sham-treated eyes (31%). Although the difference in the proportion of subjects who gained 15 letters in this trial was not statistically significant, the differences in the proportion of those who lost 15 letters and the mean visual acuity were substantial, providing support for a potential benefit of pegaptanib sodium in visual acuity of patients with macular edema secondary to CRVO. The study also found that fewer eyes in the groups treated with pegaptanib sodium showed retinal or iris neovascularization, a known and frequent complication of CRVO. However, the small sample size and short follow-up (30 weeks) would stop us from making any conclusive inference.

To summarize, almost all reports found beneficial effects of continuous VEGF suppression for macular edema from RVO. The need for repeated injections was also universally felt and the most suitable approach seems to be intervening early if central macular thickness exceeds 250 µm and follow the treat and extend approach as used in management of CNVM. The maximum duration for VEG inhibition, ideal injection interval and the effect of anti-VEGF drugs on collateral development and conversion from nonischemic to ischemic CRVO are the areas for future studies.

Radial Optic Neurotomy

Radial optic neurotomy is a surgical procedure designed to improve venous outflow in eyes with CRVO. It is proposed to relieve pressure on the occluded vein as it crosses the cribriform plate and scleral outlet.[60] After a standard pars plana vitrectomy, a single radial relaxing incision is made into the scleral ring and adjacent sclera of the optic nerve, typically nasally. The proposed theoretical basis of the procedure remains contentious, with some arguing that a single localized incision is unlikely to cause any meaningful decompression of the lamina cribrosa, which is a relatively rigid interwoven matrix of collagen and elastin.[61-63] Also, many cases of CRVO do not have an occlusion at the proposed decompression site. Initial results from a retrospective case series of 10 patients with CRVO and VA 20/400 were promising, with an initial visual improvement in 73%. Another nonrandomized prospective case series of 10 patients and a retrospective case series of five patients reported less impressive or no improvement.[64,65] Complications include severe immediate hemorrhage, postoperative neovascularization of the neurotomy site and anterior segment,[64,66] VF defects,[67] and retinal detachment (RD)[68] originating at the incision site. Some investigators have suggested that RON may facilitate the formation of chorioretinal anastomosis,[69-71] whereas others argue that the results are due to effects from the vitrectomy alone or natural history.[61]

Laser-induced Chorioretinal Venous Anastomosis

Up to 14% of eyes with CRVO can spontaneously develop chorioretinal anastomosis over a period of 3 months resulting in the resolution of retinal hemorrhages and improvement in perfusion status. Figures 10.7A to F show example of such a case. In eyes with perfused CRVO, investigators have

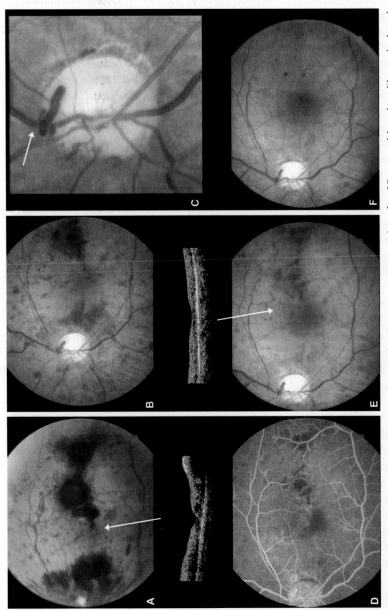

Figs. 10.7A to F: Serial fundus photographs and optical coherence tomography of a 65-year-old male with nonischemic central retinal vein occlusion. (A to F) Fundus fluorescein angiography and OCT photographs showing resolution of retinal hemorrhages and macular edema following spontaneous development of chorioretinal anastomosis (collaterals) at disk. (C) Magnified picture of optic disk showing collaterals.

attempted to bypass the occluded central retinal vein by creating a similar anastomotic outflow channel to the choroidal circulation. It has been suggested that these chorioretinal anastomoses allow transretinal retrograde flow of venous blood from the eye and prevent the development of retinal ischemia.[72,73] Visual acuity may improve as a result of the reduction or resolution of macular edema and/or maintenance of retinal perfusion. The procedure is performed using an argon or neodymium: yttrium aluminum garnet (Nd:YAG) laser to rupture Bruch's membrane and the adjacent branch retinal vein, typically nasally and 3 disk diameters away from the optic disk. A few authors have attempted to create chorioretinal anastomoses surgically through a variety of techniques including transretinal venipuncture, especially in an ischemic CRVO, with variable results.[74-76]

Meanwhile, the results of The Central Retinal Vein Bypass Study (CVBS) from Australia were also available in 2010.[76] This was a prospective, randomized, controlled, multicenter clinical trial on 113 consecutive patients with a nonischemic CRVO of more than 3 months' duration and visual acuity of less than or equal to 20/50. A total of 53 control patients and 55 treatment patients completed the study. The two groups were comparable for most parameters. A Laser chorioretinal anastomosis (L-CRA) was successfully created in 76.4% of treated patients. Over the 18-month follow-up period, treated eyes had an 8.3 letter mean improvement from baseline compared with control eyes (P = 0.03). Treated eyes that developed a functional L-CRA achieved an 11.7 letter mean improvement from baseline over the control group after 18 months (P = 0.004). Conversion to the ischemic CRVO category occurred in 20.8% of control eyes and in 9.6% of treated eyes overall (P = 0.33). Of the treated group who developed an L-CRA where the retinal ischemia was due to progression of the CRVO, 4.9% progressed to the ischemic category (P = 0.03). Incidence of complications was found to be high with 18.2% of treated patients developing neovascularization at the site of L-CRA and 9.1% of treated eyes requiring vitrectomy surgery because of macular traction or nonresolving vitreous hemorrhage. All complications were successfully managed. The authors have strongly recommended this procedure after suggesting that the risk of these complications should be weighed against the substantial visual morbidity from CRVO, as shown by the CVOS3 and supported by other studies showing that eyes similar to those enrolled in their study (nonischemic, i.e. <10 DD CNP) had a poor visual prognosis. The study, however, has few limitations like the nonavailability of OCT for assessment of benefit on macular edema and no use of anti-VEGF drugs to address neovascularization associated with L-CRA. Also the purpose-built HGM K3 laser that was used in this study is no longer available. More trials with modern solid-state green wavelength lasers, OCT, and anti-VEGF seem in order.

Pars Plana Vitrectomy and Arteriovenous Sheathotomy

Arteriovenous sheathotomy has been described as a procedure in which the retinal vein and artery are surgically separated at the arteriovenous crossing by cutting the common adventitial sheath. While many studies report no beneficial effect on visual acuity,[77,78] several case series as well as a nonrandomized controlled study have demonstrated improved CME and/or visual acuity.[79-81] The studies evaluating pars plana vitrectomy (PPV) with the removal of the posterior hyaloid, but no sheathotomy, have also found resolution of CME secondary to BRVO.[82,83] Results from a head-to-head comparison study have suggested that PPV with posterior hyaloid removal alone is as effective as combined PPV/sheathotomy in resolving CME and improving visual acuity in BRVO.[84] Complications associated with these procedures include vitreous hemorrhage, intraoperative retinal tears, rhegmatogenous retinal detachment, and cataract development.[85]

Hemodilution

The rationale for the use of hemodilution in the treatment of CRVO was based on observations of abnormal red cell deformability, increased plasma viscosity, and hematocrit and fibrinogen levels in some patients with CRVO. It was argued that reducing hematocrit levels lowers plasma viscosity, which may lead to improved retinal microcirculation and perfusion. Several studies (of the RCTs) have reported statistically significant improvements in VA, arteriovenous passage time, and clinical appearance after hemodilution.[86-91] There have been a number of adverse effects, including lethargy, fainting spells, and exertional dyspnea may occur but data from these studies indicate that the treatment is generally well tolerated even in elderly patients. Wolf et al.,[86] Hansen et al.,[89,90] Heinen et al.,[88] Poupard et al.,[91] and Hehn[92] have all reported improved VAs in patients treated with hemodilution. However, many of these studies have limitations. Most had small numbers, and the protocols, inclusion and exclusion criteria, and end points varied substantially. Small changes in the protocol can have large effects on blood hemodynamics and rheology. All the studies with improved visual outcome required a prolonged period of hospitalization, and the only randomized study that investigated hemodilution in an outpatient setting in CRVO showed no significant benefit.[93]

Isovolemic hemodilution has shown some benefits for eyes with BRVO in randomized studies.[94] This treatment strategy is often not practical, requires great care in patient selection, and is likely not appropriate for those patients with anemia, renal insufficiency, or pulmonary insufficiency.[94]

Direct Injection of Tissue Plasminogen Activator into the Retinal Vein Lumen and Other Thrombolytics

No RCT has evaluated the safety and efficacy of this intervention. Adverse effects such as vitreous hemorrhage in up to a quarter of patients and RD have been reported. Larger studies with concurrent control groups comparing the procedure with vitrectomy alone and standard care are needed before routine use of this procedure can be recommended.

There is limited evidence that any oral or systemic anticoagulation or rheological agent can significantly affect the outcome of CRVO. Although troxerutin and ticlopidine showed a trend for improvement, the evidence supporting these modalities was limited[95,96] (level B-III). Ticlopidine has uncommon (0.5–3%) but very serious hematological toxicity, including neutropenia, thrombocytopenia, and aplastic anemia requiring regular monitoring. Clopidogrel, a newer agent with an almost identical structure and mechanism of action, increasingly is used preferentially due to a reduced incidence of blood disorders and without any regular monitoring. No randomized study has assessed the role of clopidogrel in retinal venous thrombosis, and routine use of these agents is not recommended for CRVO.

REFERENCES

1. Klein R, Klein BE, Moss SE, et al. The epidemiology of retinal vein occlusion: the Beaver Dam Eye Study. Trans Am Ophthalmol Soc. 2000;98:133-41.
2. Mitchell P, Smith W, Chang A. Prevalence and associations of retinal vein occlusion in Australia: the Blue Mountains Eye Study. Arch Ophthalmol. 1996;114(10):1243-7.
3. Wong TY, Larsen EK, Klein R, et al. Cardiovascular risk factors for retinal vein occlusion and arteriolar emboli: the Atherosclerosis Risk in Communities & Cardiovascular Health Studies. Ophthalmology. 2005;112(4):540-7.
4. Sophie Rogers S, McIntosh RL, Cheung N, et al. The prevalence of retinal vein occlusion: pooled data from population studies from the United States, Europe, Asia, and Australia. Ophthalmology. 2010;117(2):313-9.
5. The Branch Vein Occlusion Study Group. Argon laser photocoagulation for macula edema in branch vein occlusion. Am J Ophthalmol. 1984;98(3):271-82.
6. Argon laser scatter photocoagulation for prevention of neovascularization and vitreous hemorrhage in BRVO. Arch Ophthalmol. 1986;104(1):34-41.
7. The Central Vein Occlusion Study Group. Natural history and clinical management of central retinal vein occlusion. Arch Ophthalmol. 1997;115(4):486-91.
8. The Central Vein Occlusion Study Group. Evaluation of grid pattern photocoagulation for macular edema in central vein occlusion. The CVOS Group M report. Ophthalmology. 1995;102(10):1425-33.
9. The Central Vein Occlusion Study Group. A randomized clinical trial of early panretinal photocoagulation for ischemic central vein occlusion. The CVOS Group N report. Ophthalmology. 1995;102(10):1434-44.
10. Funk M, Kriechbaum KF, Prager F, et al. Intraocular concentrations of growth factors and cytokines in retinal vein occlusion and the effect of therapy with bevacizumab. Invest Ophthalmol Vis Sci. 2009;50(3):1025-32.
11. McIntosh RL, Rogers SL, Lim L, et al. Natural history of central retinal vein occlusion: an evidence-based systematic review. Ophthalmology. 2010;117(6):1113-23.
12. Hayreh SS, Podhajsky PA, Zimmerman MB. Natural history of visual outcome in central retinal vein occlusion. Ophthalmology. 2011;118(1):119-33.
13. O'Mahoney PR, Wong DT, Ray JG. Retinal vein occlusion and traditional risk factors for atherosclerosis. Arch Ophthalmol. 2008;126(5):692-9.
14. Poli A, Tremoli E, Colombo A, et al. Ultrasonographic measurement of the common carotid artery wall thickness in hypercholesterolemic patients. A new model for the quantitation and follow-up of preclinical atherosclerosis in living human subjects. Atherosclerosis. 1988;70(3):253-61.

15. Nowak J, Nilsson T, Sylven C, et al. Potential of carotid ultrasonography in the diagnosis of coronary artery disease: a comparison with exercise test and variance ECG. Stroke. 1998;29(2):439-46.
16. Brown GC, Shah HG, Magargal LE, et al. Central retinal vein obstruction and carotid artery disease. Ophthalmology. 1984;91(12):1627-33.
17. Green WR, Chan CC, Hutchins M, et al. Central retinal vein occlusion: a prospective histopathologic study of 29 eyes in 28 cases. Retina. 1982;1(1):27-55.
18. Matsushima C, Wakabayashi Y, Iwamoto T, et al. Relationship between retinal vein occlusion and carotid artery lesions. Retina. 2007;27(8):1038-43.
19. Glueck CJ, Wang P, Hutchins R, et al. Ocular vascular thrombotic events: central retinal vein and central retinal artery occlusions. Clin Appl Thromb Hemost. 2008;14(3):286-94.
20. Rehak M, Rehak J, Müller M, et al. The prevalence of activated protein C (APC) resistance and factor V Leiden is significantly higher in patients with retinal vein occlusion without general risk factors. Case-control study and meta-analysis. Thromb Haemost. 2008;99(5):925-9.
21. Williamson TH. Central retinal vein occlusion: what's the story? Br J Ophthalmol. 1997;81(8):698-704.
22. Yap YC, Barampouti F. Central retinal vein occlusion secondary to protein S deficiency. Ann Ophthalmol. 2007;39(4):343-4.
23. Lahey MJ, Tunc M, Kearney J, et al. Laboratory evaluation of hypercoagulable states in patients with central retinal vein occlusion who are less than 56 years of age. Ophthalmology. 2002;109(1):126-31.
24. Janssen MC, den Heijer M, Cruysberg JR, et al. Retinal vein occlusion: a form of venous thrombosis or a complication of atherosclerosis? A meta-analysis of thrombophilic factors. Thromb Haemost. 2005;93(6):1021-6.
25. Di Capua M, Coppola A, Albisinni R, et al. Cardiovascular risk factors and outcome in patients with retinal vein occlusion. J Thromb Thrombolysis. 2010;30(1):16-22.
26. Sodi A, Giambene B, Marcucci R, et al. Atherosclerotic and thrombophilic risk factors in patients with recurrent central retinal vein occlusion. Eur J Ophthalmol. 2008;18(2):233-8.
27. McCuen BW II, Bessler M, Tano Y, et al. The lack of toxicity of intravitreally administered triamcinolone acetonide. Am J Ophthalmol. 1981;91(6):785-8.
28. Young S, Larkin G, Branley M, et al. Safety and efficacy of intravitreal triamcinolone for cystoid macular oedema in uveitis. Clin Exp Ophthalmol. 2001;29(1):2-6.
29. Martidis A, Duker JS, Greenberg PB, et al. Intravitreal triamcinolone for refractory diabetic macular edema. Ophthalmology. 2002;109(5):920-7.
30. Ip M, Kahana A, Altaweel M. Treatment of central retinal vein occlusion with triamcinolone acetonide: an optical coherence tomography study. Semin Ophthalmol. 2003;18(2):67-73.
31. Ip MS, Gottlieb JL, Kahana A, et al. Intravitreal triamcinolone for the treatment of macular edema associated with central retinal vein occlusion. Arch Ophthalmol. 2004;122(8):1131-6.
32. Bashshur ZF, Ma'luf RN, Allam S, et al. Intravitreal triamcinolone for the management of macular edema due to nonischemic central retinal vein occlusion. Arch Ophthalmol. 2004;122(8):1137-40.
33. Krepler K, Ergun E, Sacu S, et al. Intravitreal triamcinolone acetonide in patients with macular oedema due to central retinal vein occlusion. Acta Ophthalmol Scand. 2005;83(1):71-5.
34. Williamson TH, O'Donnell A. Intravitreal triamcinolone acetonide for cystoid macular edema in nonischemic central retinal vein occlusion. Am J Ophthalmol. 2005;139(5):860-6.

35. Flynn HW Jr, Scott IU. Intravitreal triamcinolone acetonide for macular edema associated with diabetic retinopathy and venous occlusive disease: It's time for clinical trials. Arch Ophthalmol. 2005;123(2):258-9.
36. Ip MS, Oden NL, Scott IU, et al. SCORE Study Investigator Group. SCORE Study report 3: study design and baseline characteristics. Ophthalmology. 2009;116:1770-7.
37. SCORE Study Research Group. A randomized trial comparing the efficacy and safety of intravitreal triamcinolone with observation to treat vision loss associated with macular edema secondary to central retinal vein occlusion: the Standard Care vs Corticosteroid for Retinal Vein Occlusion (SCORE) Study Report 5. Arch Ophthalmol. 2009;127(9):1101-14.
38. SCORE Study Research Group. A randomized trial comparing the efficacy and safety of intravitreal triamcinolone with standard care to treat vision loss associated with macular edema secondary to branch retinal vein occlusion: the Standard Care vs Corticosteroid for Retinal Vein Occlusion (SCORE) Study Report 6. Arch Ophthalmol. 2009;127(9):1115-28.
39. Kuppermann BD, Blumenkranz MS, Haller JA, et al. Dexamethasone DDS Phase II Study Group. Randomized controlled study of an intravitreous dexamethasone drug delivery system in patients with persistent macular edema. Arch Ophthalmol. 2007;125(3):309-17.
40. Haller JA, Bandello F, Belfort R Jr, et al. for the OZURDEX GENEVA Study Group. Randomized, sham-controlled trial of dexamethasone intravitreal implant in patients with macular edema due to retinal vein occlusion. Ophthalmology. 2010;117(6):1134-46.
41. Ramchandran RS, Fekrat S, Stinnett SS, et al. Fluocinolone acetonide sustained drug delivery device for chronic central retinal vein occlusion: 12-month results. Am J Ophthalmol. 2008;146(2):285-91.
42. Aiello LP, Avery RL, Arrigg PG, et al. Vascular endothelial growth factor in ocular fluid of patients with diabetic retinopathy and other retinal disorders. N Engl J Med. 1994;331(22):1480-7.
43. Rosenfeld PJ, Fung AE, Puliafito CA. Optical coherence tomography findings after an intravitreal injection of bevacizumab (avastin) for macular edema from central vein occlusion. Ophthalmic Surg Lasers Imaging. 2005;36(4):336-9.
44. Kreutzer TC, Alge CS, Wolf AH, et al. Intravitreal bevacizumab for the treatment of macular oedema secondary to branch retinal vein occlusion. Br J Ophthalmol. 2008;92(3):351-5.
45. Iturralde D, Spaide RF, Meyerle CB, et al. Intravitreal bevacizumab (Avastin) treatment of macular edema in central retinal vein occlusion: a short-term study. Retina. 2006;26(3):279-84.
46. Hsu J, Kaiser RS, Sivalingam A, et al. Intravitreal bevacizumab (avastin) in central vein occlusion. Retina. 2007;27(8):1013-9.
47. Rabena MD, Pieramici DJ, Castellarin AA, et al. Intravitreal bevacizumab (Avastin) in the treatment of macular edema secondary to branch retinal vein occlusion. Retina. 2007;27(4):419-25.
48. Ferrara DC, Koizumi H, Spaide RF. Early bevacizumab treatment of central retinal vein occlusion. Am J Ophthalmol. 2007;144(6):864-71.
49. Ferrara N, Damico L, Shams N, et al. Development of ranibizumab, an anti-vascular endothelial growth factor antigen binding fragment, as therapy for neovascular age-related macular degeneration. Retina. 2006;26:859-70.
50. Spaide RF, Cang LK, Klancnik JM, et al. Prospective study of intravitreal ranibizumab as a treatment for decreased visual acuity secondary to central retinal vein occlusion. Am J Ophthalmol. 2009;147(2):298-306.

51. Hayreh SS, van Heuven WA, Hayreh MS. Experimental retinal vascular occlusion. I. Pathogenesis of central retinal vein occlusion. Arch Ophthalmol. 1978;96(2):311-23.
52. Ishida S, Usui T, Yamashiro K, et al. VEGF164-mediated inflammation is required for pathological, but not physiological, ischemia-induced retinal neovascularization. J Exp Med. 2003;198(3):483-9.
53. Ishida S, Yamashiro K, Usui T, et al. Leukocytes mediate retinal vascular remodelling during development and vaso-obliteration in disease. Nat Med. 2003;9(6):781-8.
54. Ng EW, Adamis AP. Targeting angiogenesis, the underlying disorder in neovascular age-related macular degeneration. Can J Ophthalmol. 2005;40(3):352-68.
55. Ng EW, Shima DT, Calias P, Cunningham ET Jr, et al. Pegaptanib, a targeted anti-VEGF aptamer for ocular vascular disease. Nat Rev Drug Discov. 2006;5(2):123-32.
56. Cunningham ET Jr, Adamis AP, Altaweel M, et al. Macugen Diabetic Retinopathy Study Group. A phase II randomized double-masked trial of pegaptanib, an anti-vascular endothelial growth factor aptamer, for diabetic macular edema. Ophthalmology. 2005;112(10):1747-57.
57. Adamis AP, Altaweel M, Bressler NM, et al. Macugen Diabetic Retinopathy Study Group. Changes in retinal neovascularization after pegaptanib (Macugen) therapy in diabetic individuals. Ophthalmology. 2006;113(1):23-8.
58. Gragoudas ES, Adamis AP, Cunningham ET Jr, et al. VEGF Inhibition Study in Ocular Neovascularization Clinical Trial Group. Pegaptanib for neovascular age-related macular degeneration. N Engl J Med. 2004;351(27):2805-16.
59. Wroblewski JJ, Wells JA, Adamis AP, et al. Pegaptanib Sodium for Macular Edema Secondary to Central Retinal Vein Occlusion. Arch Ophthalmol. 2009;127(4):374-80.
60. Opremcak EM, Bruce RA, Lomeo MD, et al. Radial optic neurotomy for central retinal vein occlusion: a retrospective pilot study of 11 consecutive cases. Retina. 2001;21(5):408-15.
61. Hayreh SS, Opremcak EM, Bruce RA, et al. Radial optic neurotomy for central retinal vein obstruction. Retina. 2002;22:374-7.
62. Hayreh SS. Radial optic neurotomy for central retinal vein occlusion. Retina. 2002;22:827.
63. Hayreh SS. Radial optic neurotomy for nonischemic central retinal vein occlusion. Arch Ophthalmol. 2004;122(10):1572-3.
64. Weizer JS, Stinnett SS, Fekrat S. Radial optic neurotomy as treatment for central retinal vein occlusion. Am J Ophthalmol. 2003;136:814-9.
65. Martínez-Jardón CS, Meza-de Regil A, Dalma-Weiszhausz J, et al. Radial optic neurotomy for ischaemic central vein occlusion. Br J Ophthalmol. 2005;89(5):558-61.
66. Schneider U, Inhoffen W, Grisanti S, et al. Chorioretinal neovascularization after radial optic neurotomy for central retinal vein occlusion. Ophthalmic Surg Lasers Imaging. 2005;36(6):508-11.
67. Schneider U, Inhoffen W, Grisanti S, et al. Characteristics of visual field defects by scanning laser ophthalmoscope microperimetry after radial optic neurotomy for central retinal vein occlusion. Retina. 2005;25(6):704-12.
68. Samuel MA, Desai UR, Gandolfo CB. Peripapillary retinal detachment after radial optic neurotomy for central retinal vein occlusion. Retina. 2003;23(4):580-3.
69. Nomoto H, Shiraga F, Yamaji H, et al. Evaluation of radial optic neurotomy for central retinal vein occlusion by indocyanine green videoangiography and image analysis. Am J Ophthalmol. 2004;138(4):612-9.
70. García-Arumí J, Boixadera A, Martinez-Castillo V, et al. Chorioretinal anastomosis after radial optic neurotomy for central retinal vein occlusion. Arch Ophthalmol. 2003;121(10):1385-91.

71. Friedman SM. Optociliary venous anastomosis after radial optic neurotomy for central retinal vein occlusion. Ophthalmic Surg Lasers Imaging. 2003;34(4):315-7.

72. Leonard BC, Coupland SG, Kertes PJ, et al. Long-term follow-up of a modified technique for laser-induced chorioretinal venous anastomosis in nonischemic central retinal vein occlusion. Ophthalmology. 2003;110:948-54.

73. Fekrat S, Goldberg MF, Finkelstein D. Laser-induced chorioretinal venous anastomosis for nonischemic central or branch retinal vein occlusion. Arch Ophthalmol. 1998;116(1):43-52.

74. Peyman GA, Kishore K, Conway MD. Surgical chorioretinal venous anastomosis for ischemic central retinal vein occlusion. Ophthalmic Surg Lasers. 1999;30(8):605-14.

75. Mirshahi A, Roohipoor R, Lashay A, et al. Surgical induction of chorioretinal venous anastomosis in ischaemic central retinal vein occlusion: a non-randomised controlled clinical trial. Br J Ophthalmol. 2005;89(1):64-9.

76. McAllister IL, Gillies ME, Smithies LA, et al. The Central Retinal Vein Bypass Study: a trial of laser-induced chorioretinal venous anastomosis for central retinal vein occlusion. Ophthalmology. 2010;117(5):954-65.

77. Cahill MT, Kaiser PK, Sears JE, et al. The effect of arteriovenous sheathotomy on cystoid macular oedema secondary to branch retinal vein occlusion. Br J Ophthalmol. 2003;87(11):1329-32.

78. Le Rouic JF, Bejjani RA, Rumen F, et al. Adventitial sheathotomy for decompression of recent onset branch retinal vein occlusion. Graefes Arch Clin Exp Ophthalmol. 2001;239(10):747-51.

79. Mason J III, Feist R, White M Jr, et al. Sheathotomy to decompress branch retinal vein occlusion: a matched control study. Ophthalmology. 2004;111(3):540-5.

80. Mester U, Dillinger P. Vitrectomy with arteriovenous decompression and internal limiting membrane dissection in branch retinal vein occlusion. Retina. 2002;22(6):740-6.

81. Opremcak EM, Bruce RA. Surgical decompression of branch retinal vein occlusion via arteriovenous crossing sheathotomy: a prospective review of 15 cases. Retina. 1999;19(1):1-5.

82. Saika S, Tanaka T, Miyamoto T, et al. Surgical posterior vitreous detachment combined with gas/air tamponade for treating macular edema associated with branch retinal vein occlusion: retinal tomography and visual outcome. Graefes Arch Clin Exp Ophthalmol. 2001;239(10):729-32.

83. Tachi N, Hashimoto Y, Ogino N. Vitrectomy for macular edema combined with retinal vein occlusion. Doc Ophthalmol. 1999;97(3-4):465-9.

84. Figueroa MS, Torres R, Alvarez MT. Comparative study of vitrectomy with and without vein decompression for branch retinal vein occlusion: a pilot study. Eur J Ophthalmol. 2004;14(1):40-7.

85. Chung EJ, Lee H, Koh HJ. Arteriovenous crossing sheathotomy versus intravitreal triamcinolone acetonide injection for treatment of macular edema associated with branch retinal vein occlusion. Graefes Arch Clin Exp Ophthalmol. 2008;246(7):967-74.

86. Wolf S, Arend O, Bertram B, et al. Hemodilution therapy in central retinal vein occlusion: one-year results of a prospective randomized study. Graefes Arch Clin Exp Ophthalmol. 1994;232(1):33-9.

87. Brunner R, Heinen A, Konen W, et al. Therapy of retinal vascular disorders by modification of blood viscosity—a randomized double-blind study. Fortschr Ophthalmol. 1984;81(5):440-3.

88. Heinen A, Brunner R, Hossmann V, et al. Changes in hemorheologic and physiological coagulation parameters in different methods of therapy of retinal vascular disorders—a randomized double-blind study. Fortschr Ophthalmol. 1984;81(5):444-8.

89. Hansen LL, Wiek J, Wiederholt M. A randomised prospective study of treatment of non-ischaemic central retinal vein occlusion by isovolaemic haemodilution. Br J Ophthalmol. 1989;73(11):895-9.
90. Hansen LL, Danisevskis P, Arntz HR, et al. A randomised prospective study on treatment of central retinal vein occlusion by isovolaemic haemodilution and photocoagulation. Br J Ophthalmol. 1985;69(2):108-16.
91. Poupard P, Eledjam JJ, Dupeyron G, et al. Role of acute normovolemic hemodilution in treating retinal venous occlusions. Ann Fr Anesth Reanim. 1986;5(3):229-33.
92. Hehn F. Isovolaemic haemodilution and naftidrofuryl versus naftidrofuryl in treatment of retinal vein occlusion. Ophthalmology. 1995;9:309-12.
93. Luckie AP, Wroblewski JJ, Hamilton P, et al. A randomised prospective study of outpatient haemodilution for central retinal vein obstruction. Aust N Z J Ophthalmol. 1996;24(3):223-32.
94. Chen HC, Wiek J, Gupta A, et al. Effect of isovolaemic haemodilution on visual outcome in branch retinal vein occlusion. Br J Ophthalmol. 1998;82(2):162-7.
95. Glacet-Bernard A, Coscas G, Chabanel A, et al. A randomized, double-masked study on the treatment of retinal vein occlusion with troxerutin. Am J Ophthalmol. 1994;118(4):421-9.
96. Houtsmuller AJ, Vermeulen JA, Klompe M, et al. The influence of ticlopidine on the natural course of retinal vein occlusion. Agents Actions Suppl. 1984;15:219-29.

CHAPTER 11

Current Concepts in Central Serous Chorioretinopathy

Neha Sinha, Sandeep Saxena

INTRODUCTION

Central serous chorioretinopathy (CSCR) is a disease in which a serous detachment of the neurosensory retina occurs over an area of leakage from the choriocapillaris through the retinal pigment epithelium (RPE). It may be divided into two distinct clinical presentations:

1. *Acute CSCR*: The acute form is classically unilateral and characterized by one or more focal leak at the level of RPE in fluorescein angiography (FA). The neurosensory detachment contains clear subretinal fluid, but may be cloudy or have subretinal fibrin in some cases. This form is self-limiting and does not lead to gross visual deficit after resolution (Figs. 11.1 and 11.2).
2. *Chronic CSCR*: The chronic form is believed to be due to diffuse RPE disease and is usually bilateral. It presents with diffuse RPE atrophic changes, varying degrees of subretinal fluid, RPE alterations, and RPE tracks (Figs. 11.3A and B). It is characterized by diffuse areas of RPE leakage in FA. It has a relatively poor visual prognosis.

PATHOPHYSIOLOGY

Previously, it was thought that CSCR occurs due to focal choroidal vasculopathy and abnormal ion transport across the RPE. The discovery of indocyanine green (ICG) angiography has highlighted the importance of the choroidal circulation in the pathogenesis of CSCR. ICG angiography has demonstrated both multifocal choroidal hyperpermeability and hypofluorescent areas suggestive of focal choroidal vascular compromise. Some investigators believe that initial choroidal vascular compromise subsequently leads to secondary dysfunction of the overlying RPE.[1,2]

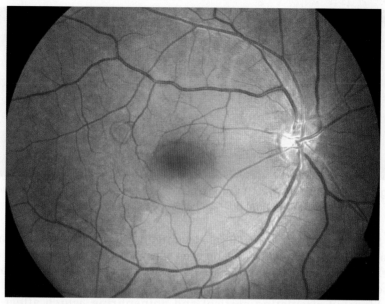

Fig. 11.1: Acute central serous chorioretinopathy: Color fundus photograph shows the neurosensory detachment of the macula along with a pigment epithelial detachment.

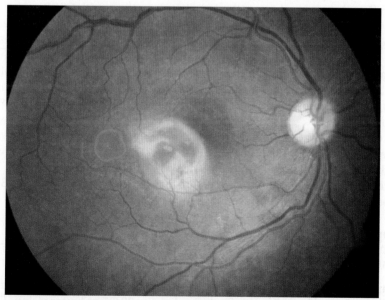

Fig. 11.2: Acute central serous chorioretinopathy: Color fundus photograph shows the neurosensory detachment of the macula along with subretinal fibrin and a pigment epithelial detachment.

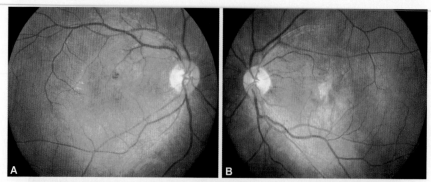

Figs. 11.3A and B: (A and B) Chronic central serous chorioretinopathy showing retinal pigment epithelial alterations and exudation.

Some studies using multifocal electroretinography have demonstrated bilateral diffuse retinal dysfunction even when CSCR was active only in one eye.[3] These studies support the belief of diffuse systemic effect on the choroidal vasculature.

Elevated circulating cortisol and epinephrine, which affect the autoregulation of the choroidal circulation, are also involved in the pathogenesis of CSCR as seen in patients of systemic hypertension, obstructive sleep apnea, and type A personalities.[4] Furthermore, Tewari et al.[5] demonstrated impaired autonomic response with significantly decreased parasympathetic activity and significantly increased sympathetic activity in patients with CSCR.

Corticosteroids have a direct influence on the expression of adrenergic receptor genes and thus contribute to the overall effect of catecholamines on the pathogenesis of CSCR. Consequently, multiple studies have conclusively implicated the effect of corticosteroids in the development of CSCR. Carvalho-Recchia et al.[6] showed in a series that 52% of patients with CSCR had used exogenous steroids within 1 month of presentation as compared with 18% of control subjects.

Cotticelli et al.[7] showed an association between *Helicobacter pylori* infection and CSCR. The prevalence of *H. pylori* infection was 78% in patients with CSCR compared with a prevalence of 43.5% in the control group. The authors proposed that *H. pylori* infection may represent a risk factor in CSCR, though no further studies have substantiated this claim.

EPIDEMIOLOGY

Visual Morbidity

Central serous chorioretinopathy typically resolves spontaneously in most of the patients (80–90%) with final visual acuity 20/25 or better vision. Even with the return of good central visual acuity, many of these patients still notice dyschromatopsia, loss of contrast sensitivity, metamorphopsia, and rarely, nyctalopia. Patients with classic CSCR have a 40–50% risk of recurrence in the same eye. The risk of choroidal neovascularization from previous CSCR is considered small (<5%) but has an increasing frequency in older patients.[8,9]

Approximately, 5–10% of patients may fail to recover 20/30 or better visual acuity. These patients often have recurrent or chronic serous retinal detachments, resulting in progressive RPE atrophy and permanent visual loss to 20/200 or worse. The final clinical picture represents diffuse retinal pigment epitheliopathy.

Otsuka et al.[10] reviewed a subset of patients who presented with a severe variant of CSCR over a mean follow-up period of 10.6 years. These patients have had multifocal lesions and bullous retinal detachments with shifting fluid and fibrin deposition. During the follow-up period, 52% of patients experienced recurrences of CSCR ranging from 1 to 5 episodes. However, 80% of eyes regained a visual acuity of better than 20/40, and 52% returned to a visual acuity of 20/20 or better. Eventually, patients reached a state of quiescent disease.

Race

Central serous chorioretinopathy is uncommon among African-Americans but appears severely among Hispanics and Asians.

Sex

This condition affects men 6–10 times more often than women.

Age

Central serous chorioretinopathy is most commonly seen in patients between the ages of 20 years and 55 years. It may manifest in older age-groups (more than 50 years). Spaide et al.[11] reviewed 130 consecutive patients with CSCR and found that their age at the first diagnosis ranged from 22.2 years to 82.9 years with a mean age of 49.8 years. Patients who presented at 50 years or later were found to have bilateral disease with a decreased male predominance (2.6:1) and showed more diffuse RPE changes. Furthermore, the patients had systemic hypertension or a history of corticosteroid use.[12]

SIGNS AND SYMPTOMS

Patients with CSCR typically present with following signs and symptoms:
1. Central visual loss
2. Metamorphopsia (especially micropsia)
3. Positive scotoma
4. Loss of color saturation
5. Loss of contrast sensitivity
6. Delayed retinal recovery time following photostress test.
   The decreased vision usually is improved by a small hyperopic correction.
   Clinical examination shows a serous retinal detachment which may be very subtle, often requiring slit-lamp biomicroscopy examination for detection.[13]

Pigment epithelial detachments, RPE mottling and atrophy, subretinal fibrin and rarely, subretinal lipid or lipofuscinoid flecks may also be seen.[14]

PATHOGENESIS

The advent of ICG angiography has highlighted the importance of choroidal circulation to the pathogenesis of central serous CSCR. Indocyanine green angiography has demonstrated both multifocal choroidal hyperpermeability and hypofluorescent areas suggestive of focal choroidal vascular compromise. Some investigators believe that the initial choroidal vascular compromise subsequently leads to a secondary dysfunction of the overlying RPE.[15]

Type-A personality and systemic hypertension may be associated with CSCR.[16]

Allibhai et al.[17] reported an association between a drug, sildenafil citrate, and CSCR. Fraunfelder and Fraunfelder[18] further evaluated the association of CSCR with sildenafil. After reviewing 1,500 cases of the ocular side effects of sildenafil, they have found 11 men had CSCR. The symptoms resolved following the cessation of sildenafil in 8 of 11 patients but recurred in 3 of these patients upon restarting the drug. A causal relationship could not be determined due to the cyclic nature of CSCR but suggested that patients with refractory CSCR should consider the cessation of sildenafil use.

Systemic associations of CSCR include organ transplantation, exogenous steroid use, Cushing syndrome, systemic hypertension, sleep apnea, systemic lupus erythematosus, pregnancy, gastroesophageal reflux disease, and the use of psychopharmacologic medications.[4,17,19-22]

Haimovici et al.[23] evaluated systemic risk factors for CSCR in 312 patients and 312 control subjects. They found that systemic steroid use and pregnancy were most strongly associated with CSCR. Other risk factors included antibiotic use, alcohol use, untreated hypertension and allergic respiratory disorders.

LABORATORY STUDIES

Laboratory tests are not very helpful in the diagnosis. An occasional elevated level of plasminogen activator inhibitor may be found in a patient with CSCR.

Fundus Fluorescein Angiography

Fundus FA of a classic case of CSCR shows one or more focal leaks at the level of the RPE (Figs. 11.4 and 11.5). Usually two types of patterns are seen. In the early stage, leakage is seen as a hyperfluorescent dot which later on expands into a large dot within the area of macular detachment called *inkblot* type. Sometimes, it rises under the neurosensory detachment as a *smokestack*. The inkblot pattern is more common than smoke stack. The smoke stack pattern is thought to be related to the increased concentration of protein in the fluid. The classic *"smokestack"* appearance of the fluorescein leak is seen only in 10–15% of cases. In this pattern, a diffuse retinal pigment epitheliopathy demonstrates focal granular hyperfluorescence corresponding to window

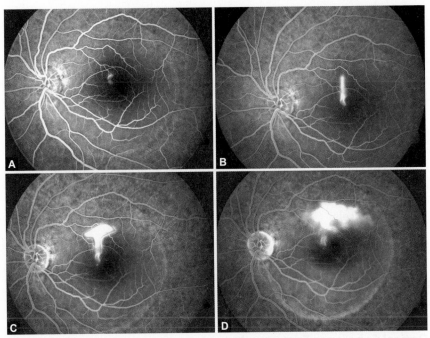

Figs. 11.4A to D: Acute central serous chorioretinopathy: Fundus fluorescein angiography showing—(A) Hyperfluorescent dot; (B) Linear expanded dot; (C and D) Increasing smoke stacks appearances (umbrella pattern).

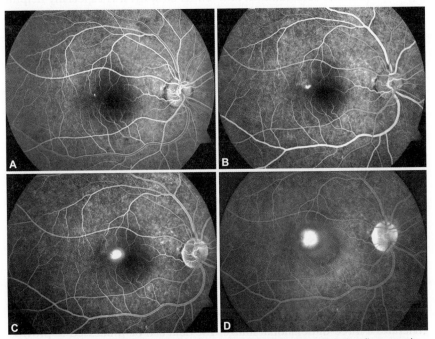

Figs. 11.5 A to D: Acute central serous chorioretinopathy: Fundus fluorescein angiography shows gradually expanding ink blot appearances.

defects and blockage caused by RPE atrophy and clumping with one or more areas of subtle continued leakage.

Indocyanine Green Angiography

Indocyanine green (ICG) angiography has shown hypofluorescent areas early in the angiogram followed by late hyperfluorescence and leakage in choroidal vasculature. Often, multiple areas of leakage are seen on ICG angiography that are not evident clinically or in FA. According to some researchers, characteristic mid-phase findings in ICG angiography allow differentiation from occult choroidal neovascularization in older individuals. Multiple patches of hyperfluorescence are presumably due to choroidal hyperpermeability which, in later phases, results in silhouetting or negative staining of larger choroidal vessels.

Scanning Laser Ophthalmoscopy

Scanning laser ophthalmoscopy is a newer technology to evaluate the retina. Ooto et al.[24] showed that adaptive optics is useful in evaluating cone abnormalities associated with visual acuity loss in eyes with CSCR.

Optical Coherence Tomography

Optical coherence tomography (OCT) can demonstrate subretinal fluid, pigment epithelial detachments, and retinal atrophy. It is especially helpful in identifying subtle or even subclinical neurosensory macular detachments. The OCT features of acute and chronic CSCR are summarized below:[25]

Acute CSCR (Figs. 11.6 to 11.8)
1. The thickening of the neurosensory retina with detachment
2. Retinal pigment epithelial detachment
3. A combination of both 1 and 2
4. The presence of moderately high reflective mass bridging the detached neurosensory retina and RPE with subretinal fibrin.

Chronic CSCR (Fig. 11.9)
1. Foveal atrophy and thinning
2. Cystoid changes at the fovea
3. Associated complications may show RPE rip and choroidal neovascularization.

Three-dimensional Optical Coherence Tomography

Three-dimensional OCT may be performed using a spectral-domain optical coherence tomography (SD-OCT) scanning protocol that achieves high sampling density in all three dimensions and acquires high-density volumetric data of the macula. Volume rendering of the three-dimensional data generates a three-dimensional image. The data can be processed to provide comprehensive structural information. The unprecedented visualization

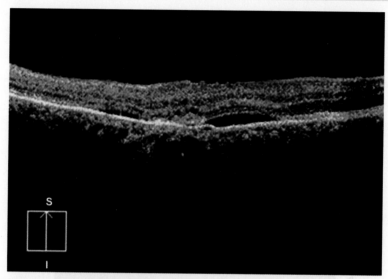

Fig. 11.6: Acute central serous chorioretinopathy: Spectral domain optical coherence tomography shows serous detachment of macula and pigment epithelial detachment.

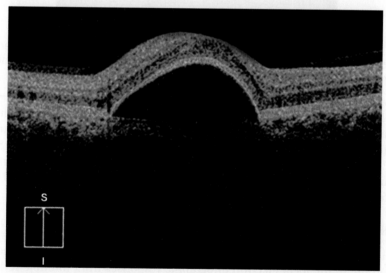

Fig. 11.7: Acute central serous chorioretinopathy: Spectral domain optical coherence tomography shows large pigment epithelial detachment.

provided by this technology enables the determination of specific alterations in the characteristics of the retinal anatomy. Three-dimensional OCT data can be used to segment measure, and map intraretinal layer thicknesses. Currently, the clinical applications of 3D retinal imaging are being evaluated for selective visualization of macular layers. SD-OCT shows morphologic alterations in the RPE elegantly.

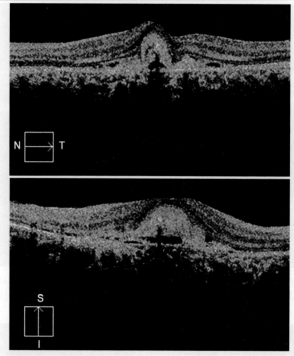

Fig. 11.8: Acute central serous chorioretinopathy: Spectral domain optical coherence tomography shows subretinal fibrin, serous detachment of macula, and pigment epithelial detachment.

The quantitative and topographic assessment of pigment epithelium detachment (PEDs) on the spectral domain single-layer retinal pigment epithelium (SD-OCT SL-RPE) map compares well with FA. SD-OCT SL-RPE map is indeed a noninvasive advanced tool for the documentation of quantitative and topographic distribution of PEDs and obviates the need for FA for monitoring the progress of PEDs in eyes with CSCR (Fig. 11.10).

Multifocal Electroretinography

Multifocal electroretinography is a technique which allows the simultaneous recording of the focal electroretinographic responses from multiple retinal locations.[26] Due to the impairment of the central macular function in CSCR, first-order mfERG responses will demonstrate reduced response amplitude, especially in the rings arising from the central macula. Delayed implicit times may also be observed in the area of serous macular detachment but, in some, it might be seen in areas without retinal detachment and even in unaffected fellow eyes, suggesting more widespread retinal dysfunction in CSCR. Chappelow and Marmor[27] first described the persistently reduced focal electrical responses on multifocal electroretinography in eyes with resolved CSCR. Furthermore, investigators including Lai et al.[28] are using multifocal

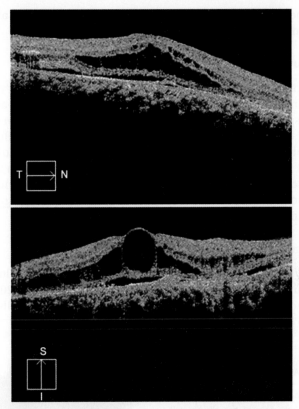

Fig. 11.9: Chronic central serous chorioretinopathy: Spectral domain optical coherence tomography shows serous detachment of macula, pigment epithelium detachment, cystic changes in retina, and proliferating cells on retinal pigment epithelium and back surface of neurosensory retina.

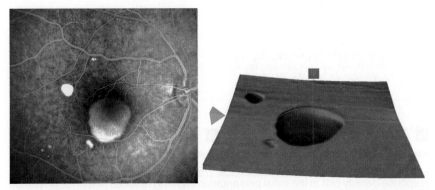

Fig. 11.10: Central serous chorioretinopathy: Three-dimensional spectral domain optical coherence tomography retinal pigment epithelium map shows topographic and quantitative distribution of pigment epithelial detachments in 512 × 128 macular cube when compared to fundus fluorescein angiography.

electroretinography as a means of assessing the efficacy and safety of new treatment modalities for CSCR (Figs. 11.11A to D).

Fundus Autofluorescence

Fundus fluorescein is a noninvasive imaging technique which evaluates the structural and metabolic condition of the RPE cells at macula. In acute CSCR, a localized spot of reduced autofluorescence may be observed corresponding to the area of focal RPE defect. Mild diffuse increase in autofluorescence might be observed due to the increased metabolic activity of RPE cells (Figs. 11.12 and 11.13).[29-31] In chronic CSCR, an irregularity in the level of autofluorescence might be seen, with both areas of reduced and increased autofluorescence. Reduced activity is due to generalized RPE atrophy or the loss of photoreceptors.[29-31]

Microperimetry

Micrometry (using the Nidek MP-1 microperimeter) has shown lower retinal sensitivity in the macula even once visual acuity returned to 20/20. Ojima et al.[32,33] showed that areas of reduced sensitivity were typically focal and localized to clinically apparent regions of irregular RPE.

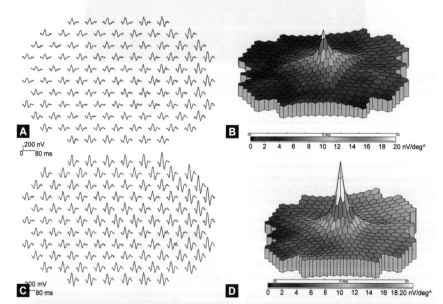

Figs. 11.11A to D: Serial first-order kernel multifocal electroretinography assessment of central serous chorioretinopathy: (A) Trace array and (B) three-dimensional response density plot at the initial presentation showing reduced response amplitude at the central macula. (C) trace array, and (D) three-dimensional response density plot after the resolution of exudative macular detachment showing recovery of the multifocal electroretinography responses, indicating recovery of macular function. *Source:* Dr Timothy YY Lai, Hong Kong.

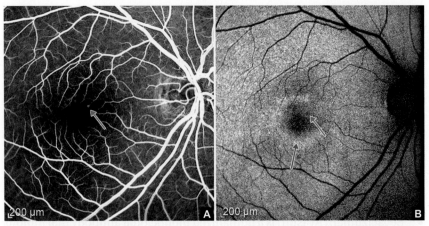

Figs. 11.12A and B: (A) Early phase fluorescein angiography showing a focal point of leakage (red arrow) in acute central serous chorioretinopathy, (B) Fundus autofluorescence image of the same eye showing a localized spot of hypofluorescence due to focal loss of retinal pigment epithelium (RPE) corresponding to the leakage site on fluorescein angiography (FA) (red arrow). An area of increased autofluorescence (green arrow) can also be seen surrounding the macula due to the increased metabolic activity of the RPE cells.
Source: Dr Timothy YY Lai, Hong Kong.

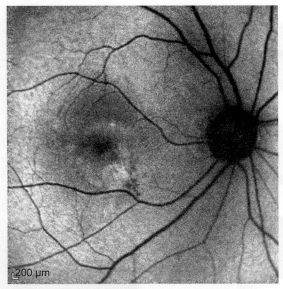

Fig. 11.13: Fundus autofluorescence image of a chronic central serous chorioretinopathy showing irregular level of autofluorescence signals. Areas of reduced autofluorescence are suggestive of retinal pigment epithelial atrophy, whereas areas of increased autofluorescence are suggestive of increased RPE activity.
Source: Dr Timothy YY Lai, Hong Kong.

TREATMENT

Medical

- The efficacy of tranquilizers or β-blockers is unknown. Furthermore, an evaluation of 230 consecutive patients with CSCR found that the use of psychopharmacologic agents (e.g. anxiolytics, antidepressants) was a risk factor for CSCR. Use of corticosteroids in the treatment of CSCR should be avoided because it may result in exacerbation of serous detachments.
- Tatham and Macfarlane[34] described a case series of patients who were treated with propranolol for CSCR. They suggested that β-blockade had a hypothetical mechanism in treating CSCR. Further evidence is needed to substantiate this potential treatment.
- Mifepristone was used in the treatment of chronic CSCR by Nielsen et al.[35]
- Bevacizumab (Avastin) is a humanized monoclonal antibody that inhibits all active isoforms of vascular endothelial growth factor (VEGF) and is approved by the US Food and Drug Administration (USFDA) since 2004 for the treatment of metastatic colorectal cancer. It has been used to successfully treat the rare complication of choroidal neovascularization following CSCR.[36-38] Variable reports are available in literature about the efficacy of intravitreal therapy (Figs. 11.14 and 11.15).
- Finasteride (phosphodiesterase inhibitor) may represent a novel medical treatment for chronic CSCR.[39]

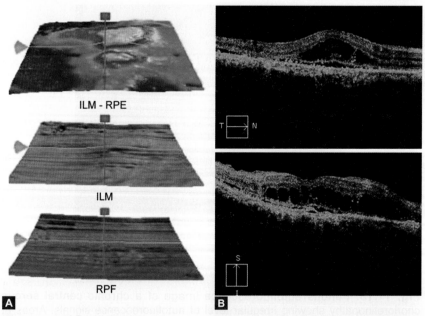

ILM - RPE

ILM

RPF

Figs. 11.14A and B: Intravitreal bevacizumab in chronic central serous chorioretinopathy: Pre-treatment: (A) Macular topography in internal limiting membrane-retinal pigment epithelium (ILM-RPE), ILM and RPE maps; and (B) Neurosensory detachment and cystic changes in the macula.

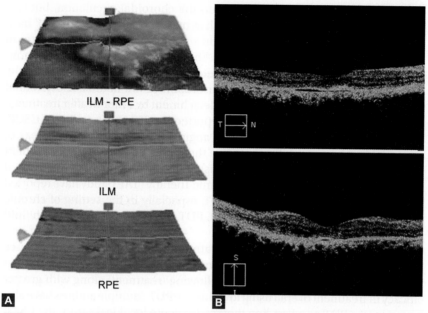

Figs. 11.15 A and B: Intravitreal bevacizumab in chronic central serous chorioretinopathy: Post-treatment: (A) Macular topography in ILM-RPE, ILM and RPE maps; and (B) Residual neurosensory detachment, resolution of cystic changes in macula, and the reappearance of foveal contour.

Laser Photocoagulation

Laser photocoagulation should be considered under the following circumstances:

1. The persistence of a serous retinal detachment for more than 4 months
2. Recurrence in an eye with visual deficit from previous CSCR
3. The presence of visual deficits in the opposite eye from previous episodes of CSCR
4. Occupational or other patient's needs requiring the prompt recovery of vision.

Laser treatment also may be considered in patients with recurrent episodes of serous detachment with a leak located more than 300 μm from the center of the fovea.[40,41] Laser treatment does not appear to improve the final visual prognosis but it shortens the course of the disease and decreases the risk of recurrence for CSCR.[42,43] It affects the final contrast sensitivity which was found to be lesser in patients treated with early laser as compared to patients kept on the conservative management. Some evidences suggest that patients with chronic CSCR (diffuse retinal pigment epitheliopathy) may have better prognosis with laser treatment.

Photodynamic Therapy

Photodynamic therapy (PDT) has growing support in the literature as a treatment of chronic CSCR and recently in acute phases of this condition.

PDT is known to have a direct effect on the choroidal circulation, but was limited by potential adverse effects, such as macular ischemia. Lai et al.[28] have described that a half dose of verteporfin significantly decreased the rates of adverse events with these modifications. They proposed 3 mg/m^2 of verteporfin infused over 8 minutes, followed 2 minutes later with ICG-guided PDT. Of the eyes treated, 85% showed complete resolution of the neurosensory retinal detachment and/or pigment epithelial detachment by 1 month after treatment. Use of verteporfin and PDT was first reported in 2003 in the setting of CSCR. Yannuzzi et al.[44] described using ICG angiography to first identify areas of choroidal hyperpermeability that were then targeted with PDT. Subsequent studies using the PDT protocols established by the Treatment of Age-related Macular Degeneration with Photodynamic Therapy (TAP) study have reported case series that support the use of PDT, especially in the setting of chronic CSCR with neurosensory detachments. PDT is believed to hasten both fluid reabsorption and visual recovery.

Reibaldi et al.[45] evaluated the treatment efficacy of standard-fluence PDT versus low-fluence PDT using microperimetry. The study found an improvement of macular sensitivity following treatment, along with greater efficacy in treatment overall using low-fluence PDT. Multiple authors have also begun to use PDT as a first-line therapy for acute focal leaks from the CSCR with reported success. Most papers describe the resolution of subretinal fluid within 1 month of treatment.

Chan et al.[46] demonstrated that there is evidence of choroidal vascular changes in ICG with regard to choroidal permeability and vascular remodeling. ICG-mediated photothrombosis is a technique using a low-intensity laser combined with ICG dye infusion to treat focal areas of hyperpermeability in the choroid. Like PDT, it addresses treatment to the level of the choroidal vasculature.[47] An 810 nm laser is applied after infusion of ICG dye.

Transpupillary Thermotherapy

Without prior ICG dye, investigators have also used the 810 nm laser as transpupillary thermotherapy (TTT) with moderate anecdotal success.[48,49] However, Penha et al.[50] described severe retinal thermal injury in a 31-year-old man following this treatment modality and recommended caution for this adverse event following ICG-mediated TTT treatment.

Micropulse Yellow Laser Therapy

Micropulse yellow laser therapy is one of the newer treatment modalities which resolves leakage and retinal detachment without scarring or retinal damage. The IQ 577 (Iridex Corporation, Mountain View, CA, United States) laser is a solid-state, multimode laser. In micropulse mode, the laser energy is delivered in short pulses. The laser stays on only 10–15% of the time (depending on the duty cycle selected), generating less heat and producing less damage to the retina than continuous-wave photocoagulation. The 577 nm yellow wavelength is ideal for CSR and other retinal applications because it is highly selective for the RPE. The oxyhemoglobin in the RPE absorbs yellow light better than any other wavelength, while xanthophylls have negligible uptake of yellow light, localizing the effects to the RPE and further protecting the fovea.[51] The results from a small series of patients with central serous retinopathy treated with the yellow laser have been very encouraging.

Follow-up

Most patients with CSCR receive follow-up care for 3 months to determine whether the fluid resolves spontaneously.

COMPLICATIONS

- Retinal pigment epithelial decompensation from recurrent attacks leads to RPE atrophy and subsequent retinal atrophy. RPE decompensation is a manifestation of CSCR but may also be considered as a long-term complication.[52]
- A minority of patients develop choroidal neovascularization at the site of the leakage and laser treatments. A retrospective review of cases shows that one-half of these patients may have had signs of occult choroidal neovascularization at the time of treatment. In the other patients, the risk of choroidal neovascularization may have been increased by the laser treatment.[9]
- Acute bullous retinal detachment may occur in otherwise healthy patients with CSCR. This appearance may mimic Vogt-Koyanagi-Harada disease, rhegmatogenous retinal detachment or uveal effusion. A case report also has implicated the use of corticosteroids in CSCR as a factor increasing the likelihood of subretinal fibrin formation. Reducing the corticosteroid dose frequently will lead to the resolution of the serous retinal detachment.[53]

PROGNOSIS

- Serous retinal detachments typically resolve spontaneously in most patients (80–90%) returning to 20/25 or better vision.[54,55]
- Patients with classic CSCR (characterized by focal leaks) have a 40–50% risk of recurrence in the same eye.[13,54,55]
- In spite of the return of good central visual acuity, many of these patients still notice dyschromatopsia, loss of contrast sensitivity, metamorphopsia, or nyctalopia.[56]
- These patients often have recurrent or chronic serous retinal detachments, resulting in progressive RPE atrophy and permanent visual loss to 20/200 or worse. The final clinical picture represents diffuse retinal pigment epitheliopathy.
- The risk of choroidal neovascularization from previous CSCR is considered small (<5%) but has an increasing frequency in older patients diagnosed with CSCR.[8,13]

REFERENCES

1. Okushiba U, Takeda M. Study of choroidal vascular lesions in central serous chorioretinopathy using indocyanine green angiography. Nippon Ganka Gakkai Zasshi. 1997;101(1):74-82.
2. Iijima H, Iida T, Murayama K, et al. Plasminogen activator inhibitor 1 in central serous chorioretinopathy. Am J Ophthalmol. 1999;127(4):477-8.
3. Marmor MF, Tan F. Central serous chorioretinopathy: bilateral multifocal electroretinographic abnormalities. Arch Ophthalmol. 1999;117(2):184-8.
4. Leveque TK, Yu L, Musch DC, et al. Central serous chorioretinopathy and risk for obstructive sleep apnea. Sleep Breath. 2007; 11(4):253-7.
5. Tewari HK, Gadia R, Kumar D, et al. Sympathetic-parasympathetic activity and reactivity in central serous chorioretinopathy: a case-control study. Invest Ophthalmol Vis Sci. 2006;47(8):3474-8.
6. Carvalho-Recchia CA, Yannuzzi LA, Negrao S, et al. Corticosteroids and central serous chorioretinopathy. Ophthalmology. 2002;109(10):1834-7.
7. Cotticelli L, Borrelli M, D'Alessio AC, et al. Central serous chorioretinopathy and *Helicobacter pylori*. Eur J Ophthalmol. 2006;16(2):274-8.
8. Gomolin JE. Choroidal neovascularization and central serous chorioretinopathy. Can J Ophthalmol. 1989;24:20-3.
9. Matsunaga H, Nangoh K, Uyama M, et al. Occurrence of choroidal neovascularization following photocoagulation treatment for central serous retinopathy. Nippon Ganka Gakkai Zasshi. 1995;99(4):460-8.
10. Otsuka S, Ohba N, Nakao K. A Long-term follow-up study of severe variant of central serous chorioretinopathy. Retina. 2002;22(1):25-32.
11. Spaide RF, Campeas L, Haas A, et al. Central serous chorioretinopathy in younger and older adults. Ophthalmology. 1996;103(12):2070-9.
12. Polak BC, Baarsma GS, Snyers B. Diffuse retinal pigment epitheliopathy complicating systemic corticosteroid treatment. Br J Ophthalmol. 1995;79(10):922-5.
13. Gass JD. Central serous chorioretinopathy and white subretinal exudation during pregnancy. Arch Ophthalmol. 1991;109(5):677-81.
14. Piccolino FC, Borgia L. Central serous chorioretinopathy and indocyanine green angiography. Retina. 1994;14(3):231-42.
15. Yannuzzi LA. Type-A behavior and central serous chorioretinopathy. Retina 1987;7(2):111-31.
16. Jampol LM, Weinreb R, Yannuzzi L. Involvement of corticosteroids and catecholamines in the pathogenesis of central serous chorioretinopathy: a rationale for new treatment strategies. Ophthalmology. 2002;109(10):1765-6.
17. Allibhai ZA, Gale JS, Sheidow TS. Central serous chorioretinopathy in a patient taking sildenafil citrate. Ophthalmic Surg Lasers Imaging. 2004;35(2):165-7.
18. Fraunfelder FW, Franufelder FT. Central serous chorioretinopathy associated with sildenafil. Retina. 2008; 28(4):606-9.
19. Cunningham ET Jr, Alfred PR, Irvine AR. Central serous chorioretinopathy in patients with systemic lupus erythematosus. Ophthalmology. 1996;103(12):2081-90.
20. Bouzas EA, Scott MH, Mastorakos G, et al. Central serous chorioretinopathy in endogenous hypercortisolism. Arch Ophthalmol. 1993;111(9):1229-33.
21. Mansuetta CC, Mason JO III, Swanner J, et al. An association between central serous chorioretinopathy and gastroesophageal reflux disease. Am J Ophthalmol. 2004;137(6):1096-100.
22. Tittl MK, Spaide RF, Wong D, et al. Systemic findings associated with central serous chorioretinopathy. Am J Ophthalmol. 1999;128(1):63-8.

23. Haimovici R, Koh S, Gagnon DR, et al. Risk factors for central serous chorioretinopathy: a case-control study. Ophthalmology. 2004;111(2):244-9.

24. Ooto S, Hangai M, Sakamoto A, et al. High-resolution imaging of resolved central serous chorioretinopathy using adaptive optics scanning laser ophthalmoscopy. Ophthalmology. 2010;117(9):1800-9.

25. Bhende M, Nair BK. Central serous chorioretinopathy. In: Saxena S, Meredith TA (Eds). Optical Coherence Tomography in Retinal Diseases. New Delhi: Jaypee Brothers Medical Publishers (P) Ltd.; 2006. pp. 137-44.

26. Sutter EE, Tran D. The field topography of ERG components in man-I. The photopic luminance response. Vision Res. 1992;32(3):433-46.

27. Chappelow AV, Marmor MF. Multifocal electroretinogram abnormalities persist following resolution of central serous chorioretinopathy. Arch Ophthalmol. 2000;118(9):1211-5.

28. Lai TY, Chan WM, Li H, et al. Safety enhanced photodynamic therapy with half dose verteporfin for chronic central serous chorioretinopathy: a short term pilot study.Br J Ophthalmol. 2006;90(7):869-74.

29. Eandi CM, Ober M, Iranmanesh R, et al. Acute central serous chorioretinopathy and fundus autofluorescence. Retina. 2005;25(8):989-93.

30. Ruckmann A, Fitzke FW, Fan J, et al. Abnormalities of fundus autofluorescence in central serous retinopathy. Am J Ophthalmol. 2002;133(60):780-6.

31. Spaid RF, Klancnik JM Jr. Fundus autofluorescence and central serous chorioretinopathy. Ophthalmology. 2005;112(5):825-33.

32. Ozdemir H, Karacorlu SA, Senturk F, et al. Assessment of macular function by microperimetry in unilateral resolved central serous chorioretinopathy. Eye. 2008;22(2):204-8.

33. Ojima Y, Tsujikawa A, Hangai M, et al. Retinal sensitivity measured with the micro-perimeter after resolution of central serous chorioretinopathy. Am J Ophthalmol. 2008;146(1):77-84.

34. Tatham A, Macfarlane A. The use of propranolol to treat central serous chorioretinopathy: an evaluation by serial OCT. J Ocul Pharmacol Ther. 2006;22(2):145-9.

35. Nielsen JS, Weinreb RN, Yannuzzi L, et al. Mifepristone treatment of chronic central serous chorioretinopathy. Retina. 2007;27(1):119-22.

36. Huang WC, Chen WL, Tsai YY, et al. Intravitreal bevacizumab for treatment of chronic central serous chorioretinopathy. Eye. 2009;23:488-9.

37. Torres-Soriano ME, Garcia-Aguirre G, Kon-Jara V, et al. A pilot study of intravitreal bevacizumab for the treatment of central serous chorioretinopathy (case reports). Graefes Arch Clin Exp Ophthalmol. 2008;246(9):1235-9.

38. Chan WM, Lai TY, Liu DT, Lam DS. Intravitreal bevacizumab (avastin) for choroidal neovascularization secondary to central serous chorioretinopathy, secondary to punctate inner choroidopathy, or of idiopathic origin. Am J Ophthalmol. 2007;143(6):977-83.

39. Forooghian F, Meleth AD, Cukras C, et al. Finasteride for chronic central serous chorioretinopathy. Retina. 2011;31(4):766-71.

40. Watzke RC, Burton TC, Woolson RF. Direct and indirect laser photocoagulation of central serous choroidopathy. Am J Ophthalmol. 1979;88(5):914-8.

41. Robertson DM, Ilstrup D. Direct, indirect, and sham laser photocoagulation in the management of central serous chorioretinopathy. Am J Ophthalmol. 1983;95(4):457-66.

42. Burumcek E, Mudun A, Karacorlu S, et al. Laser photocoagulation for persistent central serous retinopathy: results of long-term follow-up. Ophthalmology. 1997;104(4):616-22.

43. Taban M, Boyer DS, Thomas EL, et al. Chronic central serous chorioretinopathy: photodynamic therapy. Am J Ophthalmol. 2004;137(6):1073-80.

44. Yannuzzi LA, Slakter JS, Gross NE, et al. Indocyanine green angiography-guided photodynamic therapy for treatment of chronic central serous chorioretinopathy: a pilot study. Retina. 2003;23(3):288-98.

45. Reibaldi M, Boscia F, Avitabile T, et al. Functional retinal changes measured by microperimetry in standard-fluence vs low-fluence photodynamic therapy in chronic central serous chorioretinopathy. Am J Ophthalmol. 2011;151(6):953-960.e2.

46. Chan WM, Lam DS, Lai TY, et al. Choroidal vascular remodeling in central serous chorioretinopathy after indocyanine green-guided photodynamic therapy with verteporfin: a novel treatment at the primary disease level. Br J Ophthalmol. 2003;87(12):1453-8.

47. Costa RA, Scapucin L, Moraes NS, et al. Indocyanine green-mediated photothrombosis as a new technique of treatment for persistent central serous chorioretinopathy. Curr Eye Res. 2002;25(5):287-97.

48. Hussain N, Khanna R, Hussain A, et al. Transpupillary thermotherapy for chronic central serous chorioretinopathy. Graefes Arch Clin Exp Ophthalmol. 2006;244(8):1045-51.

49. Shukla D, Kolluru C, Vignesh TP, et al. Transpupillary thermotherapy for subfoveal leaks in central serous chorioretinopathy. Eye. 2008;22(1):100-6.

50. Penha FM, Aggio FB, Bonomo PP. Severe retinal thermal injury after indocyanine green-mediated photothrombosis for central serous chorioretinopathy. Am J Ophthalmol. 2007;143(5):887-9.

51. Chen SN, Hwang JF, Tseng LF, et al. Subthreshold diode micropulse photocoagulation for the treatment of chronic central serous chorioretinopathy with juxtafoveal leakage. Ophthalmology. 2008;115(12):2229-34.

52. Yap EY, Robertson DM. The long-term outcome of central serous chorioretinopathy. Arch Ophthalmol. 1996;114(6):689-92.

53. Gass JD, Little H. Bilateral bullous exudative retinal detachment complicating idiopathic central serous chorioretinopathy during systemic corticosteroid therapy. Ophthalmology. 1995;102(5):737-47.

54. Hooymans JM. Fibrotic scar formation in central serous chorioretinopathy developed during systemic treatment with corticosteroids. Graefes Arch Clin Exp Ophthalmol. 1998;236(11):876-9.

55. Cardillo Piccolino F, Eandi CM, Ventre L, et al. Photodynamic therapy for chronic central serous chorioretinopathy. Retina. 2003;23(6):752-63.

56. Ober MD, Yannuzzi LA, Do DV, et al. Photodynamic therapy for focal retinal pigment epithelial leaks secondary to central serous chorioretinopathy. Ophthalmology. 2005;112(12):2088-94.

CHAPTER 12

Proliferative Vitreoretinopathy

Ajit Majjhi

INTRODUCTION

Proliferative vitreoretinopathy (PVR) is a complex cellular process that has many similarities to a wound healing response involving inflammation, cell migration, proliferation resulting in extracellular matrix production, fibroblastic transformation, and contraction of fibrocytes.[1] Clinically, PVR is characterized by the growth and contraction of cellular membranes within the hyaloid, the vitreous, and on both retinal surfaces.[2] These membranes result in traction, which may cause a traction retinal detachment (RD) that reopens otherwise successfully treated retinal breaks or may create new retinal breaks.[3] Membrane contraction may also cause macular pucker. Proliferative vitreoretinopathy comprises a variety of different intraocular cellular proliferations including epiretinal membranes, subretinal strands, and RDs in combination with star folds, vitreous traction, and anterior loop traction (anterior PVR).[4-6]

PATHOGENESIS

The pathogenesis of PVR is similar to wound healing consisting of inflammation, proliferation, and modulation of scar (Fig. 12.1). Proliferative vitreoretinopathy occurs when cellular migration in the presence of inflammation results in membrane formation in the vitreous and inner or outer surfaces of the retina following development of rhegmatogenous RD or ocular trauma.[2] PVR is characterized by the migration and proliferation of retinal pigment epithelial (RPE) cells along with synthesis of extracellular matrix (ECM) proteins such as collagen or fibronectin which organizes into an epiretinal or subretinal membrane.[7] Various reactions may be discerned in the development of PVR, including chemotaxis and cellular migration, cellular proliferation, membrane formation, and contraction. These membranes are composed of RPE cells, glial

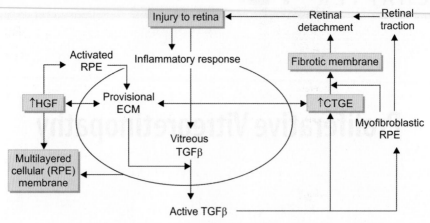

Fig. 12.1: Pathogenesis of proliferative vitreoretinopathy (PVR).

cells (primarily Müller cells and astrocytes), fibroblasts, and inflammatory cells.[8,9]

The cellular components involved in PVR include RPE cells, hyalocytes, and glial cells.[8] Proinflammatory cytokines involved in PVR include interleukin-8, monocyte chemotactic protein-1, interleukin-1, interleukin-6, tumor necrosis factor-α (TNF-α), and interferon-γ.[10,11] Growth factors involved in PVR include platelet derived growth factor (PDGF), transforming growth factor-β (TGF-β), epidermal growth factor (EGF), and fibroblast growth factor (FGF).[12,13]

The extracellular matrices involved in PVR are thrombospondin, laminin, and vetreonectin.[7,8,14] The inflammatory cells involved in PVR include macrophages, lymphocytes, and fibroblasts.[15] Proliferation and migration of the cells (mainly RPE cells and/or glial cells) form sheets of differentiated cells within a provisional ECM that contains fibronectin, laminin, and vitreonectin.[8] These cellular membranes become progressively paucicellular and fibrotic.[9] After the retinal break formation, the inflammatory cells are drawn to the lesion and secrete TNF-α.[16] TNF-α acts as a mediator of RPE activation, PDGF acts as an important mitogen, chemoattractant, and mediator of cellular contraction.[3,12] TGF-β is an important contributor for tissue fibrosis (Fig. 12.1).[17]

TERMINOLOGY AND CLASSIFICATION

Proliferative vitreoretinopathy has been termed in the past as *massive vitreous retraction* by Havener, *massive pre-retinal retraction* by Tolentino et al., and *massive pre-retinal proliferation* by Machemer and Laqua.[18] The term *PVR* was coined in 1983 by The Retina Society Terminology Committee.[19] The Retina Society Terminology Committee proposed a new classification of PVR (Table 12.1). The new classification modified the one proposed by Machemer in 1978.[18] Unlike the 1978 classification, the 1983 classification avoided any reference to the extension and/or intensity of PVR, substituting the word *massive* for the term proliferative, referred to its pathogenesis. The term

TABLE 12.1: Retina society classification of retina detachment with the proliferative vitreoretinopathy.

Grade	Name	Clinical Signs
A	Minimum	Vitreous haze, vitreous clumps (Fig. 2A)
B	Moderate	Wrinkling of the inner retinal surface, rolled edge of retinal break, retinal stiffness, vessel tortuosity (Fig. 2B)
C	Marked	Full thickness fixed retinal folds
C-1		• One quadrant (Fig. 2C)
C-2		• Two quadrants (Fig. 2D)
C-3		• Three quadrants (Fig. 2E)
D	Massive	Fixed retinal folds in four quadrants
D-1		• Wide funnel shape (Fig. 2F)
D-2		• Narrow funnel shape* (Fig. 2G)
D-3		• Closed funnel (optic nerve head not visible) (Fig. 2H)

*Narrow funnel shape exists when the anterior end of the funnel can be seen by indirect ophthalmoscopy within the 45° field of a +20D condensing lens (Nikon or equivalent).

vitreoretinopathy was selected to identify the location of the disease. The Retina Society classification is widely accepted today. This classification has been revised by the Silicone Study Group to include anterior PVR as well as quantitative assessment of amount of PVR to provide a description of PVR relevant to modern vitreoretinal surgery, which involves both anterior and posterior forms of PVR.[20]

The recognition of the anterior form of PVR is one of the most important contributions of the Silicone Study Group classification.[21] Retina Society classification has been updated (Tables 12.2 and 12.3) after the Silicone Study Group classification and results of a major randomized trial (Silicone Study results) to evaluate the efficacy of silicone oil compared to prolonged intraocular gas tamponade.[20,22]

The Silicone Study Group has evaluated the reproducibility and prognostic utility of the Retina Society and the Silicone Study classification systems of PVR.[23] The reproducibility of Silicone Study classification system was 64% for the type of contraction, 77% for the number of clock hours, 67% for the posterior PVR, 88% for the anterior and posterior PVR, and 94% for the anterior, posterior, and subretinal PVR. The reproducibility of Retina Society classification system was 99%. Thus, Retina Society classification was highly reproducible. However, the Silicone Study classification predicted post-operative visual acuity ($P = 0.004$) and incidence of hypotony ($P = 0.01$) better than the Retinal Society classification.[23] Both Silicone Study classification and Retina Society classification do not provide information about biologic activity or risk factors in progression of PVR, and number and location of retinal breaks. The individual evaluator can make an additional note of these findings to give completeness to the current classification of PVR.

TABLE 12.2: Modified retina society classification of retina detachment with the proliferative vitreoretinopathy.

Grade	Features
A	Vitreous haze; vitreous pigment clumps; pigment clusters on inferior retina
B	Wrinkling of inner retinal surface; retinal stiffness; vessel tortuosity; rolled and irregular edge of retinal break; decreased mobility of vitreous
C P 1-12	Posterior to equator; focal diffuse or circumferential full-thickness folds*; subretinal strands*
C A 1-12	Anterior to equator; focal diffuse or circumferential full-thickness folds*; subretinal strands*; anterior displacement*; condensed vitreous with strands

Expressed in the number of clock hours involved

TABLE 12.3: GRADE C PVR of modified retina society classification described by contraction type.

Type	Location (In Relation to Equator)	Features
Focal	Posterior	Star fold posterior to vitreous base
Diffuse	Posterior	Confluent star folds posterior to vitreous base. Optic disc may not be visible
Subretinal	Posterior/ Anterior	Proliferations under the retina; Annular strand near disc; linear strands; motheaten-appearing sheets
Circumferential	Anterior	Contraction along posterior edge of vitreous base with central displacement of the retina: peripheral retina stretched; posterior retina in radial folds
Anterior displacement	Anterior	Vitreous base pulled anteriorly by proliferative tissue; peripheral retinal trough; ciliary processes may be stretched, may be covered by membrane; iris may be retracted

RISK FACTORS

Retinal detachments are particularly at risk of developing PVR if they have any of the following characteristics: giant retinal tear, large or multiple retinal breaks, signs of uveitis, aphakia, vitreous hemorrhage, and pre-operative choroidal detachment.[24,25] Postoperative PVR is most strongly associated with the preoperative presence of PVR grades A and B, uveitis, vitreous hemorrhage (intraoperative or postoperative), excessive cryotherapy, diathermy or photocoagulation, repeated surgical procedures, loss of vitreous during drainage of subretinal fluid, missed or untreated retinal breaks, the use of air or SF_6, and postoperative choroidal detachment.[1,24-27] PVR is the main reason for failures of vitreoretinal surgery.[18] PVR occurs up to 20% of cases following various vitreoretinal surgical procedures.[28] PVR is found in 5–10% of rhegmatogenous RDs.[24] Of these patients, 20–40% have recurring episodes of PVR.[5] Several studies have shown that successful sealing of all retinal breaks does not necessarily provide complete protection against post-operative PVR.[24,25]

CLINICAL FEATURES

Clinical signs of PVR depend on the stage and vary from mild haze and pigment clumps in the vitreous in grade A PVR to epiretinal, vitreous, or subretinal bands and intrinsic retinal contraction in grade C (modified Retina Society classification). The different signs were detailed along with the grading of PVR in Tables 12.2 and 12.3. Grade A PVR is clinically characterized by the presence of vitreous haze and pigment clumps in the presence of rhegmatogenous RD (Fig. 12.2A). The retinal surface is undulated in the detached areas of the retina, but devoid of any surface wrinkles and the retinal breaks have sharp margins. In grade B PVR, wrinkles are observed in the surface of the detached retina with partial restricted mobility and fine pigmented membranes over the surface of the detached retina. The margins of retinal breaks characterized by rolled edges with fine pigmented membrane extending from the edge of the retinal break (Figs. 12.2B and 12.3A) over to the retinal surface in PVR grade B or more. In grade C PVR, the fine transparent pigmented membrane of grade B turns more opaque and contracted, forming either star fold if the membrane is small or a diffuse retinal fold in case of a large membrane (Figs. 12.2C to H and 12.3B). Depending upon the location of these membranes in relation to the equator, they form a part of anterior or posterior PVR. Subretinal membranes usually appear in the form of cords, extending across the quadrants. If the cord-like subretinal membrane is located in the posterior pole surrounding the disc, it forms a napkin ring configuration. Rarely, the subretinal membranes form sieve like sheets under the retina, especially when they are located anterior to the equator. PVR membranes in the region of the vitreous base form different configurations depending on the location and extent of the epiretinal membranes. They may assume a circumferential contraction sheet or as sheets of fibrous membranes pulling the vitreous base or ciliary body anteriorly. One should observe the regions anterior and posterior to equator as well as each clock hour to know the complete extent of PVR (Fig. 12.4).[21,22]

INVESTIGATIONS

Proliferative vitreoretinopathy is best diagnosed and graded by good clinical examination including indirect ophthalmoscopy and slit-lamp biomicroscopy along with Goldmann 3-mirror or 78-D or 90-D contact/non-contact lens examination. When media are cloudy, "A" or "B"-scan ultrasonography is recommended. The area between the ora serrata and the retro-iridian region is not easily visible by scleral indentation or ultrasonography, even when fundus is visible. Ultrasound biomicroscopy (UBM) is a useful tool for the examination of this region and for identifying the presence and extent of anterior PVR.[29] UBM was found to be 92% consistent with surgical observation.[29] In silicone oil-filled eye, ultrasonography images get attenuated due to reflections and attenuation of sound waves. Prone position ultrasonography is shown to yield better images in silicone oil filled eyes.[30] Silicone oil filling does not influence

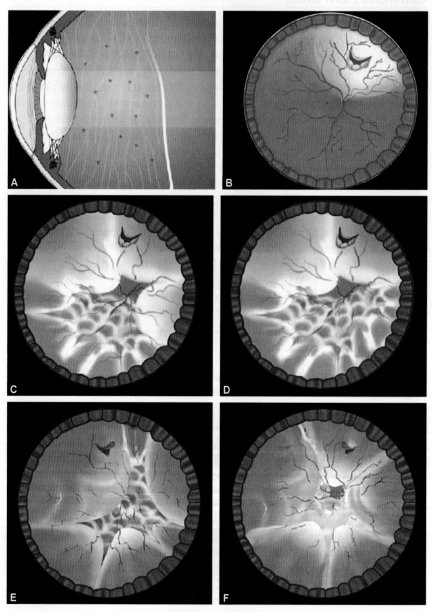

Figs. 12.2A to F

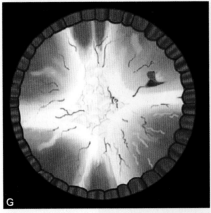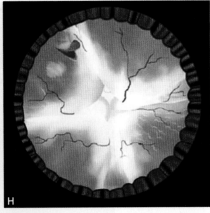

Figs. 12.2G and H

Figs. 12.2A to H: Grades of proliferative vitreoretinopathy (PVR) with rhegmatogenous retinal detachment. (A) Grade A with pigment clumps in the anterior vitreous. (B) Grade B with rolled edges of a retinal break. (C to E) Grade C with full thickness retinal fixed folds in one quadrant (PVR C1, C), two quadrants (PVR C2, D), and three quadrants (PVR C3, E). (F to H) Grade D with full thickness retinal fold in all four quadrants with wide-funnel (PVR D1, F), narrow-funnel (PVR D2, G), and closed-funnel (PVR D3, H).

UBM imaging of the eye ball wall.[29] Optical coherence tomography (OCT) is useful during post-operative period, to assess the macular attachment status and to correlate anatomic results with functional outcomes.[31-33]

MANAGEMENT

Prophylaxis

Transscleral cryopexy has been shown to release viable RPE cells and also causes inflammation and fibrin formation. All three components have been implicated in pathogenesis of PVR. To lessen the risk of PVR, one need to consider methods other than cryotherapy, to create chorioretinal adhesion in patients with a high risk of PVR.[34] In this regard, laser photocoagulation is better than cryopexy, and one should consider laser photocoagulation instead of cryopexy, whenever possible.

Any procedure that produces thermal adhesion of retina induces cell necrosis, inflammation, and fibrocellular proliferation. Efforts have been made to find non-thermal ways of retinal break closure with synthetic tissue adhesives such as cyanoacrylates, polysiloxanes, and acetate polymers or biological tissue adhesives like fibrin and recombinant cytokine TGF-β.[35,36] However, their use has been very limited in clinical setting. Recurrent RD with open retinal breaks is one of the major risk factors for the development of PVR.[24] Successful reattachment of retina with single surgical intervention avoids the development of PVR. One should aim at achieving complete attachment of retina in the first attempt.

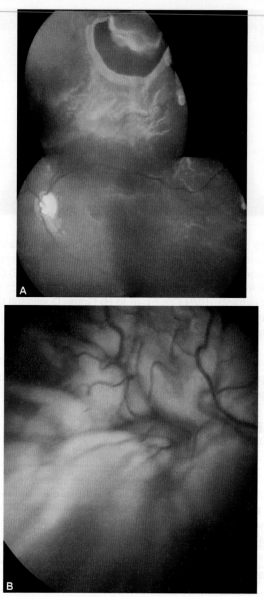

Figs. 12.3A and B: (A) Color fundus photograph showing rhegmatogenous retinal detachment with retinal break in superotemporal quadrant with rolled edges indicative of grade B proliferative vitreoretinopathy. (B) Color fundus photograph showing retinal detachment with full thickness retinal folds and closed funnel retinal detachment (RD) indicative of PVR D3.

Surgical Management

The goals of retinal reattachment surgery for PVR remain the same as those for conventional retinal re-attachment surgery, i.e. to close all retinal breaks

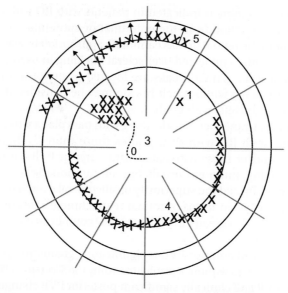

Fig. 12.4: Retina diagram to represent various types of full thickness retinal folds. Type 1: Focal = X, Type 2: Diffuse = XXX, Type 3: Subretinal = ---, Type 4: Circumferential = xxx, and Type 5: Anterior displacement = $x^\uparrow x^\uparrow x^\uparrow$.

and relieve vitreoretinal traction. However, these goals are more difficult to achieve in PVR and the difficulty increases as the severity of PVR increases. The surgical steps in PVR surgery may include scleral buckle/external encircling procedure,[37] standard pars plana vitrectomy with separation of posterior hyaloid till the vitreous base with or without the use of chromovitrectomy techniques,[8,28,38,39] peeling of epiretinal membranes,[5] release of anterior traction membranes,[40] retinotomy/retinectomy,[41-48] release of subretinal membranes,[43] intra-operative use of perfluorocarbon liquids,[49-53] internal tamponading agents (SF6/$C_3 F_8$/silicone oil/heavy silicone oil),[20,21,23,42,54-61] endophotocoagulation,[62] and the use of adjuvant antiproliferative agents.[63-66] A detailed description of each of these procedures is beyond the scope of this chapter. The readers are advised to read the relevant references given at the end of this chapter, so as to obtain an in depth understanding of surgical management.

A surgical approach to a patient with RD with PVR depends largely on grade of PVR, type, number, and location of retinal breaks and media clarity. With the advent of advances in vitreous surgery, it is preferred over scleral buckle for even initial grades of PVR especially in pseudophakic and aphakic eyes.[67] Scleral buckling technique alone may achieve a sustained retinal reattachment with good closure of retinal breaks and relief of traction in early (grades A and B) PVR. There are no clear indications for treating PVR with standard scleral buckling procedure, but PVR grades up to C_1 (Retina Society classification) can be tried if the detachment is associated with small peripheral retinal break unassociated with dynamic traction or an area of PVR.

Pars plana vitrectomy is indicated in patients with RD with early grades of PVR if there is traction from the epiretinal or subretinal membranes in patients in whom the retinal breaks cannot be appropriately sealed by scleral buckling. Vitrectomy is preferred over scleral buckling in pseudophakic and aphakic eyes or if the retinal breaks are located posterior to the equator.[68] Suture less vitrectomy without belt buckle may be considered for patients with rhegmatogenous RD with grade A or B PVR.[69-71] However, PVR grade C or worse would warranty belt buckle along with pars plana vitrectomy.[72]

In patients with RD with PVR grades more than C_1 (Retina Society classification) and/or those associated with anterior PVR, vitrectomy with membrane peeling and a gas or silicone oil tamponade is essential. The silicone study confirmed the superiority of silicone oil over SF6, but not over perfluoropropane gas in terms of retinal reattachment rates or achieving a visual acuity of 5/200 or greater in patients of RD complicated by severe grades of PVR.[73-77]

The prevalence of anterior PVR is significantly greater in eyes with prior vitrectomy than in eyes without a prior vitrectomy (88% versus 73%).[21,78,79] Eyes with anterior PVR and clinically significant posterior PVR changes (>PVR D_1) had a better visual prognosis if silicone oil rather than $C_3 F_8$ gas was used.[21] Patients with severe grades of PVR often require bimanual surgery, removal of the lens, and retinotomy or retinectomy.[40,43,80]

Vitrectomy has improved the surgical results.[81-84] The anatomic success ranges from 60% to 80% depending on the severity of PVR. Eyes with posterior PVR had better outcome at 6-month post-operative follow-up than eyes with anterior PVR.[21,37] Of the anatomically successful patients, 40–80% might recover at least ambulatory vision. Vision may be poor because of macular changes (cystoid macular edema, macular pucker, and subretinal membranes) in a high percentage of patients.[42,56,85,86] The likelihood of achieving a visual acuity of 5/200 or better was greater in eyes when the retinal reattachment was achieved with a single procedure (60%) than in those who required multiple operations (32%).[42]

In our hands, surgical intervention of either sclera buckling or pars plana vitrectomy along with other procedures has resulted in 86% (80/93) of eyes with single intervention and 95.6% (89/93) of eyes with second intervention. However, good visual outcomes have been observed only in 61.2% (57/93) of eyes (unpublished data).

Adjuvant Therapy

Intraoperative use of perfluorocarbon liquids has been widely in practice after their introduction in the 1980s.[50-52] The perfluorocarbon liquid unfolds the retinal flap in giant retinal tears, displaces the subretinal fluid or blood anteriorly, and by applying counter traction stabilizes the retina during membrane peeling in eyes with PVR.[49,87,88] Heavy silicone oil (silicone oil-RMN$_3$ mixture) with density heavier-than-water (1.03 g/cm^3 and viscosity of 3,800 cps) is useful in complicated RDs with inferior retinal tears.[89-95] Triamcinolone acetonide is shown to be useful as an adjuvant tool in delineation of posterior hyaloid and ERMs, allowing a more complete and safer removal of PVR membranes.[96,97] However, corticosteroids are not associated with improved results in terms of prevention or recurrence of PVR.[28]

Several antiproliferative agents have been considered in the treatment of PVR. 5-fluorouracil in isolation or in combination with low-molecular-weight heparin was tried with limited success.[64,65,98,99] Daunorubicin infusion was found non-toxic, but the results were not encouraging.[63,100] Gene therapy-based strategies have also been tried in animal models and were found useful in the prevention of PVR.[7,101,102] However, good clinical trials are lacking to suggest their clinical application.

REFERENCES

1. Asaria RHF, Kon CH, Bunce C, et al. How to predict proliferative vitreoretinopathy: a prospective study. Ophthalmology. 2001;108(7):1184-6.
2. Ryan SJ. The pathophysiology of proliferative vitreoretinopathy in its management. Am J Ophthalmol. 1985;100(1):188-93.
3. Pastor JC. Proliferative vitreoretinopathy: an overview. Surv Ophthalmol. 1998;43(1):3-18.
4. Lopez PF, Grossniklaus HE, Aaberg TM, et al. Pathogenetic mechanisms in anterior proliferative vitreoretinopathy. Am J Ophthalmol. 1992;114(3):257-79.
5. Aaberg TM. Management of anterior and posterior proliferative vitreoretinopathy. XLV Edward Jackson memorial lecture. Am J Ophthalmol. 1988;106:519-32.
6. Lewis H, Aaberg TM. Anterior proliferative vitreoretinopathy. Am J Ophthalmol. 1988;105:277-84.
7. Ikuno Y, Kazlauskas A. An in vivo gene therapy approach for experimental proliferative vitreoretinopathy using the truncated platelet-derived growth factor alpha receptor. Invest Ophthalmol Vis Sci. 2002;43(7):2406-11.
8. Charteris DG. Proliferative vitreoretinopathy: pathobiology, surgical management, and adjunctive treatment. Br J Ophthalmol. 1995;79(10):953-60.
9. Hiscott PS, Grierson J, Mc Leod D. Natural history of fibrocellular epiretinal membrane: a quantitative, autoradiographic and immunohistochemical study. Br J Ophthalmol. 1985;11:810-23.
10. Limb GA, Little BC, Meager A, et al. Cytokines in proliferative vitreoretinopathy. Eye. 1991;5:686-93.
11. La Heij EC, Van de Wearenburg MPH, Blaauwgeers HGT, et al. Basic fibroblast growth factor, glutamine synthetase, and interleukin-6 in vitreous fluid from eyes with retinal detachment complicated by proliferative vitreoretinopathy. Am J Ophthalmol. 2002;134(3):367-75.
12. Wiedemann P. Growth factors in retinal diseases: proliferative vitreoretinopathy, proliferative diabetic retinopathy and retinal degeneration. Surv Ophthalmol. 1992;36:373-84.
13. Ogata N, Nishikawa M, Nishimura T, et al. Inverse levels of pigment epithelium-derived factor and vascular endothelial growth factor in the vitreous of eyes with rhegmatogenous retinal detachment and proliferative vitreoretinopathy. Am J Ophthalmol. 2002;133(6):851-2.
14. Hinton DR, He S, Jin ML, et al. Novel growth factors involved in the pathogenesis of proliferative vitreoretinopathy. Eye. 2002;16(4):422-8.

15. Charteris DG, Hiscott P, Robey HL, et al. Inflammatory cells in proliferative vitreoretinopathy subretinal membranes. Ophthalmology. 1992;99:1364-7.

16. Jin ML, He S, Worpel V, et al. Promotion of adhesion and migration of RPE cells to provisional extracellular matrices by TNF-α. Invest Ophthalmol Vis Sci. 2000;41(13):4324-32.

17. Connor TB Jr., Roberts AB, Sporn MB, et al. Correlation of fibrosis and transforming growth factor-beta type 2 levels in the eye. J Clin Invest. 1989;83(5):1661-6.

18. Machemer R. Pathogenesis and classification of massive periretinal proliferation. Br J Ophthalmol. 1978;62(11):737-47.

19. The retina society terminology committee. The classification of retinal detachment with proliferative vitreoretinopathy. Ophthalmology. 1983;90(2):121-5.

20. Lean JS, Stern WH, Irvine AR, et al. Classification of proliferative vitreoretinopathy used in the silicone study. The silicone oil study group. Ophthalmology. 1989;96(6):765-71.

21. Diddie KR, Azen SP, Freeman HM, et al. Anterior proliferative vitreoretinopathy in the silicone study. Silicone study report number 10. Ophthalmology. 1996;103(7):1092-9.

22. Machemer R, Aaberg TM, Freeman HM, et al. An updated classification of retinal detachment with proliferative vitreoretinopathy. Am J Ophthalmol. 1991;112: 159-65.

23. Lean J, Azen SP, Lopez PF, et al. The prognostic utility of the silicone study classification system. Silicone study report 9. Silicone study group. Arch Ophthalmol. 1996;114(3):286-92.

24. Girard P, Mimoun G, Karpouzas I, et al. Clinical risk factors for proliferative vitreoretinopathy after retinal detachment surgery. Retina. 1994;14(5):417-24.

25. Cowley M, Conway BP, Campochiaro PA, et al. Clinical risk factors for proliferative vitreoretinopathy. Arch Ophthalmol. 1989;107(8):1147-51.

26. Tseng W, Cortez RT, Ramirez G, et al. Prevalence and risk factors for proliferative vitreoretinopathy in eyes with rhegmatogenous retinal detachment but no previous vitreoretinal surgery. Am J Ophthalmol. 2004;137(6):1105-15.

27. Mitry D, Singh J, Yorston D, et al. The predisposing pathology and clinical characteristics in the Scottish retinal detachment study. Ophthalmology. 2011;118(7):1429-34.

28. Ryan SJ. Traction retinal detachment. XLIX Edward Jackson memorial lecture. Am J Ophthalmol. 1993;115(1):1-20.

29. Liu W, Wu Q, Haung S, et al. Ultrasound biomicroscopic features of anterior proliferative vitreoretinopathy. Retina. 1999;19(3):204-12.

30. Kumar A, Sharma N, Singh R. Prone position ultrasonography in silicone filled eyes. Acta Ophthalmol Scand. 1998;76(4):496-8.

31. Odrobina DC, Michalewska Z, Michalewski J, et al. High-speed, high-resolution spectral optical coherence tomography in patients after vitrectomy with internal limiting membrane peeling for proliferative vitreoretinopathy retinal detachment. Retina. 2010;30(6):881-6.

32. Kiss CG, Richter-Müksch S, Sacu S, et al. Anatomy and function of the macula after surgery for retinal detachment complicated by proliferative vitreoretinopathy. Am J Ophthalmol. 2007;144(6):872-7.

33. Benson SE, Grigoropoulos V, Schlottmann PG, et al. Analysis of the macula with optical coherence tomography after successful surgery for proliferative vitreoretinopathy. Arch Ophthalmol. 2005;123(12):1651-6.

34. Glasser BM, Vidaurri-Leal J, Michels R, et al. Cryotherapy during surgery for giant retinal tears and intravitreal dispersion of viable retinal pigment epithelial cells. Ophthalmology. 1993;100(4):466-70.
35. Gilbert CE. Adhesives in retinal detachment surgery. Br J Ophthalmol. 1991;75(5):309-10.
36. Coleman DJ, Lucas BC, Fleischmann JA, et al. A biologic tissue adhesive for vitreoretinal surgery. Retina. 1988;8(4):250-6.
37. Hanneken AM, Michels RG. Vitrectomy and scleral buckling methods for proliferative vitreoretinopathy. Ophthalmology. 1988;95(7):865-9.
38. Farah ME, Maia M, Rodrigues EB. Dyes in ocular surgery: principles for use in chromovitrectomy. Am J Ophthalmol. 2009; 148(3): 332-40.
39. Teba FA, Mohr A, Eckardt C, et al. Trypan blue staining in vitreoretinal surgery. Ophthalmology. 2003;110(12):2409-12.
40. De Juan E, McCuen BW II. Management of anterior vitreous traction in proliferative vitreoretinopathy. Retina. 1989;9(4):258-62.
41. Machemer R, McCuen B, de Juan E. Relaxing retinotomies and retinectomies. Am J Ophthalmol. 1986;102(1):7-12.
42. Blumenkranz MS, Azen SP, Aaberg T, et al. Relaxing retinotomy with silicone oil or long-acting gas in eyes with severe proliferative vitreoretinopathy. Silicone Study report 5. The Silicone Study Group. Am J Ophthalmol. 1993;116(5):557-64.
43. Federman JL, Eagle RC. Extensive peripheral retinectomy combined with posterior 360 degrees retinotomy for retinal reattachment in advanced proliferative vitreoretinopathy cases. Ophthalmology. 1990;97(10):1305-20.
44. Tan HS, Mura M, Oberstein SY, et al. Primary retinectomy in proliferative vitreoretinopathy. Am J Ophthalmol. 2010;149(3):447-52.
45. Tsui I, Schubert HD. Retinotomy and silicone oil for detachments complicated by anterior inferior proliferative vitreoretinopathy. Br J Ophthalmol. 2009;93(9): 1228-33.
46. Banaee T, Hosseini SM, Eslampoor A, et al. Peripheral 360 degrees retinectomy in complex retinal detachment. Retina. 2009;29(6):811-8.
47. Lim AK, Alexander SM, Lim KS. Combined large radial retinotomy and circumferential retinectomy in the management of advanced proliferative vitreoretinopathy. Retina. 2009;29(1):112-6.
48. Tseng JJ, Barile GR, Schiff WM, et al. Influence of relaxing retinotomy on surgical outcomes in proliferative vitreoretinopathy. Am J Ophthalmol. 2005;140(4):628-36.
49. Scott IU, Flynn HW Jr., Murray TG, Fewer WJ. The perfluoron study group. Outcomes of surgery for retinal detachment associated with proliferative vitreoretinopathy using perfluoro-n-octane: A multicenter study. Am J Ophthalmol. 2003;136:454-63.
50. Chang S, Zimmerman NJ, Iwamoto J, et al. Experimental vitreous replacement with perfluorotributylamine. Am J Ophthalmol. 1987; 103(1):29-37.
51. Chang S. Low viscosity liquid fluorochemicals in vitreous surgery. Am J Ophthalmol 1987;103(1):38-43.
52. Chang S, Ozmert E, Zimmerman NJ. Intraoperative perfluorocarbon liquids in the management of proliferative vitreoretinopathy. Am J Ophthalmol 1988;106(6): 668-74.
53. Sirimaharaj M, Balachandran C, Chan WC, et al. Vitrectomy with short term postoperative tamponade using perfluorocarbon liquid for giant retinal tears. Br J Ophthalmol. 2005;89(9):1176-9.
54. Norton EWD. Intraocular gas in the management of selected retinal detachment. Trans Am Acad Ophthalmol Otolaryngol. 1973;77(2):85-98.

55. Hutton WL, Azen SP, Blumenkranz MS. The effects of silicone oil removal. Silicone study report 6. Arch Ophthalmol. 1994;112(6):778-85.
56. Silicone study group. Macular pucker after successful surgery for proliferative vitreoretinopathy. Silicone study report 8. Ophthalmology. 1995;102:1884-91.
57. Lincoff IT, Coleman J, Kreissig I, et al. The perfluorocarbon gases in the treatment of retinal detachment. Ophthalmology. 1983;90(5):546-51.
58. Schwartz SG, Flynn HW Jr, Lee WH, et al. Tamponade in surgery for retinal detachment associated with proliferative vitreoretinopathy. Cochrane Database Syst Rev. 2009;(4):CD006126.
59. Rizzo S, Genovesi-Ebert F, Vento A, et al. A new heavy silicone oil (HWS 46-3000) used as a prolonged internal tamponade agent in complicated vitreoretinal surgery: a pilot study. Retina. 2007;27(5):613-20.
60. Wong D, Van Meurs JC, Stappler T, et al. A pilot study on the use of a perfluorohexyloctane/silicone oil solution as a heavier than water internal tamponade agent. Br J Ophthalmol. 2005;89(6):662-5.
61. Tognetto D, Minutola D, Sanguinetti G, et al. Anatomical and functional outcomes after heavy silicone oil tamponade in vitreoretinal surgery for complicated retinal detachment: a pilot study. Ophthalmology. 2005;112(9):1574.
62. Parke DW, Aaberg TM. Intraocular argon laser photocoagulation in the management of severe proliferative vitreoretinopathy. Am J Ophthalmol. 1984;97(4):434-43.
63. Wiedemann P, Hilgers RD, Bauer P, et al. Adjunctive daunorubicin in the treatment of proliferative vitreoretinopathy: results of a multicenter clinical trial. Daunomycin study group. Am J Ophthalmol. 1998;126:550-9.
64. Asaria RHY, Kon CH, Bunce C, et al. Adjuvant 5-fluorouracil and Heparin prevents proliferative vitreoretinopathy: Results from a randomized, double-blind, controlled clinical trial. Ophthalmology. 2001;108(7):1179-83.
65. Blumenkraz MS, Ophir A, Claflin AJ, et al. Fluorouracil for the treatment of massive periretinal proliferation. Am J Ophthalmol. 1982;94(4):458-67.
66. Tano Y, Sugita G, Abrams G, Machemer R. Inhibition of intraocular proliferations with intravitreal corticosteroids. Am J Ophthalmol. 1980;89(1):131-6.
67. Ahmadieh H, Moradian S, Faghihi H, et al. Pseudophakic and Aphakic Retinal Detachment (PARD) Study Group. Anatomic and visual outcomes of scleral buckling versus primary vitrectomy in pseudophakic and aphakic retinal detachment: six-month follow-up results of a single operation—report no. 1. Ophthalmology. 2005;112(8):1421-9.
68. Martínez-Castillo V, Boixadera A, Verdugo A, García-Arumí J. Pars plana vitrectomy alone for the management of inferior breaks in pseudophakic retinal detachment without facedown position. Ophthalmology. 2005;112(7):1222-6.
69. Mura M, Tan SH, De Smet MD. Use of 25-gauge vitrectomy in the management of primary rhegmatogenous retinal detachment. Retina. 2009;29(9):1299-304.
70. Horozoglu F, Yanyali A, Celik E, et al. Primary 25-gauge transconjunctival sutureless vitrectomy in pseudophakic retinal detachment. Indian J Ophthalmol. 2007;55(5):337-40.
71. Oyagi T, Emi K. Vitrectomy without scleral buckling for proliferative vitreoretinopathy. Retina. 2004;24(2):215-8.
72. Weichel ED, Martidis A, Fineman MS, et al. Pars plana vitrectomy versus combined pars plana vitrectomy-scleral buckle for primary repair of pseudophakic retinal detachment. Ophthalmology 2006; 113(11): 2033-40.

73. McCuen BW, Azen SP, Stern W, et al. Vitrectomy with silicone oil or perfluoropropane gas in eyes with severe proliferative vitreoretinopathy. Silicone study report 3. Retina. 1993;13(4):279-84.
74. The Silicone Study Group. Vitrectomy with silicone oil or perfluoropropane gas in eyes with severe proliferative vitreoretinopathy: results of a randomized clinical trial. Silicone study report 2. Arch Ophthalmol. 1992;110(6):780-92.
75. The Silicone Study Group. Vitrectomy with silicone oil or sulfur hexafluoride gas in eyes with severe proliferative vitreoretinopathy: results of a randomized clinical trial. Silicone study report 1. Arch Ophthalmol. 1992;110(6):770-79.
76. Alexander P, Prasad R, Ang A, et al. Prevention and control of proliferative vitreoretinopathy: primary retinal detachment surgery using silicone oil as a planned two-stage procedure in high-risk cases. Eye. 2008;22(6):815-8.
77. Quiram PA, Gonzales CR, Hu W, et al. Outcomes of vitrectomy with inferior retinectomy in patients with recurrent rhegmatogenous retinal detachments and proliferative vitreoretinopathy. Ophthalmology. 2006;113(11):2041-7.
78. Yang CM, Hsieh YT, Yang CH, et al. Irrigation-free vitreoretinal surgery for recurrent retinal detachment in silicone oil-filled eyes. Eye. 2006;20(12):1379-82.
79. Lesnoni G, Rossi T, Gelso A, et al. Patient satisfaction and vision improvement after multiple surgery for recurrent retinal detachment. Eur J Ophthalmol. 2005;15(1):102-8.
80. Bourke RD, Cooling RJ. Vascular consequences of retinectomy. Arch ophthalmol. 1996;114:155-60.
81. Pastor JC, Fernández I, Rodríguez de la Rúa E, et al. Surgical outcomes for primary rhegmatogenous retinal detachments in phakic and pseudophakic patients: the Retina 1 Project—report 2. Br J Ophthalmol. 2008;92(3):378-82.
82. Lam RF, Cheung BT, Yuen CY, et al. Retinal redetachment after silicone oil removal in proliferative vitreoretinopathy: a prognostic factor analysis. Am J Ophthalmol. 2008;145(3):527-33.
83. Heimann H, Bartz-Schmidt KU, Bornfeld N, et al. Scleral buckling versus primary vitrectomy in rhegmatogenous retinal detachment: a prospective randomized multicenter clinical study. Scleral Buckling versus Primary Vitrectomy in Rhegmatogenous Retinal Detachment Study Group. Ophthalmology. 2007; 114(12):2142-54.
84. Brazitikos PD, Androudi S, Christen WG, et al. Primary pars plana vitrectomy versus scleral buckle surgery for the treatment of pseudophakic retinal detachment: a randomized clinical trial. Retina. 2005;25(8):957-64.
85. James M, O'Doherty M, Beatty S. The prognostic influence of chronicity of rhegmatogenous retinal detachment on anatomic success after reattachment surgery. Am J Ophthalmol. 2007;143(6):1032-4.
86. Doyle E, Herbert EN, Bunce C, et al. How effective is macula-off retinal detachment surgery. Might good outcome be predicted? Eye. 2007;21(4):534-40.
87. Glasser BM, Carter JB, Kuppermann BD, et al. Perfluoro–Octane in the treatment of giant retinal tears with proliferative vitreoretinopathy. Ophthalmology. 1991;98:1613-21.
88. Ang GS, Townend J, Lois N. Epidemiology of giant retinal tears in the United Kingdom: the British Giant Retinal Tear Epidemiology Eye Study (BGEES). Invest Ophthalmol Vis Sci. 2010;51(9):4781-7.
89. Wolf S, Schon V, Meier P, et al. Silicone oil–RMN 3 Mixture (Heavy silicone oil) as internal tamponade for complicated retinal detachment. Retina. 2003;23:335-42.
90. Joussen AM, Wong D. The concept of heavy tamponades-chances and limitations. Graefes Arch Clin Exp Ophthalmol. 2008;246(9):1217-24.

91. Heimann H, Stappler T, Wong D. Heavy tamponade 1: a review of indications, use, and complications. Eye. 2008;22(10):1342-59.
92. Sandner D, Herbrig E, Engelmann K. High-density silicone oil (Densiron) as a primary intraocular tamponade: 12-month follow up. Graefes Arch Clin Exp Ophthalmol. 2007;245(8):1097-105.
93. Scott IU, Flynn HW Jr, Murray TG, et al. Outcomes of surgery for retinal detachment associated with proliferative vitreoretinopathy using perfluoro-n-octane: a multicenter study. Am J Ophthalmol. 2003;136(3):454-63.
94. Duan A, She H, Qi Y. Complications after heavy silicone oil tamponade in complicated retinal detachment. Retina. 2011;31(3):547-52.
95. Drury B, Bourke RD. Short-term intraocular tamponade with perfluorocarbon heavy liquid. Br J Ophthalmol. 2011;95(5):694-8.
96. Furino C, Ferrari TM, Boscia F, et al. Triamcinolone-assisted pars plana vitrectomy for proliferative vitreoretinopathy. Retina 2003; 23(6): 771-6.
97. Ahmadieh H, Feghhi M, Tabatabaei H, et al. Triamcinolone acetonide in silicone-filled eyes as adjunctive treatment for proliferative vitreoretinopathy: a randomized clinical trial. Ophthalmology 2008;115(11):1938-43.
98. Sundaram V, Barsam A, Virgili G. Intravitreal low molecular weight heparin and 5-Fluorouracil for the prevention of proliferative vitreoretinopathy following retinal reattachment surgery. Cochrane Database Syst Rev. 2010;(7):CD006421.
99. Charteris DG, Aylward GW, Wong D, et al. A randomized controlled trial of combined 5-fluorouracil and low-molecular-weight heparin in management of established proliferative vitreoretinopathy. PVR Study Group. Ophthalmology 2004;111(12):2240-5.
100. Shinohara K, Tanaka M, Sakuma T, et al. Efficacy of daunorubicin encapsulated in liposome for the treatment of proliferative vitreoretinopathy. Ophthalmic Surg Lasers Imaging. 2003;34:299-305.
101. Sakamoto T, Kimura H, Scuric Z, et al. Inhibition of experimental proliferative vitreoretinopathy by retroviral vector mediated transfer of suicide gene. Can proliferative vitreoretinopathy be a target of gene therapy? Ophthalmology. 1995;102:1417-24.
102. Mori K, Gehlbach P, Ando A, et al. Intraocular adenoviral vector-mediated gene transfer in proliferative retinopathies. Invest Ophthalmol Vis Sci. 2002;43:1610-5.

CHAPTER 13

Diagnostic Procedures in Retinopathy of Prematurity

Yog Raj Sharma, Parijat Chandra, Rajni Sharma, Rajvardhan Azad

INTRODUCTION

Retinopathy of prematurity (ROP) is a vasoproliferative disorder of the retina and is an important cause of childhood blindness in preterm infants. There are multiple risk factors[1] that are associated with the development and severity of ROP like low birth weight, early gestational age, multiple birth, hyperoxia, hypoxemia, hypercarbia, hypocarbia, respiratory distress syndrome, apnea, blood transfusions, sepsis, intraventricular hemorrhage (IVH), prolonged parenteral nutrition, etc.

With improvement in neonatal care, smaller babies continue to survive, and the incidence of ROP is on the rise, especially in developing countries like India.[2] This is compounded by the lack of awareness about ROP among pediatricians and ophthalmologists, which leads to late presentation of these babies with advanced disease, thereby causing blindness. The timely diagnosis of ROP is important to prevent the progression of the disease, and to treat it in a timely manner to prevent blindness.

The understanding of pathogenesis, screening and management of retinopathy of prematurity has markedly changed since Terry first described it. Guided initially by the Multicenter Trial of Cryotherapy for Retinopathy of Prematurity (Cryo-ROP)[3] and now the Early Treatment Retinopathy of Prematurity (ETROP)[4] study, there are now clear national and international guidelines for the screening and treatment of ROP.

RETINOPATHY OF PREMATURITY CLASSIFICATION

During normal retinal development, the retinal vessels start to develop at the optic disk at approximately 16 weeks of gestation and migrate towards the ora serrata. They reach the nasal ora serrata by 36 weeks of gestation and the temporal ora serrata by 39–41 weeks of gestation. The interruption of this normal vasculogenesis leads to ROP. The retinal ischemia in avascular retina leads to the development of neovascularization at the junction, which can advance to retinal detachment in advanced stages of ROP.

The International Classification of Retinopathy of Prematurity (ICROP)[3] was devised by an international group of retinopathy of prematurity experts.[5] This classification divided the ROP presentation by zones and stages, and thereby helped in communication between ophthalmologists and neonatologists.

Zones

The coordinated developmental sequence permits the retina to be subdivided into 3 concentric zones (Fig. 13.1):
1. *Zone 1:* Circle from the center of the disk with a radius of twice the distance from the disk to the macula.
2. *Zone 2:* From the nasal edge of zone 1 to the ora nasally and up to the equator temporally.
3. *Zone 3:* From temporal crescent of retina anterior to zone II.

Stages

The different stages described by ICROP are as follows:
1. *Stage 1–Demarcation line:* The earliest feature of ROP in a premature baby is the development of a flat white line at the junction of vascularized and avascular retina (Fig. 13.2). The demarcation line can develop in any zone depending upon the level of prematurity.
2. *Stage 2–Demarcation ridge:* The demarcation line gains height and width and progresses to a ridge which is pink or white, with elevation of the thickened tissue (Fig. 13.3). Some neovascular tufts can be seen posterior to this ridge.
3. *Stage 3–Extraretinal fibrovascular proliferation:* Neovascular growth occurs into and above the ridge (Fig. 13.4). The vessels also grow into the vitreous and can lead to vitreous hemorrhage.

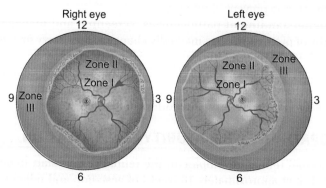

Fig. 13.1: Zones of retinopathy of prematurity.

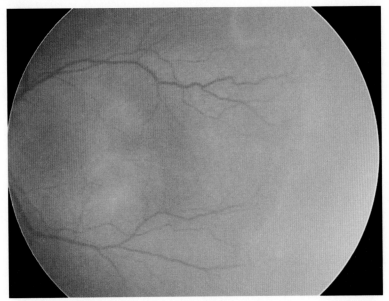

Fig. 13.2: Stage 1 retinopathy of prematurity (ROP): Demarcation line.

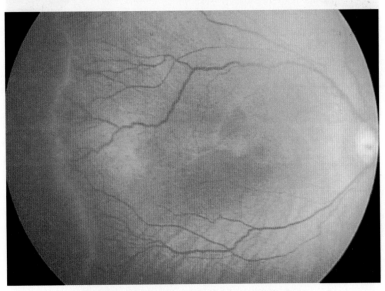

Fig. 13.3: Stage 2 ROP: Demarcation ridge.

4. *Stage 4–Partial retinal detachment:* With progressive growth into the vitreous, the contraction of the fibrovascular proliferation exerts traction on the retina, leading to partial retinal detachment, Stage 4 ROP (Fig. 13.5), either without foveal involvement or with foveal involvement.

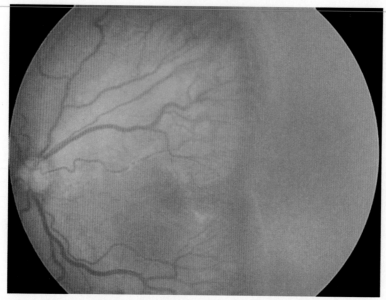

Fig. 13.4: Stage 3 ROP: Extraretinal neovascularization.

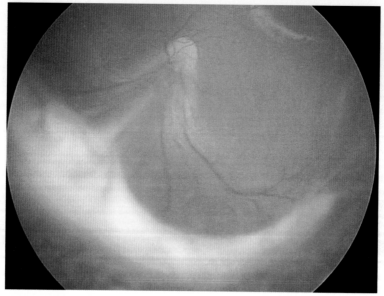

Fig. 13.5: Stage 4 ROP: Subtotal retinal detachment.

5. *Stage 5–Total retinal detachment:* These retinal detachments are mostly funnel-shaped (Fig. 13.6) and their configuration can further be described as open and closed anteriorly, and open or closed posteriorly.

    Some other important terminologies associated with ROP are discussed here.

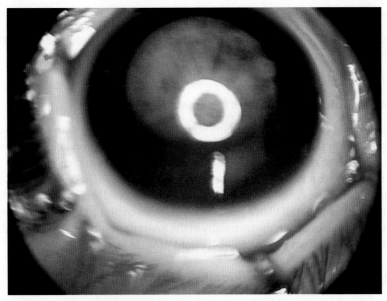

Fig. 13.6: Stage 5 ROP: Total retinal detachment.

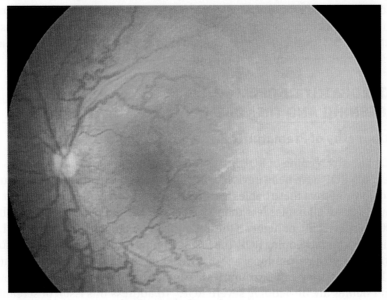

Fig. 13.7: Plus disease.

Plus Disease

Plus disease is defined as the dilated and tortuous blood vessels at the posterior pole along with pupillary rigidity and media haze (Fig. 13.7). It is an indicator of activity of ROP, and an important criterion for the treatment and regression of the disease.

Threshold Retinopathy of Prematurity

Threshold ROP is defined as stage 3 + ROP in zone-I or -II, or zone-I any stage with no plus, occupying at least 5 contiguous clock hours or 8 noncontiguous clock hours of retina.

Prethreshold Retinopathy of Prematurity

Prethreshold ROP is defined as any stage of ROP in zone-1 with plus disease and ROP stage 3 plus with 3 contiguous or 5 noncontiguous clock hours of involvement of retina in zone-II, but less than threshold stage.

Recently, the ICROP classification was updated.[6] They introduced the concept of a more virulent form of retinopathy observed in the smallest babies, aggressive posterior ROP or APROP. They also described an intermediate level called pre-plus in which the tortuosity of the posterior pole vessels is more than normal but less than plus disease. It could progress to plus disease.

Aggressive Posterior Retinopathy of Prematurity

Aggressive posterior ROP is a severe form of ROP which is characterized by posterior zone, severe plus disease, fast progression to stage 5, a featureless junction of vascular and avascular retina, and a high rate of progression to blindness. It is important to have a high index of suspicion for aggressive posterior ROP, ensure its timely detection by ROP screening programs, and perform complete treatment when indicated at the earliest.

RETINOPATHY OF PREMATURITY SCREENING AND TREATMENT

Retinopathy of Prematurity Screening Guidelines

To facilitate screening of ROP in a standardized manner, clear guidelines for screening ROP have been devised which has helped experts across the world to screen and treat these babies in time. The American guidelines[7] suggest we should screen all babies less than 30 weeks of gestational age and less than 1500 g birth weight, or higher if the attending neonatologist believes the child is high-risk for developing ROP. The first screening of all babies should be done at 31 weeks postconceptional age or 4 weeks after birth, whichever was later.

However, in developing countries like India, due to poor neonatal care, even larger babies are developing severe ROP.[8] To address this issue of screening bigger babies, the National Neonatology Forum (NNF) of India guidelines[9] suggests that ROP screening should be performed in all preterm neonates who are less than 34 weeks gestation age and/or less than 1,750 g birth weight. Larger babies between 34 weeks and 36 weeks gestational age or birth weight between 1,750 grams and 2,000 grams can also be screened if they have risk factors for ROP. The first screening should be performed not later than 4 weeks of age. However, in very small infants born less than 28 weeks or less than 1200 g birth weight, they can be screened as early as 2–3 weeks of age, for early detection of APROP.

Retinopathy of Prematurity Screening Procedure

Screening is best performed at the Neonatal ICU under the supervision of a trained neonatology staff to monitor the vital parameters during examination. Pupillary dilation can be achieved by 2.5% phenylephrine and 0.5% tropicamide eye drops instilled twice at an interval of 15 minutes. ROP screening is performed with a binocular indirect ophthalmoscope with a 28D/20D lens by an experienced ophthalmologist, preferably a retina expert or a pediatric ophthalmologist. Both the anterior and the posterior segments of the eye are examined and all clock hours of the retina are examined with indentation to detect the disease. Scleral indentation helps examine the retinal periphery, to rotate the eye to see areas of interest, and contrast structures by gentle indentation. It is necessary to record all the screening findings accurately and correctly in a detailed form to prevent ambiguity, and ensure correct data recording for medical documentation, referral and follow-up.

Retinopathy of Prematurity Treatment

The ETROP group[4] gave clear guidelines for laser treatment of the avascular retina in ROP and classified ROP into type I and type II ROP. They suggested that the early laser treatment should be done for type 1 ROP defined as: (a) Any stage of ROP in zone-I with plus disease (b) Stage 3 ROP in zone-I with or without plus disease and (c) Stage 2/3 ROP in zone-II with plus disease. In cases of type-II ROP, based on the zone, stage, plus disease, the babies are followed up at an interval of 1–2 weeks.

Recently, anti-VEGF drugs like bevacizumab have found renewed interest as an adjunct to laser treatment in progressive diseases, and in some cases as a primary treatment for zone 1 APROP, but its safety profile still needs to be established.[10] Stage 4–5 ROP are advanced stages of the disease and need vitreoretinal surgery. The surgical outcomes in stage IV ROP are good, as only subtotal retinal detachment has occurred[11] but the surgical results in stage V ROP are poor[12] as complete retinal detachment is difficult to operate and is often associated with secondary glaucoma, corneal opacity, etc.

There are various diagnostic modalities which are helpful in understanding the disease process of ROP and improving its outcomes like, wide-field retinal screening, fluorescein angiography, ultrasound biomicroscopy, B-scan ultrasound, hand-held optical coherence tomography (OCT), etc. Let's elaborate the role of some of these modalities.

Wide-field Retinal Screening

Wide-field pediatric retinal imaging systems are useful to screen the eyes of preterm babies for ROP. Retcam (Clarity Medical Systems, Inc., United States) is a popular tool that offers a quicker, faster way to examine these babies with much less stress compared to indirect ophthalmoscopy. In fact, it is possible to document the entire retina in as few as five images. The second-generation ROP lens provides a wide-angle view of the retina with a field of 130°. It has several interchangeable lenses to capture images in different magnifications. A coupling medium is required and the hand-held camera is placed directly over the cornea, changing the focus and brightness using the foot switch to record high-quality images. It allows real-time imaging, storage, and image retrieval, and allows easy access of patient data and images for review, opinion, and teaching.

Retcam 3 is the latest version with benefits like flat monitor, frame-by-frame video review, 20-second video capture and is especially useful for performing fluorescein angiography (Fig. 13.8). It is a useful tool for training residents, counseling parents and can be performed by a trained technician or nurse in any location like the neonatal ICU or the operation theatre if needed.

A major use of wide-field imaging has been for tele-screening purposes. Retcam examination performed by technicians can be transmitted to a central reading center where ROP experts can review the images and advise necessary action. The development of ROP-specific mobile applications allows images to be reviewed by ROP experts on their mobile phones anywhere in the world. Digital photography has a high degree of specificity and sensitivity for detecting and referral-warranted ROP is a very cost-effective option. Stanford University Network for Diagnosis of Retinopathy of Prematurity (SUNDROP)[13] and the Karnataka Internet Assisted Diagnosis of Retinopathy of Prematurity

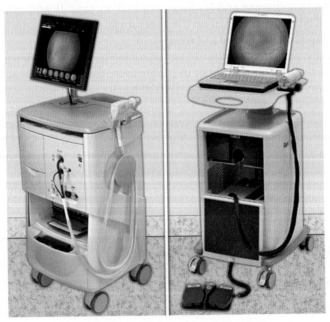

Fig. 13.8: Retcam 3 and Retcam shuttle.

(KIDROP)[14] program in Karnataka are examples of successful tele-screening models.

A major limitation of the Retcam is that it is very expensive. The growing popularity of wide-field imaging has led to the development of many cheaper wide-field indigenous cameras like 3nethra Neo (Forus Health Pvt Ltd), which have similar specifications, yet are more portable and cheaper. Some have even tried out ultra-wide-field imaging of ROP using Optomap-200TX, an imaging equipment providing 200° field of view, and that too by a noncontact mechanism, but this is difficult to perform in preterm babies.[15]

Tele-screening is expected to become mainstream in the coming years to meet the ROP screening needs of the growing number of NICUs, and neonatologists might take a lead to conduct ROP screening in future.[16]

Fluorescein Angiography

Fluorescein angiography is a very useful tool[17,18] to study in detail the vascular status of ROP eyes. Fluorescein angiography is performed with the help of the fluorescein angiography module of the Retcam. Before performing fluorescein angiography, it is essential to take informed consent from the parents. The vitals monitoring is done by the attending neonatologist.

The Retcam is prepared by switching to the blue light source, then the yellow filter is inserted into the camera hand piece, and the timer is set when the procedure is to be started. An intravenous cannula is inserted in the baby, flushed with saline, and prepared before dye injection. The child's eye is topically anesthetized with proparacaine eye drops, then the lid speculum is inserted, and the coupling gel media is poured over the cornea. To start the fluorescein angiography procedure, the neonatologist injects the sodium fluorescein dye via the intravenous cannula, and simultaneously the timer is started on the Retcam, and the hand-held camera is placed over the cornea and the fluorescein angiography is performed. Sodium fluorescein dye 20% is used in the dose of 4 mg/kg. All phases of the fluorescein angiography are recorded, with images being taken every 10 seconds initially, and then every consecutive minute till about 10 minutes.

Fluorescein angiography is especially useful in the diagnosis and management of cases of aggressive posterior ROP. It helps visualize areas of flat neovascularization, which are not seen easily by the naked eye. Though these areas may appear featureless, and the demarcation junction may be difficult to visualize, fluorescein angiography helps clearly visualize the junction and also shows extensive dye leakage in areas of neovascularization (Figs. 13.9A and B), which might help experts make early decision for treatment.

Sometimes there are vascular loops which confuse residents regarding the posterior extent of laser treatment. Incomplete laser treatment sparing a large area of posterior retina will eventually lead to ROP progression. Thus, detecting avascular areas behind these vascular loops, and treating these areas completely with the laser is essential, and fluorescein angiography provides a clear visualization of these areas helping residents perform the complete laser treatment.

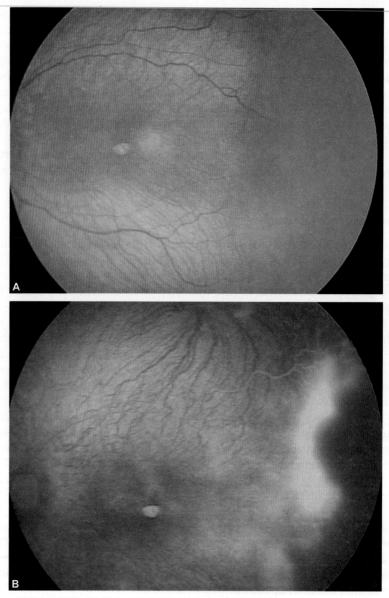

Figs. 13.9A and B: (A) Retcam photo of left eye showing faint ridge. (B) which leaks heavily on fluorescein angiography, suggestive of extensive neovascularization.

Even with ROP experts managing cases of aggressive posterior ROP, sometimes the plus disease persists despite the best of laser treatment. Fluorescein angiography helps detect skip areas of treatment, or identify new areas of avascular retina which were not visible to the naked eye earlier, thereby ensuring that complete laser treatment is performed and prevent ROP sequelae like macular dragging.

However, fluorescein angiography has some limitations. In nondilating pupils, not much information can be elicited. In cases of aggressive posterior ROP, with severe plus disease, the dye may leak quickly into the anterior chamber and vitreous chamber, making visualization very difficult. Therefore, there is a small window of time to record all the useful information from fluorescein angiography. In some cases, the dye takes a long time to transit across the eye, leading to late venous filling; while in other cases, there may be early dye wash out, making the late phase information of not much use.

Ultrasound Biomicroscopy

Ultrasound biomicroscopy is a very useful tool[19] to study the lens, ciliary body, anterior vitreous, pars plana in babies with ROP (Fig. 13.10). UBM is helpful particularly in cases of advanced stage-5 ROP which undergo complex vitreoretinal surgery.

Since advanced cases of ROP are associated with extensive anterior vitreoretinal traction and retrolental membranes, there is little space behind the lens and in the anterior vitreous for surgical instrument entry and movement. The UBM helps determine the anterior surgical space in all quadrants, and finds the maximum space where it will be easier to insert the surgical instruments, without trauma and associated complications. UBM in ROP babies is also a useful tool for decision-making for lensectomy in surgery for stage 5 ROP. UBM can clearly define landmarks related to the lens, tractional retina, vitreous membranes, ciliary body and adjacent spaces.

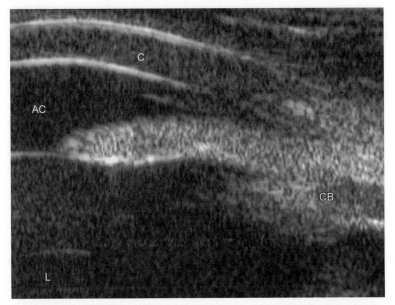

Fig. 13.10: Ultrasound biomicroscopy showing area of surgical access in stage 5 ROP. (C: cornea; AC: anterior chamber; L: lens; CB: ciliary body)

Performing a UBM examination in preterm babies is difficult. Although the UBM settings are mostly the same, it is difficult to make children cooperate for the procedure. After topical anesthesia, a lid speculum is inserted, followed by a UBM cup to hold the viscous gel. Sometimes, the eyes are so small that there is no space to insert a UBM cup, and in such cases it might be useful to create small well using cotton, and then pour the coupling medium inside the cotton well. Since these children constantly move their eyes, performing UBM examination is not easy, and areas of interest are difficult to capture.

Interpreting UBM images requires a thorough understanding of the pathoanatomy of ROP, its development and progression through different stages. Reviewing the UBM images before surgery for advanced ROP can provide useful information for the surgeon.

Ultrasonography

Ultrasound examination is a useful investigative tool for the examination of cases with advanced ROP, especially in stage 5 ROP (Fig. 13.11).[20] Usually these cases carry a very poor prognosis for surgical intervention, and B-scan ultrasound helps examine the posterior segment of the eye when the anterior segment limits the visibility of the fundus, in cases with shallow anterior chamber, posterior synechiae, cataract, dense retrolental fibrovascular proliferation, etc.

From a surgical point-of-view, an ultrasound helps determine the funnel configuration of the tractional retinal detachment in stage 5 ROP and it can

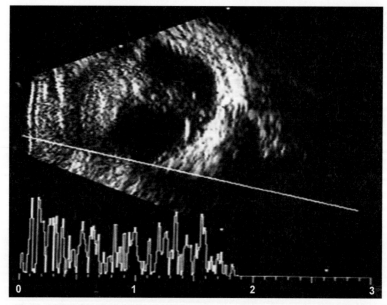

Fig. 13.11: Ultrasound showing anterior open and posterior closed funnel retinal detachment in stage 5 ROP.

be divided into various categories like open–open, narrow–narrow, open–narrow and narrow–open funnel configurations. On the basis of the funnel configuration, the surgeon gets a good idea about the posterior segment and then decides whether to operate or not, or plan the surgical steps, and advise the parents regarding the prognosis of the case and the possible outcomes.

Optical Coherence Tomography

Recently, optical coherence tomography (OCT) technology has also been found to be useful in the management of preterm babies with ROP. Using OCT, it has been reported that the choroidal thickness decreases, and CME increases with the severity of ROP,[21,22] while total retinal thickness is often increased in preterm babies.[23] While many studies have been conducted to see the effect of ROP and prematurity on the retinal structure using the standard OCT, this can be performed only in bigger children who are cooperative or in younger children under sedation with proper positioning.

However, the main advantage of OCT in preterm babies is using the hand-held OCT, which allows rapid high resolution imaging of the retina in premature babies to detect retinal structural anomalies. Much like the wide-field imaging systems, the handheld OCT system is much easier to use in preterm babies. It is possible to get real-time images and full 3D volumetric data analysis of the retina, which is useful to assess retinal changes and call it with visual outcomes after ROP regression, laser or surgical management.

Leica Envisu C-Class OCT (Fig. 13.12) is one such hand-held OCT equipment which captures high-resolution images till 3 µm, allows acquisitions

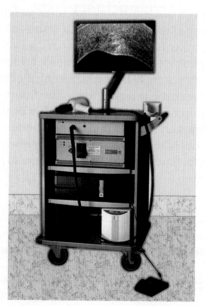

Fig. 13.12: Leica Envisu C-class optical coherence tomography (OCT).

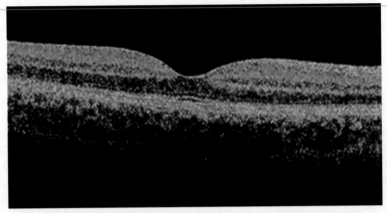

Fig. 13.13: Optical coherence tomography macular line scan of a preterm baby with ROP.

of 22,000 scans per second, thereby compensating for pediatric eye movements, and uses various interchangeable lenses. A general retina lens has a 70° field of view, while other lenses allow variable field of view. Performing OCT in preterm babies with small eyes under topical anesthesia is challenging and it requires considerable experience to effectively perform this procedure, as well as to interpret the observed changes (Fig. 13.13).

CONCLUSION

ROP is becoming an important cause of childhood blindness worldwide because of the improved survival of very low-birth-weight babies developing ROP, compounded with a lack of facilities for ROP screening and management. Wide-angle imaging systems like the Retcam have revolutionized the way we screen and follow-up cases of ROP, and with the development of cheaper and portable cameras, community ROP tele-screening models will soon become common. Newer diagnostic imaging tools like fluorescein angiography, UBM, and OCT help in better understanding of ROP, leading to optimized management strategies and better outcomes. There is an urgent need to spread awareness about ROP among ophthalmologists and neonatologists in developing countries for timely referral and management to prevent childhood blindness due to ROP.

REFERENCES

1. Kumar P, Sankar MJ, Deorari A, et al. Risk factors for severe retinopathy of prematurity in preterm low birth weight neonates. Indian J Pediatr. 2011;78(7): 812-6.
2. Blencowe H, Lawn JE, Vazquez T, et al. Preterm-associated visual impairment and estimates of retinopathy of prematurity at regional and global levels for 2010. Pediatr Res. 2013;74(Suppl 1):35-49.

3. Cryotherapy for Retinopathy of Prematurity Cooperative Group. Multicenter trial of cryotherapy for retinopathy of prematurity: ophthalmological outcomes at 10 years. Arch Ophthalmol. 2001;119(8):1110-8.

4. Good WV, Early Treatment for Retinopathy of Prematurity Cooperative Group. Final results of the early treatment for retinopathy of prematurity (ETROP) randomized trial. Trans Am Ophthalmol Soc. 2004;102:233-50.

5. An international classification of retinopathy of prematurity. The Committee for the Classification of Retinopathy of prematurity. Arch Ophthalmol Chic Ill. 1984;102(8):1130-4.

6. International Committee for the Classification of Retinopathy of Prematurity. The International Classification of Retinopathy of Prematurity revisited. Arch Ophthalmol. 2005;123(7):991-9.

7. Fierson WM, American Academy of Pediatrics Section on Ophthalmology, American Academy of Ophthalmology, American Association for Pediatric Ophthalmology and Strabismus, American Association of Certified Orthoptists. Screening examination of premature infants for retinopathy of prematurity. Pediatrics. 2013;131(1):189-95.

8. Vinekar A, Dogra MR, Sangtam T, et al. Retinopathy of prematurity in Asian Indian babies weighing greater than 1250 grams at birth: ten year data from a tertiary care center in a developing country. Indian J Ophthalmol. 2007;55(5):331-6.

9. NNF. Clinical Practice Guidelines [online]. Available from: http://v2020eresource. org/content/files/NNF.html [Accessed December, 2016].

10. Mintz-Hittner HA, Kennedy KA, Chuang AZ. BEAT-ROP cooperative group. Efficacy of intravitreal bevacizumab for stage 3+ retinopathy of prematurity. N Engl J Med. 2011;364(7):603-15.

11. Xu Y, Zhang Q, Kang X, et al. Early vitreoretinal surgery on vascularly active stage 4 retinopathy of prematurity through the preoperative intravitreal bevacizumab injection. Acta Ophthalmol (Copenh). 2013;91(4):e304-10.

12. Gopal L, Sharma T, Shanmugam M, et al. Surgery for stage 5 retinopathy of prematurity: the learning curve and evolving technique. Indian J Ophthalmol. 2000;48(2):101-6.

13. Wang SK, Callaway NF, Wallenstein MB, et al. SUNDROP: six years of screening for retinopathy of prematurity with telemedicine. Can J Ophthalmol. 2015;50(2):101-6.

14. Vinekar A, Gilbert C, Dogra M, et al. The KIDROP model of combining strategies for providing retinopathy of prematurity screening in underserved areas in India using wide-field imaging, tele-medicine, non-physician graders and smart phone reporting. Indian J Ophthalmol. 2014;62(1):41-9.

15. Theodoropoulou S, Ainsworth S, Blaikie A. Ultra-wide field imaging of retinopathy of prematurity (ROP) using Optomap-200TX. BMJ Case Rep. 2013;2013:bcr2013200734.

16. Gilbert C, Wormald R, Fielder A, et al. Potential for a paradigm change in the detection of retinopathy of prematurity requiring treatment. Arch Dis Child Fetal Neonatal Ed. 2016;101(1):6-9.

17. Azad R, Chandra P, Khan MA, et al. Role of intravenous fluorescein angiography in early detection and regression of retinopathy of prematurity. J Pediatr Ophthalmol Strabismus. 2008;45(1):36-9.

18. Lepore D, Molle F, Pagliara MM, et al. Atlas of fluorescein angiographic findings in eyes undergoing laser for retinopathy of prematurity. Ophthalmology. 2011;118(1):168-75.

19. Azad R, Mannan R, Chandra P. Role of ultrasound biomicroscopy in management of eyes with stage 5 retinopathy of prematurity. Ophthalmic Surg Lasers Imaging Off J Int Soc Imaging Eye. 2010;41(2):196-200.
20. Muslubas IS, Karacorlu M, Hocaoglu M, et al. Ultrasonography findings in eyes with stage 5 retinopathy of prematurity. Ophthalmic Surg Lasers Imaging Retina. 2015;46(10):1035-40.
21. Erol MK, Coban DT, Ozdemir O, et al. Choroidal thickness in infants with retinopathy of prematurity. Retina 2016;36(6):1191-8.
22. Erol MK, Ozdemir O, Turgut Coban D, et al. Macular findings obtained by spectral domain optical coherence tomography in retinopathy of prematurity. J Ophthalmol. 2014;2014:468653.
23. Park KA, Oh SY. Analysis of spectral-domain optical coherence tomography in preterm children: retinal layer thickness and choroidal thickness profiles. Invest Ophthalmol Vis Sci. 2012;53(11):7201-7.

CHAPTER 14

Macular Dystrophies

Nidhi Relhan, Subhadra Jalali

INTRODUCTION

There are several forms of hereditary disorders that affect the macular area in children, teenagers, and young adults. These macular dystrophies often present with a failing vision that progresses variably and results often in a severe loss of central vision and rarely, the peripheral vision. Patients can progress to legal blindness. Peripheral residual vision is very often preserved even in late stages of the macular dystrophies. Common conditions include X-linked retinoschisis, Best's vitelliform dystrophy, Stargardt's with or without fundus flavimaculatus, pattern dystrophy, macular cone dystrophy, dominant cystoid macular edema (CME). Some of the generalized retinal dystrophies can have associated changes in the macular area and are not discussed here. These include Leber's congenital amaurosis (LCA) that can have macular colobomas or macular atrophy, and retinitis pigmentosa (RP) that can have a variety of macular changes including CME, macular holes, epiretinal membrane, atrophy, and rarely, a central pigmentary retinopathy or central RP.

DEFINITION OF HEREDITARY MACULAR DYSTROPHIES

A group of hereditary disorders that are defined as bilaterally symmetrical, usually present during childhood or early adulthood involving the macular area and sparing the peripheral retina, and characterized by a typical fundus picture, especially in moderately advanced stages of the condition that almost always has normal retinal vessels often with associated electrophysiological test abnormalities.[1-4] Figures 14.1 to 14.4 show normal visual electrophysiology waveforms of retinal pathways for understanding the subsequent abnormal electrophysiogy.[4] The diseases involve early and premature cell changes

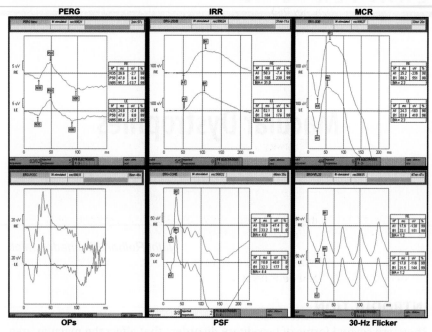

Fig. 14.1: Normal Flash electroretinogram (ERG) in an emmetropic subject with visual acuity 20/20.
(PERG: pattern ERG for macular function; IRR: isolated rod inner retinal response; MCR: maximal combined rod-cone response; OPs: oscillatory potentials from inner retina; PSF: photopic single flash cone response)

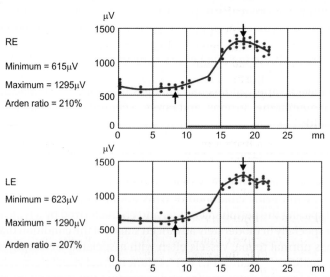

Fig. 14.2: An electrooculogram (EOG) graph with the light rise and normal Arden ratio of greater than 200% in each eye.

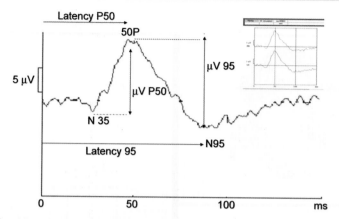

Fig. 14.3: A pattern electroretinogram (PERG) measurements inset shows actual PERG recording.

and cell death for which no clearly demonstrable cause except genetic abnormalities has been determined.

CLASSIFICATION

Macular dystrophies can be classified on the basis of:
1. Anatomical layers of the retina (Box 14.1) or
2. Inheritance pattern (Box 14. 2).
   Some of the important macular dystrophies are described below:

AUTOSOMAL DOMINANT MACULAR DYSTROPHIES

Best's Vitelliform Dystrophy

Best's vitelliform macular dystrophy[1-7] (Figs. 14.5 and 14.6) is a commonly seen autosomal dominant dystrophy of the retinal pigment epithelium characterized by a distinctive, if not pathognomonic "egg yolk cyst" in the foveal area, and is associated with a normal Flash electroretinogram (ERG) but an abnormal light peak/dark trough ratio on the electrooculogram (EOG).

Genetic Mutation

Bests' disease results from a mutation in the *vitelliform macular dystrophy 2 (VMD2) gene*. In families in which the EOG is a distinguishing marker, all members of the family bearing the gene can be identified by EOG testing and at least one member would show the "egg-yolk cyst" phenotype.

Ophthalmoscopic Staging and Visual Function[5]

There is wide phenotypic variability in the expression of the fundus lesions, both in the fovea and in the extra-foveal retina. The five stages of the disease and the sequalae are:
1. Carrier state
2. Vitelliform

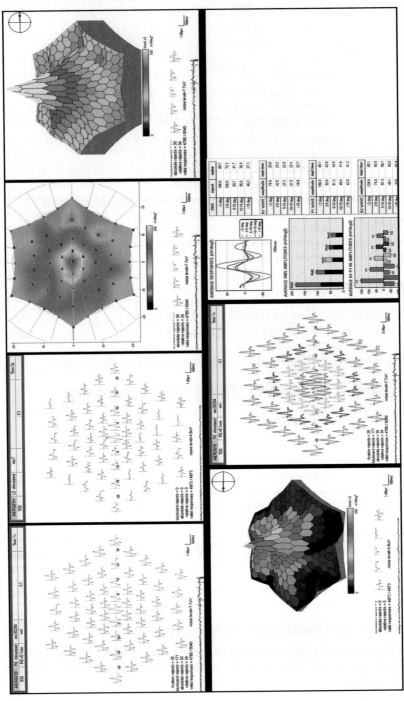

Fig. 14.4: Various displays available for mfERG in a normal eye. Clockwise from top left: trace arrays of two eyes, colored density plot, 3D scalar plot, scalar plot compared to normative data base, ring averages, average values of N1, P1, and P2.

BOX 14.1: Classification of hereditary macular dystrophies based on retinal layers affected.

- Nerve fiber layer
  - X-linked juvenile retinoschisis

- Photoreceptors and retinal pigment epithelium (RPE)
  - Stargardt's disease (atrophic macular dystrophy with fundus flavimaculatus)
  - Pericentral retinitis pigmentosa
  - Progressive atrophic macular dystrophy
  - Cone (-rod) dystrophy

- Retinal pigment epithelium
  - Best's vitelliform dystrophy
  - Fundus flavimaculatus
  - Butterfly-shaped pigment dystrophy, or pattern dystrophy
  - Reticular dystrophy
  - Dominant cystoid macular dystrophy (DCMD)
  - Familial grouped pigmentations
  - Benign concentric annular macular dystrophy
  - Dominant drusen

- Bruch's membrane
  - Pseudoinflammatory dystrophy
  - Angioid streaks
  - Age-related macular dystrophy
  - Myopic macular degeneration

- Choroid
  - Central areolar choroidal dystrophy

BOX 14.2: Classification of heredomacular dystrophies based on inheritance patterns.

- Autosomal dominant
  - Best's disease
  - Pattern dystrophy
  - Adult onset vitelliform macular dystrophy
  - Central areolar dystrophy
  - Dominantly inherited drusens
  - North Carolina macular dystrophy
  - Progressive foveal dystrophy
  - Cystoid macular edema

- Autosomal recessive
  - Stargardt's disease (fundus flavimaculatus)
  - Sjögren reticular dystrophy
  - Bietti's crystalline dystrophy

- X-linked
  - X-linked familial foveal retinoschisis
  - Familial foveal hypoplasia

- Hereditary cone and rod dysfunction syndromes
  - Dominantly inherited cone dysfunction syndrome
  - Autosomal recessive cone dysfunction syndrome
  - X-linked cone dysfunction syndrome

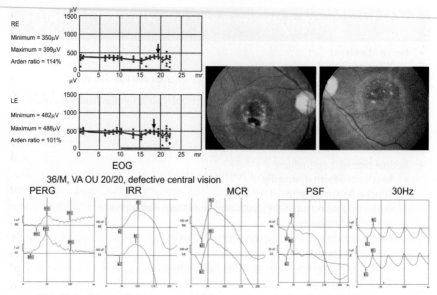

Fig.14.5: Absent light-rise on EOG and normal ERG in Best's disease.

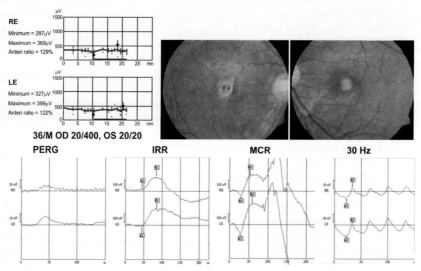

Fig. 14.6: Atrophic stage in the right eye and egg-yolk stage in the left eye in Best's disease.

3. Scrambled egg
4. Pseudohypopyon
5. Atrophic
6. Cicatricial or choroidal neovascular.

In most infants and children, the fundus is normal at birth, although some individuals could demonstrate an appearance of foveal hypoplasia appearing as an abnormal neuroretinal light reflex (stage 0). This is possibly similar to the "carrier state" in older adults who can genetically transmit the disease to their offspring, have an abnormal EOG, but who themselves have no visible ophthalmoscopic lesions.

The earliest visible lesion, the "previtelliform stage" (stage 1) shows a fine yellow speckled pigment disturbance under the central fovea. This can appear as early as 1 week of age. A subtle window defect on fundus fluorescein angiography (FFA) may be present at this point. Thereafter, usually between 4 years and 10 years of age, but occasionally later, a yellow–orange "cyst" like an "intact egg yolk" evolves (stage 1). This is centered in and under the foveal neuroepithelium and ultimately progresses to about one disc-diameter in size. Although usually bilateral and symmetrical, asymmetries of both extent and size can be seen. FFA may show blocked choroidal fluorescence. Usually, there are no visual complaints at this stage.

The vitelliform "cyst" may remain intact into middle age with little disturbance in visual function, and most patients may retain visual acuity of better than 20/40. The intact vitelliform cyst may sometimes "break up" and flatten, having the appearance of a "scrambled egg" (stage 2a) often with the slight reduction of visual acuity. Alternatively, it may evolve into a secondary macular retinal detachment with layering of the yellow material as a pseudohypopyon (stage 3). This yellow lipofuscin-like material gravitates inferiorly in the subretinal space and shifts with the changing head positioning and is compatible with good (including 20/20) visual acuity. Peripheral visual fields and dark adaptation remain normal.

A disparity between fundus appearance and visual function should raise the suspicion of Bests' diseases.

Following the pseudohypopyon stage, a variety of alternatives may occur. Resorption of the yellow material may leave an indistinct area of retinal pigment epithelial (RPE) atrophy, orange to red in color due to the increased visibility of the choroidal vasculature resembling central areolar choroidal sclerosis and can occur in middle-aged and older individuals. In FFA, large choroidal vessels may become visible in the atrophic stage. Sometimes, choroidal neovascular membrane (CNVM) with subretinal pigment epithelium or subretinal hemorrhagic detachment of macula may occur even as early as at 6–10 years of age. FFA and optical coherence tomography (OCT) help to delineate and monitor the treatment of CNVM. A fibrous white central disciform scar may develop that sometimes can retain remarkably good visual function, sometimes in the 20/40 to 20/60 range. Some eyes may have severe reduction of central vision.

Extrafoveal vitelliform lesions, unilaterally or bilaterally, may develop in some patients. Variations include drusen-size lesions, sometimes in clusters and belts, to large vitelliform cysts eccentric to the fovea, single or multiple. Uncommonly, pseudohypopyon and eccentric disciform scars develop in these extrafoveal lesions.

Because of the wide variability of phenotypic expression, family screening by retinal examination and EOG may help to establish the diagnosis.

Pathology

A retinal pigment epithelium defect leads to the accumulation of lipofuscin granules in the RPE cells and macrophages in the subretinal space and periodic acid–Schiff (PAS) positive, finely granular material in the photoreceptors.

Electrooculogram and Flash ERG

For Bests' disease both flash ERG[6] and EOG always need to be performed. The disparity between the presence of a normal flash ERG and an abnormal, distinctly pathological, light peak/dark trough ratio on EOG is an important diagnostic criterion for Bests' disease. Only butterfly epithelial dystrophy of the fovea has similar coincidentally normal responses on flash ERG with abnormal EOG. In virtually, all other diseases, the EOG is abnormal only when the ERG is abnormal. Thus, there is no merit in performing an EOG if the ERG is abnormal, since no useful information can be derived from such an abnormal EOG. The EOG abnormality may precede ophthalmoscopic findings and can help to identify genetic "carriers" with normal retinal examination who can transmit disease to the next generation but do not express the macular change.

Pattern Dystrophy

Pattern dystrophy[1,2,7-11] is an autosomal dominant macular dystrophy that usually starts in midlife. A variety of patterns of deposits of yellow, orange, and gray pigment in the macular area have been described. Rarely, these could be associated with systemic conditions like myotonic dystrophy and pseudoxanthoma elasticum.

The following four groups of pattern dystrophy have been described, all characterized by normal Flash ERG and EOG:
1. *Group 1*: Adult onset foveomacular vitelliform dystrophy
2. *Group 2*: Butterfly-shaped pigment dystrophy
3. *Group 3*: Reticular dystrophy of the pigment epithelium
4. *Group 4*: Coarse pigment mottling in the macula.

Foveomacular Vitelliform Dystrophy: Adult Type

Foveomacular vitelliform dystrophy—adult type is an autosomal dominant disease with mild symptoms of decreased visual acuity and metamorphopsia beginning in the fourth and fifth decades in one or both eyes, although rarely as early as at 20 years of age. It progresses slowly. Clinically, one can see pseudovitelliform lesions approximately one-quarter to one-third disc diameter in size. It is a horizontally oval, slightly elevated, yellowish subretinal lesion with a surrounding ring of white or gray depigmentation and a central brown to gray dot of hyperpigmentation. There may be a few small yellow flecks paracentrally.

The histopathology in pattern dystrophies shows that the central pigmented spot consists of a clump of large pigment-laden cells and extracellular melanin, while the surrounding white/gray ring consists of granular, eosinophilic, PAS-positive material lying between the atrophic RPE and Bruch's membrane.

Color vision, ERG and EOG are normal for the patient's age and are not diagnostic. Fluorescein angiography shows a blocked center corresponding to the gray–brown central pigment dot and a ring of surrounding fluorescence without secondary retinal detachment. Other reported findings are eccentric, nonfoveal lesions which on FFA block fluorescein centrally and may have a small surrounding halo window defect. Progression to severe vision loss is rarely reported.

Butterfly-shaped Pigment Pattern Dystrophy

Gray or yellow pigment is seen arranged in a well-organized tri-radiate pattern confined to the center of the macula in the shape of a butterfly. FFA reveals the hyperfluorescent margin of the nonfluorescent pigment figure. The disease is moderately progressive with most patients having moderate loss of vision.

Reticular Dystrophy of the Pigment Epithelium

The pigmentation starts in the foveal area and slowly extends into the periphery of the macula in a knotted fishnet fashion. It can be seen in 10–20% of patients of pseudoxanthoma elasticum.

Coarse Pigment Mottling in the Macula

The macular area shows prominent, coarse mottling of the pigment epithelium in the central macular area. The condition leads to a moderate loss of central vision.

Central Areolar Choroidal and Pigment Epithelial Atrophy

Central areolar dystrophy[1-4] is commonly seen after 45–50 years of age. The visual acuity, fields, ERG and EOG are normal initially. Later they develop mild to moderate visual loss. Retinal examination shows fine, mottled depigmentation in the macular region. This slowly evolves into symmetric, sharply outlined, bull's eye oval or round areas of geographic atrophy of the RPE in the absence of flecks/drusen. FFA shows varying degree of loss of choriocapillaris within the area of RPE atrophy. Multifocal ERG would show a corresponding reduction of amplitudes (Fig. 14.7).

Familial Dominant Drusen

Familial dominant drusen[1,2,12] is an autosomal dominant disease. It is characterized by widespread drusen extending beyond the macula, especially nasal to the optic disc. It is commonly seen during routine dilated retinal screening in the fourth to fifth decades. It is generally a benign condition but some patients can develop macular atrophy or CNVM, leading to a central scotoma on visual field evaluation. FFA shows the atrophy of RPE and the drusen appear more extensive than seen clinically. Dark adaptation and ERG remain normal while EOG may be subnormal in some cases.

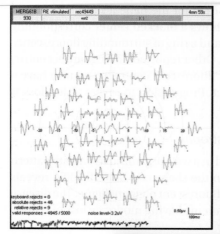
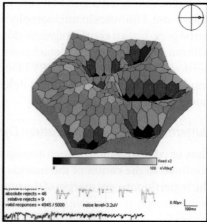
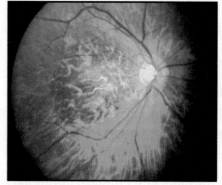

Fig. 14.7: Central areolar atrophy.

Histopathology shows round accumulation of hyaline in the pigment epithelium that is continuous with the inner layer of Bruch membrane. Later on, the choroid and the neural retina show atrophy. The disease gene has been mapped to chromosome 2.

North Carolina Macular Dystrophy

North Carolina macular dystrophy[1,2] is a rare autosomal dominant macular degeneration. It is characterized by macular coloboma with a well-demarcated atrophy of the RPE and choriocapillaris, and pigment deposition in macular area. Visual acuity remains relatively better and can range from 6/6 to 6/60 (mean 6/18). The gene has been mapped to chromosome 6q.

Progressive Foveal Dystrophy[1,2]

Progressive foveal dystrophy[1,2] has a dominant mode of inheritance. It shows the atrophy of the pigment epithelium in the macula and flecks similar to those seen in fundus flavimaculatus. The visual loss varies from mild to severe and the disease progresses with age. There is normal cone and rod ERG and EOG. Color defects also present later in life.

Autosomal Dominant Inherited Cystoid Macular Edema

Autosomal dominant inherited CME[1,2,7] is seen in hyperopic patients at a young age. Progressive decrease in VA (<6/36) is found in 50% of cases by the fourth decade. It progresses to atrophy and pigmentary changes in macula which can be confirmed on FFA. Normal ERG and abnormal EOG suggest poor prognosis.

AUTOSOMAL RECESSIVE MACULAR DYSTROPHIES

Stargardt's Disease and Fundus Flavimaculatus

This group of diseases[1-4,13,14] is characterized by the bilateral presence of peculiar yellowish flecks within the RPE. Most commonly, school-going children complain of a recent reduction of central vision. They are unable to copy from the school board while earlier they were able to do so. The correction of refractive error does not provide 20/20 vision. At the very early stage, the flecks may be difficult to visualize ophthalmoscopically and patients may be subjected to various tests for macular and optic nerve diseases, and indeed may be labeled as malingerers. Males and females are equally affected.

Classically, when flecks were distributed throughout the fundus and the onset was in adulthood, it was called as *fundus flavimaculatus*. If the flecks were confined to the posterior pole and were present relatively early in life, it was called as *Stargardts' disease*. Pathology shows excessive accumulation of lipofuscin within the RPE that prevents the visualization of choroidal details. The condition has in recent years been divided into following four groups:

1. *Group 1*: Vermilion fundus and hidden choroidal fluorescence
2. *Group 2*: Atrophic maculopathy with or without flecks
3. *Group 3*: Atrophic maculopathy with late signs and symptoms of RP
4. *Group 4*: Flecks not associated with macular atrophy.

Vermilion Fundus and Hidden Choroidal Fluorescence (Fig. 14.8)

The heavily-pigmented RPE obscures choroidal details. The FFA shows prominent retinal vessels, especially the retinal capillary network against a dark background of minimal choroidal fluorescence called as the *"silent choroid."* The optic disc and retinal vessels are normal.

Atrophic Maculopathy with or without Flecks (Fig. 14.9)

The degree and pattern of atrophy of the central macular RPE vary. It may show a beaten metal (bronze) appearance or marked geographic atrophy often as a diffuse oval lesion and very rarely as a bull's eye pattern. The optic disc and retinal vessels are normal.

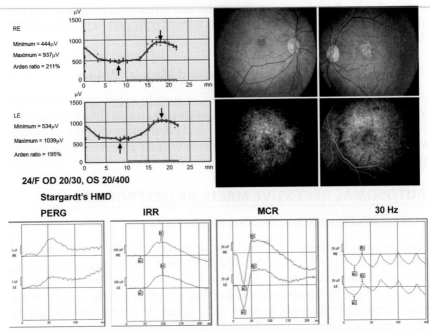

RE
Minimum = 444μV
Maximum = 937μV
Arden ratio = 211%

LE
Minimum = 534μV
Maximum = 1039μV
Arden ratio = 195%

24/F OD 20/30, OS 20/400

Stargardt's HMD

PERG   IRR   MCR   30 Hz

Fig. 14.8: Vermilion fundus and silent choroid in FFA with normal flash ERG, and EOG in Stargardt's dystrophy. Pattern ERG is abnormal in both eyes, more in the left eye that has developed atrophic changes around the fovea.

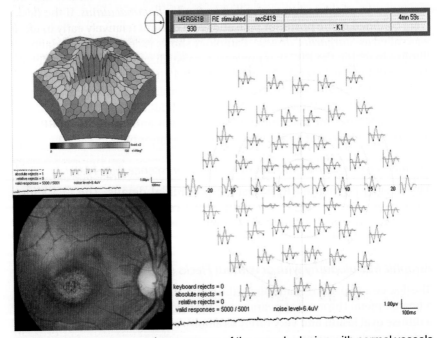

Fig. 14.9: The beaten-metal appearance of the macular lesion with normal vessels and surrounding retina. Corresponding multifocal ERG in Stargardt's dystrophy.

Atrophic Maculopathy with Late Signs and Symptoms of Retinitis Pigmentosa

The fundus appearance is similar to atrophic maculopathy with or without flecks. In addition, there are signs and symptoms of RP. This includes nyctalopia, a loss of pigment from the RPE, narrowing of the retinal vessels, pigment migration, and abnormal scotopic and photopic ERG.

Flecks not Associated with Macular Atrophy

Paracentral and central flecks are associated with minimal biomicroscopic and angiographic evidence of atrophy of the RPE. The visual acuity may be normal if the center of the fovea is not involved by a fleck. FFA shows blocked fluorescence due to flecks and minimal hyperfluorescence due to the RPE atrophy. FFA shows more flecks than visible clinically.

The progression of symptoms in this group of disorders is variable. Visual acuity slowly decreases till it reaches around 20/40 after which there is a relative rapid progression till it reaches 20/200. By 50 years of age, almost 50% of patients have 20/200 visual acuity. Eventually, visual acuity usually stabilizes between 20/200 and 20/400 in all cases. Autofluorescence is a very useful noninvasive tool to diagnose early disease, and monitor its severity and progression. Multifocal ERG is also very useful for the functional assessment of these eyes.

Genetics and clinical trials: Flecks not associated with macular atrophy is an autosomal recessive condition. It is due to mutations in the *ABCA 4 gene*, which normally causes the production of a protein involved in the visual cycle. The dysfunctional protein produced due to *ABCA 4* mutation leads to lipofuscin accumulation in the RPE cells. Gene therapies with a normal *ABCA 4 gene* are just starting that are believed to help in the restoration of the production of the normal proteins. The administration of the drugs that slow down the lipofuscin buildup in retina is likely to delay the visual loss in the various stages of development of the disease.

Bietti's Crystalline Dystrophy

Bietti's crystalline dystrophy[1,2,15,16] is characterized by crystalline deposits in all the layers of retina. It has autosomal recessive inheritance. There are varying degrees of choriocapillary and RPE loss especially in the macula. Some eyes would show associated superficial limbal corneal crystals. The crystals are cholesterol and complex lipid deposits. It is a slowly progressive disorder. We recently reported tortuous vessels and subfoveal neurosensory detachment (Fig. 14.10) in this condition.[16]

Sjögren's Reticular Dystrophy of the RPE

Sjögren's reticular dystrophy of the RPE[1,2] is a rare autosomal recessive condition characterized by the accumulation of pigment in a fishnet-like network at the level of the RPE. It often starts centrally and slowly extends to the periphery in later stages. Visual acuity is affected minimally. The EOG and flash ERG are normal. FFA shows blocked choroidal fluorescence due to the pigment.

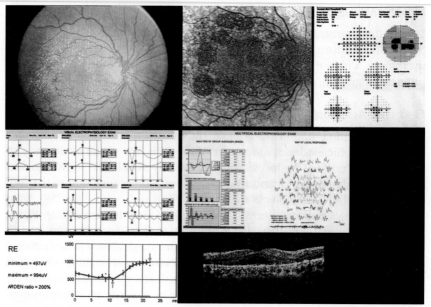

Fig. 14.10: Fundus photo, autofluorescence visual field, visual electrophysiology and optical coherence tomography (OCT) in Bietti's crystalline retinal dystrophy

Source: Padhi TR, Kesarwani, Jalali S. Bietti crystalline retinal dystrophy with subfoveal neurosensory detachment and congenital tortuosity of retinal vessels: case report. Documenta Ophthalmologica. 2011;122(3):199-206.

X-LINKED RECESSIVE DISEASES

Juvenile X-linked Retinoschisis

Juvenile X-linked retinoschisis[1-4,17] is characterized by typical stellate, radial schisis of the foveal tissue, often associated with surrounding radial retinal striae. One half of all patients may also have peripheral retinoschisis cavities, usually not extending to the ora serrata. These peripheral retinoschises are seen at presentation or develop later in life.

Clinical Features

Juvenile X-linked retinoschisis has been reported across races and ethnic groups including Asian Indians. It may be one of the most common causes of subnormal vision due to macular disease in male children and adolescents. Clinically, a bimodal age of presentation is seen in 6–10-year-old schoolboys or in 30–50-year-old adults. In schoolboys, the common mode of presentation is an inability to read the classroom board or in current times, being detected during school vision screening programs. The visual acuity cannot often be corrected beyond 20/40 to 20/60 and deteriorates slowly over the next three decades to about 20/200. Sometimes a severe congenital or infantile retinoschisis, which may evolve rapidly into retinal detachment in the first year of life, can be seen. This may sometimes present as a leukocoria or esotropia, and be mistaken for retinoblastoma or congenital retinal dysplasia. Careful ultrasonography and a detailed examination of both eyes under anesthesia can usually make the diagnosis apparent.

Fundus changes are seen in the fovea and in the periphery (Figs. 14.11 and 14.12). The foveal lesion called *foveal schisis* initially appears as a cluster of small radially-arranged patterns of "cysts" (Figs. 14. 12 and 14.13). Occasionally, a few radial folds of the inner limiting membrane are also seen. FFA typically shows no leakage from the macular area (Fig. 14.12). OCT shows typical cystic changes and splitting of the nerve fiber layer and ganglion cell layers, involving the fovea with the thinning of the superficial layers. Autofluorescence imaging also highlights the foveal cystic lesions in a noninvasive manner (Fig. 14. 12).

With increasing age, the characteristic radial folds in the fovea disappear as the microcysts enlarge or coalesce, forming an irregular shredded appearance, occasionally resembling a foveal hole. In late stages, foveal atrophy and thinning is seen with nonspecific pigmentary change and retinal vascular pattern changes around the fovea. Diagnosis may be difficult in such eyes. A high degree of suspicion, the presence of peripheral lesions, family screening, pedigree charting, and ERG provide useful clues to the disease condition.

True peripheral retinoschisis is commonly present in the inferior temporal quadrant (Fig. 14.11) and never extends to the ora serrata, unlike retinal detachments. Silver-gray, glistening spots are also seen scattered throughout the retina and may represent the first pathological changes in the retinal periphery due to splitting of the Müller cells across the retinal split (Fig. 14.13).

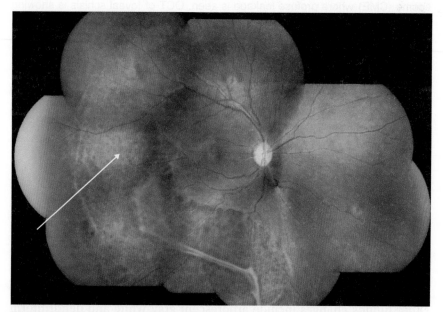

Fig. 14.11: X-linked retinoschisis with foveal and peripheral schisis. Note the dark-brown, pinhead-sized, rounded appearance of the split retinal layers in area of the schisis, due to rupture of the Müller cells across the schisis cavity (arrow). Retinoschisis does not extend to the ora.

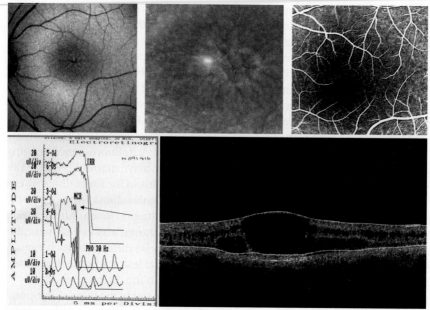

Fig. 14.12: Area of altered autofluorescence in low and high magnification depicting cystoid and stellate pattern of foveal schisis changes. Fundus fluorescein angiography (FFA) shows minimal pooling of dye in the schitic stellate lesions without any obvious leakage that helps to differentiate from inflammatory cystoid macular edema (CME) where profuse leakage is seen. OCT of foveal schisis is showing a split in the inner retina and thinning of the overlying retinal layers. Flash ERG shows a negative ERG with much reduced scotopic b-wave of inner retina (arrow) and nearly normal photoreceptor a-wave (star).

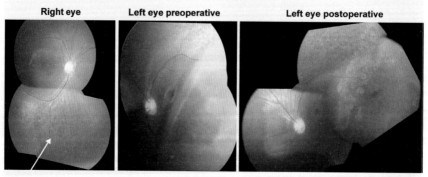

Fig. 14.13: Infantile retinoschisis presenting with recent-onset left esotropia due to retinal detachment. Esotropia disappeared after surgical reattachment. The arrow shows early peripheral schisis in the right eye. Foveal schisis is seen in both eyes.

Other fundus changes include arborescent gray-white and dendritiform figures particularly within areas of peripheral schisis, perivascular phlebitis, vitreous veils with or without enclosed retinal vessels, "pseudopapilledema" or "pseudoneuritis," apparently caused by glial tissues spreading onto the borders of the disc. Later, clumped pigmentation suggestive of an old chorioretinitis or a spontaneously attached retinal detachment is observed.

Other long-term complications include vitreous hemorrhage, avulsed retinal vessels, vitreous veils, peripheral cysts with intracystic or vitreous hemorrhages, and both inner and outer retinal holes with resultant rhegmatogenous retinal detachment (Fig. 14.13). These would need surgical intervention in many cases. Female carriers have normal retina, normal electrophysiology, and normal psychophysiology and are hence difficult to detect.

Visual Fields

Nonspecific and nondiagnostic field changes include relative central scotoma and some mild concentric constriction; peripheral visual field reduction is seen often in the superonasal quadrant from the inferotemporal schisis. Rhegmatogenous retinal detachment would cause an absolute field defect while retinoschisis causes a relative field defect.

ERG and EOG

In flash ERG, the a-wave is generally intact but the b-wave is characteristically subnormal. The scotopic recordings are more disturbed than the photopic. ERG shows a "negative ERG" with reduced amplitudes and a prolonged implicit time of the scotopic b-wave, normal a-wave, and reduced oscillatory potentials (Fig. 14.12). Other causes of inner retinal dysfunction can also appear as "negative ERG" and need to be excluded, such as congenital stationary night blindness (CSNB). With the progression of the retinal pathology, all Ganzfeld voltages deteriorate and rarely, the ERG becomes nonrecordable at which stage the normal EOG of retinoschisis eyes also becomes abnormal. EOG is hence not a useful diagnostic procedure.

Nonsex-linked Foveal Schisis

Nonsex-linked foveal schisis[18] that affects females and males from pedigrees with autosomal dominant inheritance are also reported. In such eyes, the foveal changes resemble the CME of RP rather than of retinoschisis, though peripheral retina also shows schisis in some eyes.

Hereditary Cone and Rod Dysfunction Syndromes

Noncongenital dominantly inherited, autosomal recessively inherited and X-linked recessive cone dysfunction syndromes have been described.[1–4,7,19]

The dominantly inherited disease is most widely studied. The syndrome is characterized by a gradual, progressive reduction of visual acuity starting often in the second decade. There is no nystagmus and patients are not symptomatic in earlier years. There are associated abnormal color vision (often hue) problems and photo aversion or hemeralopia. In the initial stages, the retina looks normal and visual acuity is often 20/30 or so. This is followed by early temporal disc pallor and the patient may undergo visual-evoked potential (VEP) and neuroimaging to rule out optic nerve diseases. Macular ERG (multifocal/focal or pattern ERG) techniques can diagnose the condition to be retinal in origin at an early stage. Later stages of the disease show classical pigment stippling in the perifoveal area that evolves into a round or ovoid bull's-eye like lesion. FFA can show diffuse stippled hyperfluorescence in patients with pigment stippling. In the bull's-eye lesion, a zone of hyperfluorescence is seen that surrounds a hypofluorescent center. Some of the dystrophies may be confined to the macular area (macular cone dystrophies, Fig. 14.14) or be associated with a more generalized cone dysfunction (Fig. 14.15) as diagnosed by flash and macular ERG techniques. Rod responses are usually normal or subnormal with stable waveforms. Peripheral visual fields remain normal while central fields may show scotoma corresponding to the clinical lesions. Prognosis is generally better than in RP and cone-rod dystrophy. Often the patient gets benefit by tinted glasses worn according to the lighting conditions. Some patients report relief from glare with antioxidants such as beta carotene and lutein. Late-onset X-linked patients have a tapetal-like bright sheen in the inferior retina.

MANAGEMENT OF HEREDOMACULAR DYSTROPHY

Initially and on each subsequent visit, all patients with heredomacular dystrophy (HMD) must have a detailed comprehensive eye examination including refraction, slit-lamp biomicroscopy, ocular motility and alignment, pupillary reactions, intraocular pressure measurement, and dilated lens and fundus evaluation. Fundus evaluation should include optic nerve, macula, peripheral retina, vitreous, and retinal vasculature. It should not be forgotten

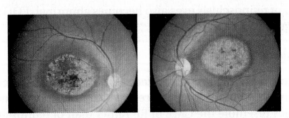

36/M, VA 20/200, Color Blind, Amsler–central scotoma

Macular cone dystrophy

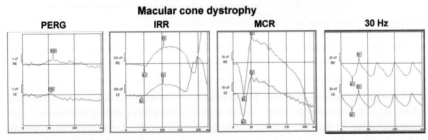

| PERG | IRR | MCR | 30 Hz |

Fig. 14.14: Well-circumscribed ovoid macular lesions with markedly reduced PERG and normal peripheral cone ERG responses showing localized macular cone dystrophy.

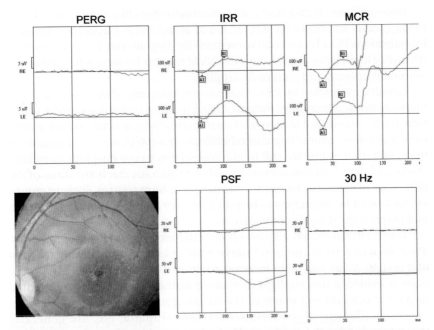

Fig. 14.15: Macular changes with absent PERG, absent photopic cone ERG and normal rod waveforms in a 47-year-old female with VA of 20/400, central scotoma and defective color vision due to generalized cone dystrophy.

that patients with HMD can develop any other ocular pathology including glaucoma, central nervous system (CNS) tumors, neovascular pathologies, etc. that need to be diagnosed and treated. A question often asked is what the frequency of eye evaluations should be after the diagnosis is confirmed. In children and teenagers, we usually follow-up every year to evaluate their visual status and address their functional, educational, social, and vocational needs in tandem with the low-vision specialists. In adulthood, we see every 2–3 years if the condition is stable and no complications are envisaged. In conditions that are known to develop complications like RD or CNVM, evaluations could be more frequent and a discussion about sign/symptoms is reinforced.

While making a diagnosis especially in the early stages of HMD, it may be required to exclude optic nerve diseases, generalized retinal degenerations like RP,[1-4,20] solar retinopathy, drug toxicity and other acquired disorders including nutritional problems, trauma and drug abuse. Proper pedigree charting, family history of consanguinity and vision problems, and evaluation of family members are desirable.

Detailed visual functional history should include information about nyctalopia, color vision, especially matching colors, peripheral vision, light sensitivity, impaired contrast sensitivity, and current and past eye poking behavior. The history of the onset and progression of visual disturbance should be noted. A general review of systems including skeletal, auditory, balance, skin, neurology, and gastroenterology is mandatory.

Investigations should start with noninvasive ones like color vision, visual fields, fundus autofluorescence, OCT, and visual electrophysiology. Invasive investigations like FFA are used sometimes for diagnosis such as in Stargardts' disease or to evaluate the presence of CNVM that can be seen in Best's disease, dominant drusens and pattern dystrophy.

Detailed evaluation by a low-vision specialist is critical in these patients as there are limited treatment options. Using modern technological low-vision aids, most patients are able to lead near-normal educational and vocational lives. Vocational counseling and rehabilitation services are now available in many larger cities but are still to percolate down to eye hospitals in smaller towns and cities. An optometrist or vision technician can learn some of the basic skills of managing low vision through short-term courses. Support groups are facilitated by physicians to help in advocacy and the educational, social, and psychological needs of the patient.

The physician should discuss a proper diet rich in vitamins and minerals. Avoidance of retinal and optic nerve toxic substances, including tobacco and certain drugs may help to avoid additional causes of visual loss. There is some evidence that sunlight may cause further harm to eyes with retinal degenerations and so the use of UV blocking sunglasses or sun-protection measures like use of umbrellas/hats/caps/dupatta, etc. are generally recommended for the outdoors. Dark glasses reduce the contrast and are generally not preferred by most patients with retinal diseases, except those with a predominant cone dysfunction.

Counseling and explanation are a very important aspect in the management of these potentially incurable diseases. Unfortunately, most physicians either do not have the time or patience to talk in detail to the patient, or are more often embarrassed to talk about a condition where they can offer no "treatment"! Patients and caregivers are often upset and shocked that except for saying that the disease is genetic, incurable, and progressive, no further explanation or support was provided by the physician who diagnosed the condition. Realistic and correct information on the nature of condition, the underlying etiology, rate of progression, long-term prognosis, and recent advances toward cure must be conveyed to the patient and family members. Genetic counseling regarding the mode of inheritance and risk to other family members is required but unfortunately only a few trained genetic counselors are available in larger cities in India currently.

REFERENCES

1. Newsome DA. Retinal degenerations and dystrophies. New York: Raven Press; 1998.
2. Heckenlively JR, Arden GB. Principles and Practice of Clinical electrophysiology of vision, 2nd edition. Cambridge, Massachusetts: MIT Press; 2006.
3. Krill AE, Deutman AF. Hereditary retinal and choroidal dystrophies. Hagerstown: Harper and Roy; 1977.
4. Jalali S, Holder GE, Ram LSM, et al. Visual electrophysiology in the clinic: a basic guide to recording and interpretation. AIOS CME series number 17. Delhi: AIOS; 2009.

5. Mohler CW, Fine SL. Long-term evaluation of patients with Best's vitelliform dystrophy. Ophthalmology. 1981;88(7):688-92.
6. Deutman AF. Electro-oculography in families with vitelliform dystrophy of the fovea. Arch Ophthalmol. 1969;81(3):305-16.
7. Shetty NS, Sharma T, Shanmugam MP, et al. The Sankara Nethralaya atlas of fundus fluorescein angiography, New Delhi: Jaypee Brothers Medical Publishers (P) Ltd.; 2004.
8. Bloom IH, Swanson DE, Bird AC. Adult vitelliform macular degeneration. Br J Ophthalmol. 1981;65:800-1.
9. Hsieh CR, Fine BS, Lyons JS. Patterned dystrophies of the retinal pigment epithelium. Arch Ophthalmol. 1977;95(3):429-35.
10. Marmor MF, Byers B. Pattern dystrophy of the pigment epithelium. Am J Ophthalmol. 1977;84:32-44.
11. Ayazi S, Fagan R. Pattern dystrophy of the pigment epithelium. Retina. 1981;1: 287-9.
12. Deutman AF, Jansen LM. Dominantly inherited drusen of Bruch's membrane. Br J Ophthalmol. 1970;54(6):373-82.
13. Fishman GA, Farber M, Patel BS, et al. Visual acuity loss in patients with Stargardts' Macular Dystrophy. Ophthalmology. 1987;94(7):809-14.
14. Glazer LC, Dryja TP. Understanding the etiology of Stargardt's disease. Ophthalmol Clin N Am. 2002;15(1):93-100.
15. Welch RB. Bietti's tapetoretinal degeneration with marginal corneal dystrophy and crystalline retinopathy. Trans Am Ophthalmol Soc. 1977;75:164-79.
16. Padhi TR, Kesarwani S, Jalali S. Bietti Crystalline retinal dystrophy with subfoveal neurosensory detachment and congenital tortuosity of retinal vessels. Doc Ophthalmol. 2011;122(3):199-206.
17. Kellner U, Brummer S, Forester MH, et al. X-linked congenital retinoschisis. Graefes' Arch Clin Exp Ophthalmol. 1990;228(5):432-7.
18. Noble KG, Carr RE, Siegel IM. Familial foveal retinoschisis associated with a rod-cone dystrophy. Am J Ophthalmol. 1978;85(4):551-7.
19. Heckenlively JR. RP cone-rod degeneration. Trans Am Ophthalmol Soc. 1987;85:438-70.
20. Jalali S. Retinitios Pigmentosa. In: Dutta LC (Ed). Modern Ophthalmology, 3rd edition. New Delhi: Jaypee Brothers Medical Publishers (P) Ltd.; 2005.

CHAPTER 15

Management of Age-related Macular Degeneration

Nazimul Hussain, Supriya Dabir, Anjali Hussain

INTRODUCTION

Age-related macular degeneration (AMD) is the leading cause of blindness in the world.[1] For many patients, the visual impairment associated with AMD means a loss of independence, depression, increased financial concerns, and the need to adapt to vision loss at a time when they are likely suffering from other debilitating conditions.[2]

Clinically, AMD is classified into the nonexudative "dry" or atrophic form (Fig. 15.1) and the exudative "wet" or neovascular form (Fig. 15.2). A more severe vision loss is typically associated with the "wet" form that occurs in about 10% of all patients with AMD, but up to 20% of legal blindness from AMD is due to the "dry" form.[3] However, recent advances in clinical research have led to a better understanding of genetics and the pathophysiology of AMD, as well as the discovery of new therapies designed to treat and prevent different forms of AMD.

The classification of dry AMD is shown in Table 15.1 and a more comprehensive clinical staging is shown in Table 15.2.[4,5]

DEMOGRAPHIC FACTORS

The incidence, prevalence, and progression of all forms of AMD increase with advancing age.[6] Women have only a slightly higher prevalence of the disease and this risk is confined to those above 75 years of age.[7] However, recent analyses from the Blue Mountains Eye Study suggest that the 5-year incidence of neovascular AMD among women is double that of men (1.2% vs 0.6%).[8] All forms of AMD are more prevalent in the white population than in the more darkly pigmented races,[9,10] leading to the belief that melanin may

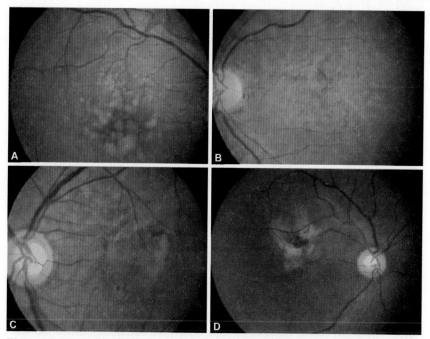

Figs. 15.1A to D: Dry age-related macular degeneration (AMD) forms: (A) Intermediate category 3 AMD; (B) Advanced category 4 AMD and wet or neovascular AMD; (C) Active choroidal neovascular membrane (CNV); (D) Disciform scar.

TABLE 15.1: Classification of AMD (Age-related Eye Disease Study).	
Category	Clinical features
Category 1	No drusen or nonextensive small drusen only, in both eyes
Category 2	Extensive small drusen, nonextensive intermediate drusen, or pigment abnormalities in at least one eye
Category 3	Large drusen, extensive intermediate drusen, or noncentral geographical atrophy in at least one eye
Category 4	Geographical atrophy in at least one eye
Category 5	(Neovascular) evidence suggesting CNVM or RPE detachment, (serous/hemorrhagic) in one eye

be protective against the development of choroidal neovascular membrane (CNVM). The presence of melanin also seems to protect against the formation of RPE lipofuscin, a marker of cellular senescence and a promoter of oxidative damage.[11,12] A recent study found no differences in macular or melanin pigment densities between eyes with and without early AMD.[13] In sum, the data seem to suggest that racial differences in AMD prevalence may be due to factors other than pigmentation.

TABLE 15.2: The clinical age-related maculopathy staging system (CARMS).

Grade of maculopathy	Clinical features
1.	No drusen or <10 small drusen without pigment abnormalities
2.	Approximately >10 small drusen or <15 intermediate drusen, or pigment abnormalities associated with ARM
	A. Drusen
	B. RPE changes (hyperpigmentation and hypopigmentation)
	C. Both drusen and RPE changes
3.	Approximately >15 intermediate drusen or any large drusen
	A. No drusenoid RPED
	B. Drusenoid RPED
4.	Geographic atrophy with involvement of the macular center, or noncentral geographic atrophy at least 350 μm in size
5.	Exudative AMD, including nondrusenoid pigment epithelial detachments, CNVM with subretinal or sub-RPE hemorrhages or fibrosis, or scars consistent with treatment of AMD
	A. Serous RPED, without CNVM
	B. CNVM or disciform scar

(AMD: age-related macular degeneration; ARM: age-related maculopathy; CNVM: choroidal neovascular membrane; RPE: retinal pigment epithelium; RPED: retinal pigment epithelial detachment). *SMALL, drusen <63 μm in diameter located within 2 disc diameters (DDs) of the center of the macula; INTERMEDIATE, drusen >63 μm but <125 μm, located within 2 DDs of the center of the macula; LARGE, drusen >125 μm in diameter located within 2 DDs of the center of the macula; drusenoid RPED, confluent soft drusen >500 μm in size.*

MANAGEMENT OF DRY AGE-RELATED MACULAR DEGENERATION

Smoking

Smoking has been associated with an increased risk of developing AMD in most population-based studies.[14-16] Both prior and current smokers are at increased risk for AMD,[17,18] with these individuals developing AMD 5–10 years before nonsmokers, respectively.[19] This may be due to smoking's effects on antioxidant metabolism and choroidal blood flow. Nicotine stimulates neovascularization by inducing endothelial cell proliferation and accelerating fibrovascular growth.[20] The first step in the management of any smoker with AMD should therefore be a discussion of the risks of smoking and encouragement to quit. This is especially important if the patient wishes to commence the Age-Related Eye Disease Study (AREDS) formulation vitamins because the doses of β-carotene used in this study have been associated with an increased risk of lung cancer in smokers.[21]

Genetic Factors

Over the past decade, researchers have begun to focus their attention on determining the genetic component of AMD. This task has been inherently difficult due to the nature of the disease. AMD onset occurs late in life, and therefore often only one generation in the appropriate age range is available for study.

An increased incidence of AMD has been noticed in patients with a family history,[22] although inheritance is unclear. This may be more important in earlier-onset disease. In a number of families with a dominant pattern, late-onset retinal degeneration (LORD), the gene mutation has been identified on chromosome 1. Other candidate genes include fibulin 5, where a missense mutation is causal in a small number of people with AMD.[23] Recently, genetic variation in a major regulator of the alternative complement pathway, factor H (HF1), has been proposed to underlie a major proportion of AMD.[24] HF1 is synthesized by the retinal pigment epithelium and accumulates in drusen. A statistically significant association of manganese superoxide dismutase gene polymorphism with AMD has been reported.[25] Whole genome linkage scans have implicated the most replicated signals residing on 1q25-31 and 10q26. Recent reports suggest that PLEKHA1/LOC387715 and the BF/C2 regions may be major risk loci for AMD as well.[24,25]

Age-related macular degeneration is a late-onset complex disorder with multifactorial etiologies. Both genetic and environmental factors play a role in the disease pathogenesis.[26] AMD is the third leading cause of blindness in the elderly. Familial aggregation, segregation studies, and linkage analysis have provided both qualitative and quantitative evidence on the genetic basis in AMD. Several candidate loci have been earlier mapped in AMD but variants in the genes, viz. *APOE*, *ABCA4*, *FBLN6* and *EFEMP1* harboring these loci have accounted for only a small proportion of cases. Recent screening of two major loci has led to the identification of the Complement Factor H (CFH) on 1q32 and *LOC387715* and *HTRA1* on the 10q26 gene cluster. Single nucleotide polymorphisms (SNPs) in *CFH* (Y402H), *LOC387715* (A69S), and a promoter variant in *HTRA1* have been associated with AMD in large case–control cohorts. These SNPs exhibited large effect sizes and high disease odds for the risk genotypes across different populations. Interestingly, these associations have been widely replicated across multiple ethnic groups worldwide indicating their potential role in the disease pathogenesis. In this article, we would outline the genetics of AMD with special emphasis on *CFH* followed by other genetic variants based on studies done by our group and colleagues worldwide. We would also provide a brief overview on the possible molecular mechanisms leading to AMD.

In future, more such studies are required across wider geographical regions to identify candidates that contribute to the AMD pathogenesis. The genetic typing of AMD patients would also permit clinicians to develop correlations with genotypes for estimating disease risk and progression. The identification of susceptible gene variant(s) would allow early intervention in subjects "at risk" of developing AMD for a better prognosis. While the underlying biological functions of these candidate genes and their interactions are yet to be characterized, large multicenter studies with these variants should be undertaken with respect to treatment modalities in order to understand the therapeutic mechanisms in subjects carrying the risk genotype(s).

Sunlight

There have been conflicting reports on the association of ultraviolet or visible light with AMD.[27,28] The association between cataract surgery and the development of signs of late AMD [29] may suggest a detrimental effect of increased light exposure. One study suggests that the use of hats and sunglasses may be slightly protective.[28] In the absence of conclusive evidence, it seems reasonable to advise patients that it is worth considering wearing sunglasses and avoiding excessive sunlight when practical.

Dietary Factors and Antioxidants

The high levels of certain antioxidant vitamins and minerals in the retina, and the concentration of carotenoids in the macula have led to the speculation that micronutrient supplementation may confer protection from AMD. Data from the AREDS suggest that supplementation with antioxidants (vitamin C 500 mg, and vitamin E 400 IU) plus β-carotene 15 mg; antioxidants plus zinc 80 and copper 2 mg provide a modest protective effect on the progression to advanced neovascular AMD in patients with extensive intermediate size drusen, at least one large druse, noncentral geographic atrophy in one or both eyes, or advanced AMD or vision loss due to AMD in one eye, and without contraindications such as smoking.[21] This benefit did not extend to patients without AMD or with few drusen.

The AREDS was a prospective, multicentric randomized clinical trial designed to assess the natural course and the risk factors of age-related cataract and AMD and the effects of antioxidant vitamins and minerals on these two ocular conditions. It used a factorial design in which 4,757 participants were randomized to one of four groups:
1. Antioxidant vitamins
2. Zinc
3. Combination of antioxidant vitamins and zinc (Table 15.3)
4. Placebo.

The participants were followed for a mean of 6 years and 3,640 participated in the study.

Early Age-related Macular Degeneration (Age-related Eye Disease Study Category 2)

This is characterized by a combination of multiple small drusen (<63 microns in diameter), few intermediate drusen (63–124 microns in diameter) or RPE abnormalities. The central visual acuity is usually normal in these patients. In the AREDS these patients had a 1.3% risk of progressing to advanced AMD in 5 years in either eye. The use of the combination of antioxidant vitamins and minerals did not reduce the progression of early AMD to the intermediate stage of AMD.[30]

TABLE 15.3: Antioxidant vitamin and mineral supplements used in the Age-related Eye Disease Study (AREDS).

Supplement	Daily dose
Vitamin C	500 mg
Vitamin E	400 IU
Beta-carotene	15 mg (25,000 IU)
Zinc oxide	80 mg
Cupric oxide	2 mg

The doses listed on the commercially available vitamin/mineral supplements are not the same as the above because of a change in labeling rules by the FDA, which states that the doses must reflect the amounts available at the end of the shelf life.

Intermediate Age-related Macular Degeneration (Age-related Eye Disease Study Category 3)(Fig. 15.1)

This is characterized by extensive intermediate drusen, at least one large drusen (≥125 microns in diameter) or geographic atrophy not involving the center of the fovea. According to AREDS, the rate of progression of this category to advanced AMD at 5 years is 18%.

Advanced Age-related Macular Degeneration (Age-related Eye Disease Study Category 4) (Fig. 15.1)

Characterized by one or more of the following:
• Geographic atrophy involving the foveal center
• Neovascular AMD:
    – Choroidal neovascular membrane
    – Serous or hemorrhagic PED
    – Lipid exudates
    – Disciform scar.

In patients with one eye involved, approximately 43% of the fellow eyes progress to advanced AMD in 5 years.

Intermediate Age-related Macular Degeneration, Advanced Age-related Macular Degeneration in One Eye

• Following treatment with antioxidant vitamins, zinc, and copper, the rate of development of advanced AMD at 5 years was reduced by 25%.
• The risk of losing three or more lines of vision was reduced by 19% using this combination of treatments.

Meanwhile, absent convincing evidence, patients should be cautioned that nutrient supplements are not necessarily innocuous. For instance, among male smokers, β-carotene supplementation increases the risk of lung cancer and mortality,[31] whereas multivitamin supplementation increases overall cancer mortality.[32] High serum levels of zinc are associated with Alzheimer's disease,[33] promote amyloid fibril aggregation, worsen outcomes after acute stroke, may cause RPE cell apoptosis, and exacerbate diabetes mellitus.[34,35] Higher rates of hospitalizations for genitourinary dysfunction in males taking the high-dose micronutrient supplementation were observed in AREDS.[30] AREDS II added 10 mg of lutein along with 2 mg of zeaxanthin, 1 g of docosahexaenoic acid (DHA)] and eicosapentaenoic acid as supplements. The results are awaited.

Patients should also be counseled to decrease the dietary intake of fat, maintain healthy weight and blood pressure, and to increase the dietary intake of antioxidants through foods, such as green leafy vegetables, whole grain, fish, and nuts. High intake of beta-carotene, vitamin C and E, zinc, and long-chain polyunsaturated fatty acids and fish has shown independently to decrease the risk of development of neovascular AMD.

Anecortave Acetate

Anecortave acetate is a synthetic analog of cortisol that has been chemically modified to remove the typical side effects of the glucocorticoid receptor-mediated activity. The result is a novel angiostatic "cortisene" that inhibits the development of new blood vessels by preventing the expression of extracellular proteases required for endothelial cell migration. Anecortave is delivered via a posterior subtenons or juxtascleral depot administration using a novel, curved, blunt-tipped cannula. A study is currently under way to investigate the effect of the injections every 6 months for 2 years on prevention of the development of CNV. Patients with dry AMD in the study eye and end-stage AMD from CNV in the fellow eye are being recruited.[36]

Laser Treatment

Multiple trials were conducted to evaluate the utility of prophylactic low-intensity laser treatment to drusen in preventing the complications of advanced AMD, namely, Choroidal Neovascularization Prevention Trial[37] and Drusen Laser Study.[38] The results demonstrated that CNV onset was approximately 6 months earlier in laser-treated patients compared with those with no laser treatment. The Prophylactic Treatment of AMD Study has also shown an increased risk of CNV in laser-treated fellow eyes. Subsequent multicenter randomized clinical trials like the Complications of Age-related Macular Degeneration Prevention Trial[39] are ongoing.

Rheopheresis

This is a new blood filtration method that uses novel nanopore, hollow fiber membrane technology to remove high-molecular-weight plasma components. It has been hypothesized to aid in the removal of these high-molecular-weight proteins from Bruch's membrane, which may reduce the barrier to diffusion and improve the metabolic exchange between the RPE and choriocapillaris. This may allow an improved supply of nutrients to the RPE cells and, perhaps more importantly, improved clearance of the metabolic wastes from photoreceptor turnover. An additional theory is that it may improve choroidal blood flow.[40] The Multicenter Investigation of Rheopheresis for AMD (known as MIRA-1) did not show any promising results.[41]

Low Visual Aid

The functional implications of AMD are reduced visual acuity, reduced contrast sensitivity, glare, color vision deficiency, and reduced stereopsis. Reduced visual acuity will lead to problems in reading small print in newspapers, magazines, etc., recognizing faces and facial expressions, reading road signs, orientation and mobility, driving, and using computer.

Inability to read can be managed by increasing the magnification, thereby displacing the central scotoma as shown in Figure 15.1. Magnification is increased using low vision devices (LVDs) such as high add spectacles, hand magnifiers, stand magnifiers, and electronic devices such as closed-circuit televisions (CCTVs). For viewing objects from a distance, the "telescope" is the only LVD. It can be prescribed monocularly or binocularly. The disadvantage with a telescope is that it cannot be used for mobility. Bioptic telescopes are useful for driving. Telescope can be used for face recognition but it may not be culturally accepted in few countries.

Difficulties in orientation and mobility can be managed using eccentric viewing techniques. In case of severe visual impairment, cane techniques are useful. Sighted-guide technique is other option for safe navigation, especially while crossing roads and crowded areas. Using a flashlight in dimly lit areas helps in avoiding falls especially in unfamiliar areas. In most cases, combination of these techniques is useful.

Information technology, computer literacy, and information access are of crucial importance for everyone in society, including the visually impaired. Special software helps visually impaired to use computers. Available softwares can magnify text, menus and icons on the computer screen up to 16 times. It also provides a speech output for the text displayed on screen. The Kurzweil 1000 software scans and reads printed text with accuracy, speed, and reliability. Moreover, it opens and reads a broad variety of electronic text formats, and can efficiently search, download, and read electronic books directly from the Internet. For severe visually impaired, the software JAWS is useful as it is a screen-reading program that enables the text displayed on the screen to be spoken by a speech synthesizer, making it accessible to a visually impaired user. A screen reader allows menus, dialog boxes, tool tips and system messages to be read back.

Reduced contrast sensitivity will lead to problems in driving or mobility in dimly lit areas (in the night or in the rain or fog), judging distances, walking down steps, recognizing faces, finding a telephone number in a directory, reading instructions on a medicine container, and navigating safely through unfamiliar environments.

There are limited strategies to enhance the contrast. Optimum lighting, minimizing glare, and reversing or increasing print contrast are the only interventions for enhancing contrast. If contrast sensitivity is severely impaired, nonvisual techniques such as audio books may be required. Increasing the contrast of the edges of the door frames, furniture, stairs, and walls by painting the edges in contrasting colors will help in safe navigation. Nonoptical devices such as fiber-tipped black ink pen, bold line papers, typoscopes, etc. may help in enhancing the contrast while writing. Glare is reduced by using absorptive lenses such as tinted lenses, filters, or polarizing glasses.

MANAGEMENT OF ACTIVE WET AGE-RELATED MACULAR DEGENERATION

Several treatment strategies are clinically approved and have been evaluated in clinical trials. Based on the outcome of these studies, some therapies are currently recommended for the treatment of neovascular AMD.

Laser Photocoagulation

Laser photocoagulation is done to thermally ablate a neovascular membrane and stop its further growth, limiting the size of central or paracentral visual field defect.[42,43] However, collateral damage to the adjacent neurosensory retina results in an absolute scotoma at the treated site. This approach was based on the assumption that the photoreceptor function at the CNV site may not recover but is irreversibly lost. The principle of this therapy also relies on a clear differentiation of two angiographic subtypes of CNV, including classic and occult lesions.

Photocoagulation of extrafoveal CNV resulted in a significant reduction of expected vision loss over 2 years. The primary benefit was reduced by a recurrence rate of 50%, particularly since recurrent growth usually occurred at the subfoveal border of the treated CNV. The benefit of photocoagulation therapy of juxtafoveal CNV was limited by an even higher rate of persistence and recurrence. Progression despite intervention was found in about 80% of treated eyes over a 5-year observation period.

Laser photocoagulation may be an alternative in extrafoveal small CNV or the extrafoveal recurrence of a large subfoveal lesion, with marked fibrotic or atrophic changes at the level of the foveal avascular zone where vision improvement is not an option, but merely maintenance of a useful visual field.

Photodynamic Therapy

Verteporfin (Visudyne) has been the first genuine pharmacological therapy approved for the treatment of subfoveal CNV secondary to AMD. Following intravenous administration of a chemical photosensitizer, a laser with nonthermal light intensity in the red wavelength spectrum (689 nm), which is absorbed by the sensitizer, is used to physically activate the sensitizer. Since the light absorption induces a focal photochemical oxidation that is toxic to vascular endothelial cells, the internal vascular lining is altered selectively. Intravascular thrombosis is induced, which occludes the neovascular channels, but no thermal tissue damage occurs. In contrast to laser coagulation, photoreceptor integrity and retinal function are maintained and laser-induced scotoma is usually not seen. The photodynamic therapy (PDT) strategy was the first therapy attempting to avoid nonselective tissue damage.

In the TAP (treatment of AMD with photodynamic therapy) study, subfoveal lesions, containing any proportion of a classic component, up to 5,400 mm in diameter and a visual acuity ranging from 20/40 to 20/200 were treated with verteporfin therapy. PDT reduced the risk of moderate vision loss, defined as losing more than 15 letters (three lines), from 62% in the sham-treated patients to 47% in the PDT treated patients over 2 years. Subgroup analysis revealed the largest benefit for predominantly classic lesions with 59% of treated eyes as compared to 31% of placebo-treated eyes losing less than 15 letters.[44] The Verteporfin in Photodynamic Therapy (VIP) study[45] enrolled patients with subfoveal lesions composed of occult-only CNV types without any classic component. Patients were only eligible if recent disease progression, including vision loss by at least one line, new hemorrhage or an enlargement of the CNV by at least 10% seen by angiography was documented. At 2 years, 45% of the PDT-treated eyes compared to 32% of sham-treated eyes lost less than 15 letters (Early Treatment of Diabetic Retinopathy Study chart). Subgroup analysis revealed that CNV with a lesion size of less than or equal to 4 MPS DA or an initial VA of less than or equal to 65 letters had a better outcome.

Photodynamic therapy is still used as a standard therapy for neovascular AMD (Figs. 15.2A to D) with predominantly classic CNV and occult CNV smaller than 4 MPS DA in combination with recent disease progression in many countries. In general, lesion size was identified as the most important prognostic factor with smaller lesions presenting a more favorable outcome. Another unfavorable prognostic factor is the number of PDT treatments applied; the lower the number of PDT applications, the better the visual outcome. With increasing retreatment rates, vision continuously declines, most likely due to an irreversible damage to the adjacent choriocapillaris and the overlying retinal pigment epithelium (RPE).[46] In lesions with serous detachment of the RPE, mechanical rips are a serious concern and severe vision loss was found as a rare event following PDT of occult lesions.[47]

Vascular Endothelial Growth Factor Inhibitors

Vascular endothelial growth factor (VEGF) plays a principal role in the neovascular forms of age-related degeneration. It causes endothelial proliferation, migration, and new capillary formation-inducing angiogenesis. It also enhances vascular permeability. There are six different isoforms of VEGF having 121, 145, 165, 183, 189, and 206 amino acids.[48,49] VEGF 165 is thought to be predominantly responsible for pathological neovascularization and exists in both soluble and bound forms.[48] Its function at the retinal pigment epithelial level is poorly understood. It probably plays a role as a vascular survival factor for the choriocapillaris as well as in the maintenance of fenestrations in the choriocapillaris through directed secretion from the basal portion of the pigment epithelium.[48]

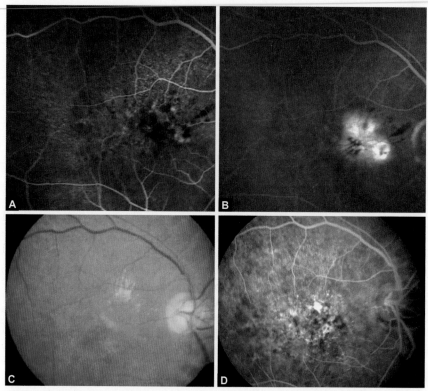

Figs. 15. 2A to D: Pre-photodynamic therapy (PDT) fluorescein angiography (FA) images (A and B) and post-PDT fundus and FA image (C and D) at the end 12 months follow-up.

Pegaptanib Sodium

Pegaptanib sodium is an aptamer composed of ribonucleic acids which competitively and selectively binds VEGF 165 and inhibits angiogenesis and pathologic leakage. It is administered intravitreally and reinjections are performed in six-weekly intervals as the molecule is rapidly degraded enzymatically by intraocular nucleases.

The VISION trial,[7] designed as two parallel phase III double-masked, sham-controlled, dose-ranging studies included a total of 1.186 patients. All lesion subtypes with subfoveal location and a total area of less than 12 DA were included. PDT could be applied to the investigator's discretion. Intravitreal injections were performed on a fixed regular schedule with 6-week intervals. After 1 year, 70% of the pegaptanib treated eyes versus 55% of control eyes lost less than 15 letters in VA, and a gain of more than 15 letters was found in 6% versus 2%, respectively. Pegaptanib patients lost a mean of nine letters during the observation period of 1 year as compared to a loss of 14 letters in the control group. At 2 years, 59% of eyes treated with a dose of 0.3 mg pegaptanib lost less than 15 letters compared to the 45% of standard care (sham) treated eyes. The therapeutic benefit of pegaptanib is comparable to the effect obtained with PDT monotherapy, but requires a continuous regimen of retreatments on a 6-weekly basis. The most frequent potential VEGF-inhibition-related adverse events, such as ischemic coronary artery disorders, vascular hypertensive disorders, thromboembolic events, heart failure, and serious hemorrhagic events, were all comparable between the treatment and control groups and all less than 10%. The most common effects were eye pain, floaters, punctate keratitis, nontraumatic cataracts, anterior segment inflammation, vitreous opacities, etc. The serious adverse effects were endophthalmitis, traumatic cataracts and retinal detachments.[7]

Ranibizumab (Figs. 15.3A and B)

Ranibizumab is a monoclonal antibody fragment (Fab) directed towards all isoforms of VEGF-A that was specifically designed to target wet AMD.[50] The human antibody fragment is produced by an *E. coli* expression system and has a molecular weight of 48 kD allowing for excellent retinal penetration. The half-lifetime of the small Fab fragment is 2–4 days, resulting in a rapid systemic clearance and high systemic safety.[50]

The FDA has approved the use of ranibizumab in the treatment of neovascular wet AMD based on 1-year clinical efficacy and safety data from the two pivotal phase III trials, ANCHOR and MARINA, and the phase I-II FOCUS trial.[51] The efficacy of ranibizumab has been studied in these clinical trials having the same primary efficacy end point, the proportion of patients losing less than 15 letters from baseline at 12 months. The multicenter, Phase III, randomized, double blind, sham-controlled, 24-month clinical trial evaluated ranibizumab 0.3 mg and 0.5 mg with minimally classic or occult choroidal neovascularization (CNV) associated with AMD.[50,51] Ranibizumab showed loss of less than 15 letters in visual acuity in 90% of the patients as compared to 53% in sham.

The findings of these three large clinical trials suggest that ranibizumab was effective and well-tolerated in patients. The benefits apply to all angiographic subtypes of neovascular AMD and across all lesion sizes. Although the pivotal phase III trials (MARINA and ANCHOR) used monthly injections of ranibizumab for 2 years, the ongoing PIER, PrONTO, and SAILOR trials are investigating less frequent dosing regimens, and preliminary results from the PrONTO study suggest that fewer injections will most likely result in visual acuity improvements similar to the results from the phase III trials. When comparing the ANCHOR results with the FOCUS results, it also becomes apparent that the combination of ranibizumab with PDT does not necessarily result in better visual acuity outcomes, and the use of PDT may even reduce the visual acuity benefits achieved with ranibizumab alone. It seems unlikely that combination therapy provides any significant advantage over ranibizumab alone unless the combination of PDT and ranibizumab can decrease the need for frequent retreatment.[52-54] The results from the PrONTO study already suggest that less frequent treatment with ranibizumab is possible by using a variable dosing regimen with optical coherence tomography (OCT).[51] Ranibizumab

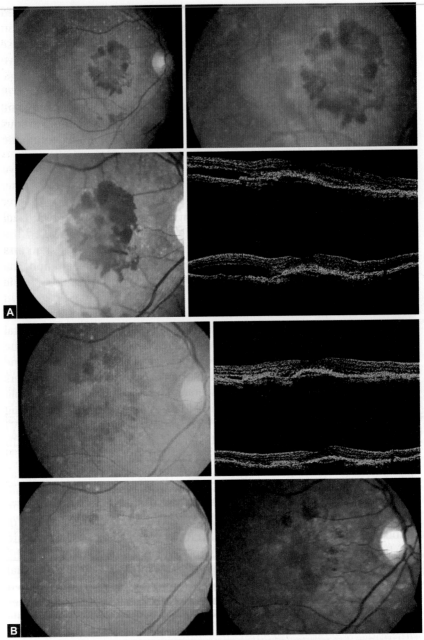

Figs. 15.3A and B: (A) Fundus and optical coherence tomography (OCT) image of subfoveal choroidal neovascular membrane (CNV) secondary to age-related macular degeneration (preintravitreal ranibizumab); (B) Fundus photo and OCT image of resolving subfoveal CNV at 6 months and resolved status at the end of 12 months following multiple injection of intravitreal ranibizumab.

also seems to be safe, with the 2-year MARINA[50,51] data showing no increase in the incidence of systemic adverse events that could be associated with anti-VEGF therapy, such as myocardial infarction and stroke. There was a hint of a safety concern, however, in the pooled 1-year safety results from the MARINA and ANCHOR trials. Although the combined rate of myocardial infarction and stroke during the first year of the ANCHOR and MARINA trials was similar in the control and the 0.3 mg ranibizumab arms (1.3% and 1.6%, respectively), these adverse events were slightly higher in the 0.5 mg ranibizumab arm (2.9%).[51] The most common ocular complaints of patients receiving ranibizumab injections in randomized clinical trials were transient conjunctival hemorrhage, vitreous floaters, intraocular inflammation, increased intraocular pressure and eye pain.[50] The rates of serious adverse events such as retinal detachment, cataract and endophthalmitis were similar to those that have been reported with other intravitreal injections, and patients should always be treated under strict aseptic conditions to reduce this risk.[50]

Appropriate studies (EXCITE trial, SUSTAIN trial) evaluating a pro re nata regimen administering treatment when needed based on the disease activity are under way. Appropriate diagnostic tools such as OCT may offer useful parameters for an optimal, i.e. individualized follow-up and retreatment decision.

Avastin

Bevacizumab is a full-length recombinant, humanized antibody of a molecular weight of 149 kDa binding to all VEGF isoforms. Since the binding affinity of bevacizumab is about 100 times lower than that of ranibizumab (N Ferrara, unpublished data), a comparison of clinical efficacy is difficult without clinical trials. The drug was originally developed to target pathologic angiogenesis in tumors and was approved by the FDA for the treatment of metastatic colorectal cancer. Avery et al.[55] described a complete resolution of retinal edema in 37% of eyes 4 weeks after initial an injection of bevacizumab and in 49% of eyes 8 weeks after the initial injection when treated monthly on an as-needed basis. Spaide et al.[56] also reported statistically significant improvement in central retinal thickness measurements for 3 months after monthly bevacizumab injections. However, an appropriate clinical trial is necessary to answer its long-term effect.

Combination Therapies

Combination of Verteporfin Therapy (Photodynamic Therapy) with Intravitreal Triamcinolone

Corticosteroids are known to exert an inhibitory effect on VEGF expression, vascular permeability and inflammatory pathways. Therefore, it has been suggested that a combination of PDT and intravitreal steroids may have a beneficial additive effect on the visual outcome and rate of recurrence.

Preliminary findings suggest that the combination is safe, reduces PDT-associated leakage and leads to a resolution of retinal edema and atrophy of the CNV.[57] Side effects of ocular steroids include cataract progression in almost every eye and an increased intraocular pressure which may not be controlled with topical therapy.

Combination Therapy of Antiangiogenic Pharmacotherapy and Verteporfin Therapy

Combining the anti-VEGF approach with PDT may have a synergetic long-term effect, potentially reducing the frequency of retreatments. Evidence was gained from the VISION trial with about 50% of patients with predominantly classic lesions receiving additional PDT treatments. The study population representing these patients showed a more beneficial course compared to eyes receiving PDT only.[58]

A phase I/II randomized sham-controlled study, the FOCUS trial,[59] compared the safety and efficacy of ranibizumab in combination with PDT vs PDT monotherapy. An intravitreal injection of 0.5 mg ranibizumab in a lyophilized formulation was given 1 week after standard PDT. An improvement by X3 lines was found in the combination arm, while only 5% of patients in the PDT monotherapy group demonstrated an improvement. A significant difference was found in the rate of PDT retreatments: a total number of 3.4 treatments were required in the monotherapy, but only 2.3 PDT treatments were needed in the combination arm. The PROTECT trial, a prospective, open-label phase I/II study, examined the safety of same-day administration of standard PDT and an intravitreal injection of the liquid formulation of ranibizumab which was routinely used in the MARINA, ANCHOR, and PIER studies. The initial treatment was followed by three subsequent monthly injections of ranibizumab. After 4 months, 92% of eyes had stable vision, improved by a mean of seven letters was found in the overall population, and 25% of patients improved by more than three lines.[60]

A combination of PDT and anti-angiogenic agents was proven to be safe and effective. The prognosis with respect to improvement, seen in a third of patients in the previously untreated FOCUS group, appears to be comparable to anti-angiogenic monotherapy. However, combination therapy may potentially reduce the need for retreatments and, therefore, might offer an alternative, which is less time- and cost-intensive than any type of monotherapy.

Surgical Treatment Approach

Various surgical approaches to the treatment of neovascular AMD have been suggested, including surgical removal of subfoveal CNV, macular translocation, transplantation of retinal pigment epithelium and removal of subretinal hemorrhage.

Macular translocation has a primary goal of relocating the central neurosensory retina or fovea during or after surgery, specifically for the management of macular disease.[61] The surgical objective of macular translocation is to:

- Reposit the neurosensory retina of the fovea in an eye with a subfoveal lesion to a new location with presumably a healthier bed of RPE–Bruch membrane–choriocapillaris complex devoid of the lesion, allowing the fovea to recover.
- Relocate the fovea overlying a lesion such as CNV to an area outside the border of the CNV, which converts the subfoveal lesion to one that is juxtafoveal or extrafoveal. This allows the destruction of the CNV with conventional laser photocoagulation without destroying the fovea, thereby preserving central vision and arresting the progression of the CNV.
- Combine with submacular surgery, allowing the fovea to be relocated to an area outside the retinal pigment epithelial defect often associated with CNV removal.

The submacular surgery trials (SSTs) research group could not demonstrate any benefit of surgery compared to observation for subfoveal CNV or hemorrhagic lesions with respect to VA, reading speed, or contrast threshold in a large randomized multicenter study.[62] Furthermore, a recently published meta-analysis did not find any relevant evidence for a beneficial outcome of any of the listed surgical procedures in neovascular AMD.[63]

Stem Cells

Stem cell technology has the exciting potential to provide the ability to repair or renew dysfunctional or dead RPE cells. Transplantation of allogeneic fetal RPE cells has been performed in patients with CNV and in those with geographic atrophy. Although these reports demonstrated the feasibility of the surgical technique, there was evidence of the rejection of the transplanted cells. This led to interest in the transplantation of autologous RPE, and a recent prospective trial of surgical excision of CNV[64] with the transplantation of autologous RPE demonstrated better results than membrane excision alone. Autologous iris pigment epithelial transplantation is an alternative technique; when transplanted into the sub-retinal space, these cells have been shown to survive for at least 6 months.[65]

Cell therapy is an exciting area of research that is aimed at regeneration tissues/organs in patients with irreparable damage to tissues or organs. Cell therapy is no longer restricted to the transfer of cells from a healthy subject to a patient, as in bone marrow transplant or corneal transplant. We can now envisage a cell therapy that involves generation of patient-specific cells for transplantation, manipulate them in vitro into the desired cell type and transplant these cells into patient for functional restoration of the damaged tissue. Although many cell therapies are right now being tested in animal models and their clinical application might take much longer, results from these studies are encouraging and suggest that regeneration of custom-made organ might indeed be possible in real life. With the advances in stem cell biology, it is also now possible to generate patient-specific pluripotent stem cells that are capable of generating all types of cells, if the correct milieu is provided. It remains to be seen whether these cells can be coaxed in vitro to differentiate into retinal cells that can integrate and restore retinal function.

Artificial Retina

As a result of building novel interfaces to the nervous system, new concepts for vision prostheses have evolved to the point where, currently, there are four approaches to a vision prosthesis.[66]

Subretinal Prosthesis

In this approach, a silicon micromanufactured device called a microphotodiode (MPD) array or semiconductor microphotodiode array (SMA) is placed behind the retina between the sclera and the bipolar cells where incident light is transformed into graded electrical potentials that stimulate the bipolar cells to form a visual sensation.

Epiretinal Prosthesis

In contrast to the subretinal approach, where the stimulating device was placed in the outer retina between the sclera and the bipolar cells, the epiretinal approach places the stimulating device on the inner retina between the vitria and the retinal ganglion cells. The epiretinal implant will likely stimulate both RGC cell bodies and passing axons from the RGC located on the periphery. This approach bypasses the damaged or missing photoreceptors, as well as any remnant retinal circuitry (amacrine, bipolar, and horizontal cells) and directly stimulates the output layer of the retina.

Optic Nerve Stimulation

In the visual pathway, the optic nerve is one place where the entire visual field is represented in a relatively small area. Multielectrode cuff electrodes are placed around the optic nerve and, by using complex patterns of electrical stimulation, they selectively stimulate subsets of axons, or even individual axons, in the optic nerve.

Intracortical Microstimulation of Visual Cortex

The final approach currently being investigated for vision prosthesis is the electrical stimulation of the primary visual cortex. Progress in intracortical microstimulation (ICMS) of the visual cortex has concentrated on establishing the safety, long-term biocompatibility, and functionality of penetrating microelectrode arrays in the brain.

New Therapies under Clinical Investigation

Anecortave Acetate for Dry Age-related Macular Degeneration

This is a novel drug, which preserves the angiostatic effect of corticosteroids, but does not exhibit clinically relevant glucocorticoid receptor-mediated activity and, thus, does not elevate intraocular pressure or induce cataract. The therapeutic level of the drug is achieved only when anecortave acetate (AA) is placed into direct contact with the posterior scleral surface. The drug is delivered as a periocular posterior juxtascleral depot using a specially designed blunt-tipped cannula to deliver the drug onto the outer surface of the sclera over the macula. Retreatment is necessary only every 6 months.[67] AA suspension (15 and 30 mg) is currently under evaluation to reduce the risk of disease progression in patients with dry AMD (the AART study). The study's objective is to determine the safety and efficacy of AA suspension when used to treat patients with nonexudative AMD who are at risk of progressing to exudative AMD.

Squalamine Lactate

Squalamine lactate is a small molecule isolated from the cartilage of the dogfish shark, *Squalus acanthus*, a species known for its resistance to bacterial and viral infections. The molecule belongs to a class of compounds called aminosterols, a steroid chemically linked to an amino acid. Squalamine has a unique combination of various mechanisms of action. It blocks the function of specific ion transporters in the cell membrane. These ion pumps control basic cell functions through regulation of intracellular pH, cell metabolism and cell volume. Squalamine can block various angiogenic cytokines such as VEGF, as well as the expression of integrin and cytoskeleton by chaperoning calmodulin. A phase III clinical trial is currently on.[68]

Small Interfering Ribonucleic Acid

Ribonucleic acid interference is a natural mechanism to inhibit the intracellular production by silencing gene coding for that specific protein, which is mediated by double stranded RNA homologous to the targeted protein. Small interfering RNA (siRNA) is a double-stranded RNA consisting of 21–22 nucleotides which is incorporated into the cell. After being further processed to an RNA-induced silencing complex (RISC) by intracellular enzymes, the fragment binds specifically to messenger RNA (mRNA), causing cleavage and further digestion of the mRNA. The RISC complex can then bind to other mRNA molecules and the process is repeated multiple times resulting in a very efficient overall inhibition of the production of the targeted protein. Clinical phase I and II studies evaluating siRNAs have already been performed.[69] The two siRNAs undergoing clinical trial are Cand5 and siRNA-027. Cand5 is an siRNA against all isoforms of VEGF. siRNA-027 is an siRNA against a VEGF receptor 1. The results are awaited.

Vascular Endothelial Growth Factor Trap

The VEGF Trap is a fully human-soluble decoy receptor protein that consists of a fusion of the second Ig domain of human VEGF receptor (VEGFR) 1 and the third Ig domain of human VEGFR2 with the constant region (Fc) of human Ig IgG1. This is used as a means of blocking the normal VEGF signaling pathway by inhibiting the binding of VEGF to its normal VEGF receptors rather than to the decoy soluble receptors.[70]

The VEGF Trap was engineered to have optimized pharmacokinetic properties and a very high affinity for all isoforms of VEGF-A (<1 pM), as well as placental growth factor, a closely related angiogenic factor. VEGF Trap has shown robust anti-tumor effects in numerous mouse models of cancer and is now in clinical trials (VIEW-2).[71,72]

Gene Therapy

Angiogenesis is a multifactorial process with multiple actors and counteractors. Several cytokines, such as pigment-epithelium-derived growth factor (PEDF), endostatin and angiostatin, are known to act as antiangiogenic agents. LentiVector, a gene delivery system, was used to introduce the angiostatic genes of endostatin and angiostatin, only being turned on under hypoxic conditions, into the retinal pigment epithelium of mice. This has potential therapeutic implications in management of progressive AMD. However, the identification of several AMD genes makes this approach more complex.

CONCLUSION

The future may include a combination approach that has the potential to decrease the recurrence, progression and also improve efficacy besides providing additional blockade of the angiogenic cascade. In a nutshell, with increasing life expectancy, we will face more patients with AMD searching for a cost-effective approach yet functionally beneficial. Limited financial resources will force us to select the best and most effective therapy for our patients. One must also understand that present scientific evidence should allow us to select therapies that can restore quality central vision and allow patients to experience the benefit of treatment.

REFERENCES

1. National Advisory Eye Council (US). Vision Research: A National Plan 1994-8.NIH Publication No.93-3186. Bethesda, MD: US Department of Health and Human Services; 1993.
2. Berman K, Brodaty H. Psychosocial effects of age-related macular degeneration. Int Psychogeriatr. 2006;18(3):1-14.
3. Sunness JS. The natural history of geographic atrophy, the advanced atrophic form of age-related macular degeneration. Mol Vis. 1999;5:25.
4. Seddon J, Sharma S, Adelman R. Evaluation of the clinical age-related maculopathy staging system. Ophthalmology. 2006;113(2):260-6.
5. Bindewald A, Bird AC, Dandekar SS, et al. Classification of fundus autofluorescence patterns in early age-related macular disease. Invest Ophthalmol Vis Sci. 2005;46(9):3309-14.
6. Klein R, Klein BE, Tomany SC, et al. Ten-year incidence and progression of age-related maculopathy: The Beaver Dam eye study. Ophthalmology. 2002;109(10):1767-79.

7. Evans JR. Risk factors for age-related macular degeneration. Prog Retin Eye Res. 2001;20(2):227-53.
8. Mitchell P, Wang JJ, Foran S, et al. Five-year incidence of age-related maculopathy lesions: The Blue Mountains eye study. Ophthalmology. 2002;109(6):1092-7.
9. Friedman DS, Katz J, Bressler NM, et al. Racial differences in the prevalence of age-related macular degeneration: The Baltimore Eye Survey. Ophthalmology. 1999;106(6):1049-55.
10. Klein R, Klein BE, Marino EK, et al. Early age-related maculopathy in the cardiovascular health study. Ophthalmology. 2003;110(1):25-33.
11. Kayatz P, Thumann G, Luther TT, et al. Oxidation causes melanin fluorescence. Invest Ophthalmol Vis Sci. 2001;42(1):241-6.
12. Sundelin SP, Nilsson SE, Brunk UT. Lipofuscin-formation in cultured retinal pigment epithelial cells is related to their melanin content. Free Radic Biol Med. 2001;30:74-81.
13. Berendschot TT, Willemse-Assink JJ, Bastiaanse M, et al. Macular pigment and melanin in age-related maculopathy in a general population. Invest Ophthalmol Vis Sci. 2002;43(6):1928-32.
14. Age-Related Eye Disease Study Research Group. Risk factors associated with age-related macular degeneration. A case-control study in the age-related eye disease study: age-related eye disease study report number 3. Ophthalmology. 2000;107(12):2224-32.
15. Delcourt C, Diaz JL, Ponton-Sanchez A, et al. Smoking and age-related macular degeneration. The POLA Study. Pathologies Oculaires Liees a l'Age. Arch Ophthalmol. 1998;116(8):1031-5.
16. Klein R, Klein BE, Moss SE. Relation of smoking to the incidence of age-related maculopathy. The Beaver Dam Eye Study. Am J Epidemiol. 1998;147(2):103-10.
17. Hyman LG, Lilienfeld AM, Ferris FL III, et al. Senile macular degeneration: a case-control study. Am J Epidemiol. 1983;118(2):213-27.
18. Smith W, Mitchell P, Leeder SR. Smoking and age-related maculopathy. The Blue Mountains Eye Study. Arch Ophthalmol. 1996;114(12):1518-23.
19. Mitchell P, Wang JJ, Smith W, et al. Smoking and the 5-year incidence of age-related maculopathy: the Blue Mountains Eye Study. Arch Ophthalmol. 2002;120(10):1357-63.
20. Heeschen C, Jang JJ, Weis M, et al. Nicotine stimulates angiogenesis and promotes tumor growth and atherosclerosis. Nat Med. 2001;7(7):833-9.
21. Omenn GS, Goodman GE, Thornquist MD, et al. Effects of a combination of beta-carotene and vitamin A on lung cancer and cardiovascular disease. N Engl J Med. 1996;334(18):1150-5.
22. Klein BE, Klein R, Lee KE, et al. Risk of incident age-related eye diseases in people with an affected sibling: the Beaver Dam Eye Study. Am J Epidemiol. 2001;154(3):207-11.
23. Stone EM, Braun TA, Russell SR, et al. Missense variations in the fibulin 5 gene and age-related macular degeneration. N Engl J Med. 2004;351(4):346-53.
24. Hageman GS, Anderson DH, Johnson LV, et al. A common haplotype in the complement regulatory gene factor H (HF1/CFH) predisposes individuals to age-related macular degeneration. Proc Natl Acad Sci USA. 2005;102(20):7227-32.
25. Kimura K, Isashiki Y, Sonoda S, et al. Genetic association of manganese superoxide dismutase with exudative age-related macular degeneration. Am J Ophthalmol. 2000;130(6):769-73.
26. Stephen H, Clara AC, Susan LS, et al. The genetics of age-related macular degeneration: a review of progress to date. Surv Ophthalmol. 2006;51(4):316-63.

27. Blumenkranz MS, Russell SR, Robey MG, et al. Risk factors in age-related maculopathy complicated by choroidal neovascularization. Ophthalmology. 1986;93(5):552-8.
28. Cruickshanks KJ, Klein R, Klein BE. Sunlight and age-related macular degeneration. The Beaver Dam Eye Study. Arch Ophthalmol. 1993;111(4):514-8.
29. Klein R, Klein BEK, Wong TY, et al. The association of cataract and cataract surgery with the long-term incidence of age-related maculopathy. The Beaver Dam Eye Study. Arch Ophthalmol. 2002;120(11):1551-8.
30. Age-related Eye Disease Study Research Group. A randomized, placebo-controlled, clinical trial of high-dose supplementation with vitamins C and E, beta carotene, and zinc for age-related macular degeneration and vision loss: AREDS report no. 8. Arch Ophthalmol. 2001;119(10):1417-36.
31. Watkins ML, Erickson JD, Thun MJ, et al. Multivitamin use and mortality in a large prospective study. Am J Epidemiol. 2000;152(2):149-62.
32. Rulon LL, Robertson JD, Lovell MA, et al. Serum zinc levels and Alzheimer's disease. Biol Trace Elem Res. 2000;75(1-3):79-85.
33. Cunningham JJ, Fu A, Mearkle PL, et al. Hyperzincuria in individuals with insulin-dependent diabetes mellitus: concurrent zinc status and the effect of high-dose zinc supplementation. Metabolism. 1994;43(12):1558-62.
34. Raz I, Karsai D, Katz M. The influence of zinc supplementation on glucose homeostasis in NIDDM. Diabetes Res. 1989;11(2):73-9.
35. Cannon CP, Braunwald E, McCabe CH, et al. Pravastatin or atorvastatin evaluation and infection therapy-thrombolysis in myocardial infarction Investigators: antibiotic treatment of Chlamydia pneumoniae after acute coronary syndrome. N Engl J Med. 2005;352:1646-54.
36. Regillo C, Jerdan J. Anecortave acetate: prevention of AMD. In: Program of the Annual Meeting of the American Academy of Ophthalmology. Retina Subspecialty Day. San Francisco, CA: American Academy of Ophthalmology. 2004;10-1.
37. Choroidal Neovascularization Prevention Trial Research Group. Laser treatment in fellow eyes with large drusen: updated findings from a pilot randomized clinical trial. Ophthalmology. 2003;110(5):971-8.
38. Owens SL, Bunce C, Brannon AJ, et al.; Drusen Laser Study Group. Prophylactic laser treatment hastens choroidal neovascularization in unilateral age-related maculopathy: final results of the Drusen Laser Study. Am J Ophthalmol. 2006;141(2):276-81.
39. Complications of Age-Related Macular Degeneration Prevention Trial Study Group. The Complications of Age-related Macular Degeneration Prevention Trial (CAPT): rationale, design and methodology. Clin Trials. 2004;1(1):91-107.
40. Pulido JS, Sanders D, Klingel R. Rheopheresis for age-related macular degeneration: clinical results and putative mechanism of action. Can J Ophthalmol. 2004;40(3):332-40.
41. Pulido JS. Multicenter Investigation of Rheopheresis for AMD (MIRA-1) Study Group. Multicenter prospective, randomized, double-masked, placebo-controlled study of rheopheresis to treat nonexudative age-related macular degeneration: interim analysis. Trans Am Ophthalmol Soc. 2002;100:85-106.
42. Macular Photocoagulation Study Group. Argon laser photocoagulation for neovascular maculopathy. Five-year results from randomized clinical trials. Arch Ophthalmol. 1991;109(8):1109-14.
43. Macular Photocoagulation Study Group. Laser photocoagulation for juxtafoveal choroidal neovascularization. Five-year results from randomized clinical trials. Arch Ophthalmol. 1994;112(4):500-9.

44. TAP Study Group. Verteporfin therapy for subfoveal choroidal neovascularization in age-related macular degeneration: four-year results of an open-label extension of 2 randomized clinical trials—TAP Report No. 7. Arch Ophthalmol. 2005;123(9):1283-5.

45. Verteporfin in Photodynamic Therapy Report 2. Verteporfin therapy of subfoveal choroidal neovascularization in age-related macular degeneration: two-year results of a randomized clinical trial including lesions with occult with no classic choroidal neovascularization—verteporfin in photodynamic therapy report 2. Am J Ophthalmol. 2001;131(5):541-60.

46. Schmidt-Erfurth U, Laqua H, Schlotzer-Shrehard U, et al. Histopathological changes following photodynamic therapy in human eyes. Arch Ophthalmol. 2002;120(6):835-44.

47. Pieramici DJ, Bressler SB, Koester JM, et al. Occult with no classic subfoveal choroidal neovascular lesions in age-related macular degeneration: clinically relevant natural history information in larger lesions with good vision from the verteporfin in photodynamic therapy (VIP) trial: VIP Report No 4. Arch Ophthalmol. 2006;124(5):660-4.

48. Ferrara N. Vascular endothelial growth factor: basic science and clinical progress. Endocr Rev. 2004;25(4):581-611.

49. Ruckman J, Green LS, Beeson J, et al. 2'-Fluoropyrimidine RNA-based aptamers to the 165-amino acid form of vascular endothelial growth factor (VEGF165): inhibition of receptor binding and VEGF-induced vascular permeability through interactions requiring the exon 7-encoded domain. J Biol Chem. 1998;273(32):20556-67.

50. Singh RP, Kaiser PK. Role of ranibizumab in management of macular degeneration. Indian J Ophthalmol. 2007;55(6):421-5.

51. Rosenfeld PJ, Brown DM, Heier JS, et al. Ranibizumab for neovascular age-related macular degeneration. N Engl J Med. 2006;355(14):1419-31.

52. Brown DM, Kaiser PK, Michels M, et al. Ranibizumab versus verteporfin for neovascular age-related macular degeneration. N Engl J Med. 2006;355(14):1432-44.

53. Kaiser PK, Brown DM, Zhang K, et al. Ranibizumab for predominantly classic neovascular age-related macular degeneration: subgroup analysis of first-year ANCHOR results. Am J Ophthalmol. 2007;144(6):850-7.

54. *Eter N. Focus Study 2-Year Results: Combination Therapy with Ranibizumab and Photodynamic Therapy with Verteporfin. Bordeaux: Club Jules Gonin; 2006.

55. Avery RL, Pieramici DJ, Rabena MD, et al. Intravitreal bevacizumab (Avastin) for neovascular age-related macular degeneration. Ophthalmology. 2006;113(3):363-72.

56. Spaide RF, Laud K, Fine HF, et al. Intravitreal bevacizumab treatment of choroidal neovascularization secondary to age-related macular degeneration. Retina. 2006;26(4):383-90.

57. Spaide RF, Sorenson J, Maranan L. Combined photodynamic therapy with verteporfin and intravitreal triamcinolone acetonide for choroidal neovascularization. Ophthalmology. 2003;110(8):1517-25.

58. Gragoudas ES. Photodynamic therapy and/or Macugen update. Presented at Academy of Ophthalmology Subspecialty Meeting, Chicago; 2005.

59. Heier JS. Lucentis Update. Presented at AAO Subspecialty Day, Retina. Chicago; 2005.

60. Schmidt-Erfurth UM, Gabel P, Hohman T. PROTECT Study Group. Preliminary results from an open-label, multicenter, phase II study assessing the effects of same

day administration of ranibizumab (Lucentis) and verteporfin PDT (PROTECT Study). ARVO. 2006;47:2960.

61. Fujii GY, Au Eong KG, Humayun MS, et al. Limited macular translocation: current concepts. Ophthalmol Clin North Am. 2002;15(4):425-36.

62. Hawkins BS, Bressler NM, Miskala PH, et al. Surgery for subfoveal choroidal neovascularisation in age-related macular degeneration: ophthalmic findings. SST Report No. 11. Ophthalmology. 2004;111(11):1967-80.

63. Falkner CI, Leitich H, Frommlet F. The end of submacular surgery for age-related macular degeneration? A meta-analysis. Graefes Arch Clin Exp Ophthalmol. 2007;245(4):490-501.

64. Binder S, Krebs I, Hilgers RD, et al. Outcome of transplantation of autologous retinal pigment epithelium in age-related macular degeneration: a prospective trial. Invest Ophthalmol Vis Sci. 2004;45(11):4151-60.

65. Semkova I, Kreppel F, Welsandt G, et al. Autologous transplantation of genetically modified iris pigment epithelial cells: a promising concept for the treatment of age-related macular degeneration and other disorders of the eye. Proc Natl Acad Sci. USA. 2002;99(20):13090-5.

66. Maynard EM. Visual prosthesis. Annu Rev Biomed Eng. 2001;3:145-68.

67. Slakter JS. Anecortave acetate for treating or preventing choroidal neovascularization. Ophthalmol Clin North Am. 2006;19(3):373-80.

68. Connolly B, Desai A, Garcia CA, et al. Squalamine lactate for exudative age related macular degeneration. Ophthalmol Clin North Am. 2006;19(3):381-9.

69. Tolentino M. Interference RNA technology in the treatment of CNV. Ophthalmol Clin North Am. 2006;19(3):393-9.

70. Rudge JS, Thurston G, Davis S, et al. VEGF trap as a novel antiangiogenic treatment currently in clinical trials for cancer and eye diseases, and VelociGene-based discovery of the next generation of angiogenesis targets. Cold Spring Harbor Symp Quant Biol. 2005;70:411-8.

71. Nambu H, Nambu R, Melia M, et al. Combretastatin A-4 phosphate suppresses development and induces regression of choroidal neovascularization. Invest Ophthalmol Vis Sci. 2003;44(8):3650-5.

72. Cheng N, Van Hoof H, Bockx E, et al. The effects of electric currents on ATP generation, protein synthesis, and membrane transport of rat skin. Clin Orthop Relat Res. 1982;171:264-72.

CHAPTER 16

Polypoidal Choroidal Vasculopathy

Lingam Gopal, Mayuri Bhargava, Su Xinyi

INTRODUCTION

Polypoidal choroidal vasculopathy (PCV) is a spectrum of disease involving the choroidal vasculature and usually affecting the adult population. Although described first in females of African-American origin,[1] it is now known to be more common in the Asian population. The clinical presentations were initially described as "posterior uveal bleeding syndrome".[2] We now know that while hemorrhage is an important component of the manifestation, it is not a *sine qua non* of the disease entity. The incidence of PCV can be grossly underestimated if retinal surgeons do not routinely use indocyanine green angiography for evaluating serosanguinous maculopathy in adults.

DEMOGRAPHICS

The prevalence has been reported to be 22–25% among the Japanese, Koreans and Chinese,[3-5] while in countries like Italy, Belgium, Greece, and the United States, the prevalence has been reported to range from 4% to 9%.[6-8] In a report from Japan, up to 58.5% of the eyes presenting with neovascular age-related macular degeneration (AMD) was shown to have PCV.[9] Contrary to the original description, PCV has been shown to occur in both genders and perhaps with equal frequency. The age at presentation is one to two decades earlier than the typical AMD. PCV tends to be bilateral, although the presentation can be quite asymmetrical.

CLINICAL PRESENTATION

Polypoidal choroidal vasculopathy is primarily a disease of the inner choroidal circulation. Two angiographic features, the polyps and the branching vascular network (BVN), characterize PCV. Secondary features include the collection of fluid/blood/lipids in various spaces.

SYMPTOMATOLOGY

Polypoidal choroidal vasculopathy and neovascular AMD can share common presenting symptoms such as reduced visual acuity, especially for near and metamorphopsia. However, the incidence of sudden significant drop in vision is more common with PCV in view of its propensity to lead to large hemorrhagic detachments of the retina and retinal pigment epithelium. PCV can also remain asymptomatic if the lesions are extramacular. The extent of vision disturbance obviously is related to the extent and location of the serous exudation and hemorrhage.

Ophthalmoscopic Features

- *Choroidal polyp*: Ophthalmoscopically, choroidal polyps can be seen as orange—red nodules of variable size, most commonly located in the macular area (69.5%).[10] However, the lesions can also occur near arcades and in peripapillary area.
- *Serous exudation*: The hyperpermeability of the lesions leads to the production of serous pigment epithelial detachments, retinal detachments as well as intraretinal fluid. The extent of these serous detachments can vary from subtle lesions that are only detected on optical coherence tomography (OCT) to large retinal detachments involving several quadrants of the fundus. Large serous retinal detachments are usually associated with an episode of massive hemorrhage.
- *Hemorrhage*: The hallmark of PCV is the occurrence of a hemorrhage in the subretinal pigment epithelial space; subretinal space; and sometimes breakthrough vitreous hemorrhage. Massive hemorrhages are more often seen as a feature of PCV rather than AMD.
- Fibrotic sequelae: Contrary to AMD, PCV does not form large disciform scars, at least to start with.[11,12] Multiple hemorrhages lead to variable degree of fibrosis.
- *Role of anti-platelet agents and anticoagulants*: Patients who are on anticoagulants are at an increased risk of massive hemorrhages, sometimes resulting in no perception of light. Patients on anti-platelet drugs (aspirin, clopidogrel) are also at increased risk of hemorrhage. These drugs may not cause the hemorrhage but perpetuate the same resulting in large bleeds.

TYPES

Yuzawa et al.[19] classified PCV into two types based on indocyanine green (ICG) characteristics:
1. Polypoidal choroidal neovascularization (CNV), or type 1 PCV, characterized by visible feeder and draining vessels and numerous network vessels or "interconnecting channels" on ICG video angiography. This type is considered to be the representative of CNV beneath the RPE.

2. In typical PCV, or type 2 PCV, neither feeder nor draining vessels is detectable, and the number of network vessels is small similar to BVN. Mean subfoveal choroidal thickness is also noted to be thicker in typical PCV than in polypoidal CNV.

The concept of late geographic hyperfluorescence (LGH): Kang et al.[20] have identified well-demarcated hyperfluorescent lesions in late-phase indocyanine green angiography (ICGA) and believe that they are highly characteristic of PCV. These lesions typically are seen as clearly demarcated geographic areas of hyperfluorescence seen about 10 minutes after the injection of the dye. In contrast, in late-onset hyperfluorescence due to AMD, the borders of the lesions are fuzzy. They believe that these areas of LGH may be predictive of future lesions and need a close watch. On the flipside, the disappearance of these lesions is believed to be a good prognostic indicator.

INVESTIGATIONS

Currently, multimodal imaging including fundus fluorescein angiography (FA), ICGA and optical coherence tomography (OCT) are becoming essential in differentiating PCV from choroidal neovascularization (CNV) secondary to age-related macular degeneration and lesions of retinal angiomatous proliferation (RAP).[13]

Fluorescein Angiography

On the fluorescein angiography (FA), PCV usually appears as a leak similar to "occult choroidal neovascular membrane" (CNVM), since the branching vascular networks are located in Bruch's membrane and are thus subretinal pigment epithelium (RPE). Sometimes however, PCV can also present like a "classic" CNV with early well-defined hyperfluorescence. This can be due to increased hyperfluorescence from atrophy of overlying RPE; subretinal fibrinous exudation or the occurrence of type 2 CNV secondary to PCV. The polyps can look like small PEDs on FA. Thus, macular PCV can be misdiagnosed as AMD if FA alone is performed.[14,15]

Indocyanine Green Angiography

It is considered the gold standard for definitive diagnosis of PCV, since it is primarily a pathology of the choroidal vasculature. ICG has a high protein-binding capacity and fluoresces in the infrared range (790–805 nm). Considering this emission spectrum, lesions under RPE are better detected with ICG angiography.[16] The main characteristics of PCV on ICGA are the polyps and the BVN. On ICGA, polyps (which are aneurysmal dilatations arising from inner choroidal vessels) are seen as hyperfluorescent spots with a halo seen in the first six minutes. In the late phase, the leak beyond the lesion remains, while the lesion itself can become hypofluorescent. The washout phenomenon describes total disappearance of the dye from the lesion in the very late phase. However, leaky lesions can retain the dye as hyperfluorescent rings.[17] Polyps may be single or multiple and when multiple can be seen as a cluster or at the terminals of a BVN.

BVN are seen as radiating vessels deep to RPE. Early-stage ICG video angiograms show a filling of the network vessels, and pulsatile polypoidal lesions are often observed in up to 10% of patients. Choroidal vascular hyperpermeability, (detected on ICGA as multifocal spots of hyperfluorescence in the mid and late phases) is more often seen in eyes with PCV than with exudative AMD. ICG can also identify areas of pigment epithelial detachments (PEDs). A notch in the PED can often represent the location of the polyp. Tan et al.[18] described two varieties of abnormal vasculature in relation to PCV:

1. A network of crisscrossing vessels that have no specific identifiable origin
2. The typical branching vascular network (BVN) that have a point of origin and subsequent sequential branching.

Optical Coherence Tomography

B-scan imaging with OCT shows the polypoidal lesions as steep dome-like elevations of highly reflective RPE layers with moderate reflectivity of the lesion. The elevations are sharper than what are noted in PEDs.[21] The BVN is identifiable as two hyper-reflective lines (the double layer sign), representing separation of RPE from Bruch's membrane by the BVN and generally corresponds to LGH on ICGA.[22] Treatment of BVN does not eliminate the double-layer sign due to the presence of fibrosis beneath RPE. A common feature noted is a notch in the PED where the polyps usually lie. PCV also tends to produce more serous retinal detachment and less intraretinal fluid compared to CNV–AMD.[23]

Choroidal hyperpermeability is very often associated with an increased thickness of the choroid, termed "pachychoroid." Chung et al. have demonstrated a thickened subfoveal choroid in eyes with PCV compared to those with AMD.[24,25] Pachychoroid has also been noted in conditions such as central serous chorioretinopathy (CSCR). The interpretation of the thickened choroid can be difficult when the overall thickness is affected by the relative thinning of one layer (choriocapillaris) along with the thickening of another. Agarwal et al. have described the choroidal vascularity index (CVI) to define the ratio of luminal area to the total choroidal area.[26] This index is more robust. Vortex vein engorgement has also been noted to be more often seen in PCV eyes compared to controls.[27]

There is a suggestion that PCV could be a disease of choroidal congestion considering the observations of increased choroidal thickness and vortex vein engorgement.

En-face Optical Coherence Tomography Imaging

High-speed scanning with present day machines permits en-face imaging. To visualize the PCV complex, it is ideal to scan below the RPE and above the

Bruch membrane using slabs of 10 μm to 30 μm. Polyps are seen as round, ring-like structure and BVNs appear as mesh-like configuration.[28] PCV complexes may appear larger on en face imaging due to the ability of this technique to detect areas that may have no flow, and due to the imaging of tissue that extends over and around the PCV vessels. Studies have demonstrated some correlation of en face OCT and ICGA in their ability to detect PCV complexes permitting en face imaging to be used in lieu of ICGA in follow up studies.

Optical Coherence Tomography Angiography

Optical coherence tomography angiography is a noninvasive form of investigation that permits the imaging of blood flow without a contrast dye being injected. In a study by Srour et al.,[29] BVN was detected as a hyperflow lesion consistently, but the polyps were seen as hyperflow round lesions only in 25% and as hypoflow round structures in 75% indicating unusual blood flow through the polyps.

Fundus Autofluorescence

The polyps show a central hypo-autofluorescence with a circumferential hyper-autofluorescent ring, while the BVN shows granular hyper-autofluorescence. The disappearance of the hyper-autofluorescent ring tends to correspond with closure of polyps on follow-up studies.[30] FAF is a useful addendum but does not replace the other investigations in the routine diagnosis and management of PCV.

DIAGNOSIS

The Japanese study group of polypoidal choroidal vasculopathy[31] defined the types of PCV as:
- *Definite PCV:* As presence of clinically evident orange red nodules or polyps identified with characteristic features on ICGA.
- *Probable PCV:* As abnormal vascular network or recurrent RPE detachments of hemorrhagic or serous nature.

An expert panel developed evidence-based guidelines for the clinical diagnosis of PCV.[32] The summary of the guidelines are as follows:
1. *Clinical suspicion:* Serous/serosanguinous or notched PED; massive sub-macular hemorrhage; presence of subretinal orange nodule; and non-antivascular endothelial growth factor (VEGF) responder.
2. *Confirmatory (after ICGA):* Single or multiple focal nodular areas of hyperfluorescence from choroidal circulation within first 6 minutes after ICG injection. Nodular appearance on stereoscopic viewing; hypofluorescent halo; association with the BVN; pulsatile filling of polyp on dynamic ICGA; focal hyperfluorescence corresponding to the orange nodule seen on clinical examination; and association with massive submacular hemorrhage.

AGE-RELATED MACULAR DEGENERATION AND POLYPOIDAL CHOROIDAL VASCULOPATHY

There is some confusion about AMD and PCV. Some questions remained unanswered:

1. Whether AMD and PCV represent two different and distinct entities
2. Are they variants of the same disease?
3. What causes the polypoidal lesions to develop and how do we explain the observed racial differences?
4. What exactly is the role of the pachychoroid?
5. Is the treatment approach different for the two?
6. Is the long-term prognosis different?

However, neovascular AMD and PCV present differences in epidemiology and their clinical manifestations (Table 16.1).

MANAGEMENT

Considering the spectrum of manifestations, the confusion in clearly differentiating it from AMD, and the variable natural course. The approach to the treatment is also fuzzy.

The treatment can be discussed under the following heads:

1. Management of PCV
2. Management of subretinal hemorrhage.

TABLE 16.1: Differences between neovascular AMD and PCV.

	CNV-AMD	PCV
Race	More in Caucasians	More in Japanese, Chinese, Blacks
Age	Occurs at 65 years and above usually	Occurs one decade earlier
Drusen	Important feature	Usually absent
Orange nodules	Absent	Pathognomonic
Large hemorrhagic PEDs	Less common	More common
Fluorescein angiography	Occult/Combined occult classic CNVM	Appearance similar to occult CNVM
ICG angiography	Plaque or ill-defined hyperfluorescence	Polyps and BVN
Fibrosis as sequelae	More common	Less common
Intraocular VEGF levels	Higher	Lower than in AMD but higher than controls

(CNV: choroidal neovascularization; AMD: age-related macular degeneration; PCV: polypoidal choroidal vasculopathy; PED: pigment epithelial detachment; CNVM: chroidal neovascular membrane; ICG: indocyanine green; BVN: branching vascular network; VEGF: vascular endothelial growth factor)

Management of Polypoidal Choroidal Vasculopathy

The options available are thermal laser photocoagulation, photodynamic therapy (PDT) and intravitreal injection of anti-VEGF agents.

Thermal Laser[33,34]

Laser using green or yellow laser can be used to target the polyps directly. However, the collateral damage to the overlying and surrounding retina limits its use to extramacular lesions. Being an orange–red lesion, the diode laser is not ideally suited.

Photodynamic Therapy[35]

Photodynamic therapy involves intravenous infusion of the photosensitive dye 'Verteporfin' followed by the treatment of the lesion of interest with a 689 nm laser of low fluency. This results in damage to the vascular endothelium by liberation of free oxygen radicals and not by heat generation. Hence, collateral damage is avoided. This makes it possible to treat lesions within the macular area as well. The relative choroidal ischemia caused by the PDT is expected to reduce perfusion to the PCV lesion and encourage thrombosis and occlusion. While it is relatively straightforward to treat polyps, treating BVNs can pose a problem if the size of the BVN is large. The potential complications of PDT specific to PCV include tears in the RPE, choroidal ischemia, and perceived increased risk of subretinal hemorrhage.[36,37] The larger the area treated, the more the risk of damage due to choroidal ischemia.

Antivascular Endothelial Growth Factor Drugs[38]

Currently, experience is accumulating with use of both ranibizumab and aflibercept in PCV. There is general agreement on the role of anti-VEGF drugs, although the levels of VEGF were found to be less than in AMD. The reduction in edema and subretinal fluid is prominently seen but polyp regression is less often noted.

Combination Therapy

It appeals to the logic that a combination of PDT to the lesions, combined with anti-VEGF drugs may perhaps give the best result in terms of recovery from this episode as well as reducing the risk of future recurrent hemorrhages. However, this is not a consistent observation clinically.

Figure 16.1 shows a case of choroidal polyp identified on ICG, but seen as occult CNVM on the fundus fluorescein angiography (FFA). The effect of direct laser photocoagulation is evident in Figure 16.2. Figures 16.3 to 16.9 show the features of PCV on ICG and OCT in the form of multiple polyps and BVN. The partial closure of some of the polyps on PDT is also evident in the Figure 16.9.

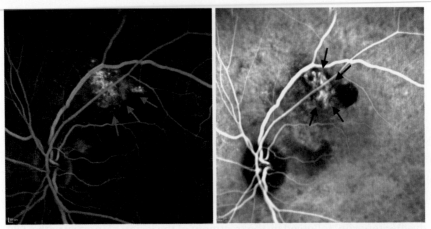

Fig. 16.1: Case 1: A case of extramacular polypoidal choroidal vasculopathy (PCV). The right half of the figure shows a fundus fluorescein angiogram that mimics occult choroidal neovascular membrane (blue arrows). The left half shows indocyanine green angiogram clearly depicting the polyps (black arrows).

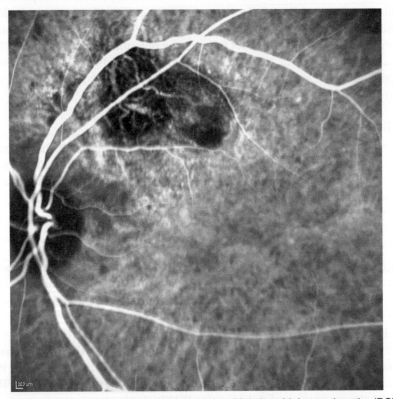

Fig. 16.2: Case 1: A case of extramacular polypoidal choroidal vasculopathy (PCV). Postfocal laser indocyanine green (ICG) angiogram demonstrating successful closure of the polyps.

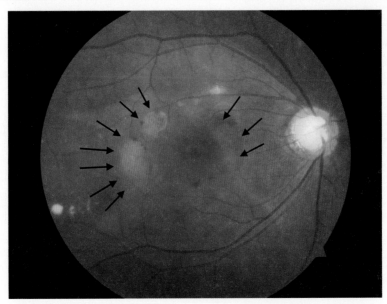

Fig. 16.3: Case 2: A case with multifocal polyps around macula. Typical orange nodules are seen around the macula along with serous retinal detachment.

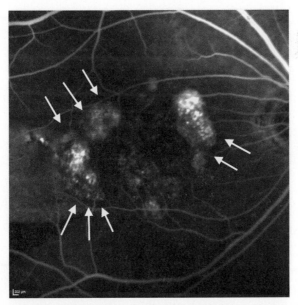

Fig. 16.4: Case 2: A case with multifocal polyps around macula. Fundus fluorescein angiography reveals leaks corresponding to the nodules.

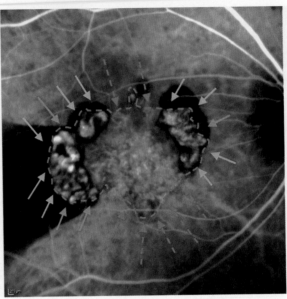

Fig. 16.5: Case 2: A case with multifocal polyps around macula. The ICG angiogram clearly demarcates the polyps (green arrows) as well as the central branching vascular network (blue arrows). The whole PCV complex is outlined by the blue dotted line.

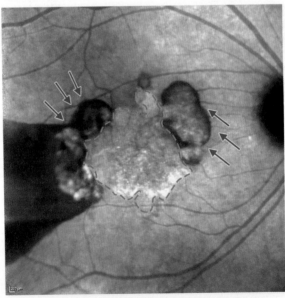

Fig. 16.6: Case 2: A case with multifocal polyps around macula. In the late-phase ICG angiogram showing the branching vascular network (BVN) more prominently, and some of the polyps show fading of fluorescence while others retain the dye.

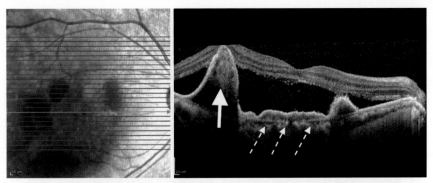

Fig. 16.7: Case 2: A case with multifocal polyps around macula. The optical coherence tomography features of the polyps (sharp dome-shaped elevation of retinal pigment epithelium with moderate intralesional reflectivity) and BVN (double layer sign). Note also the serous retinal detachment across the entire scan.

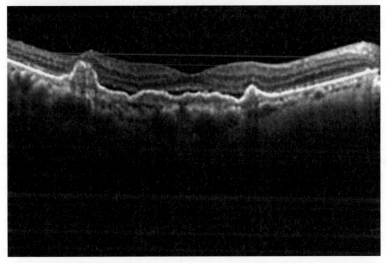

Fig. 16.8: Case 2: A case with multifocal polyps around macula. The OCT after photodynamic therapy depicting reduction in serous retinal detachment but persistence of the polyps and double layer sign of the BVN.

Management of Subretinal Hemorrhage

The evaluation of the eye should include the extent of subretinal versus sub-RPE hemorrhage and their location in relation to center of macula. The principles of management are as follows:

1. If the hemorrhage is not extensive, especially in terms of subfoveal thickness, it is best to ignore the hemorrhage and manage the PCV.
2. Sub-RPE hemorrhage is not amenable to be shifted away from posterior pole or removal surgically since the removal of these clots is associated with loss of RPE.

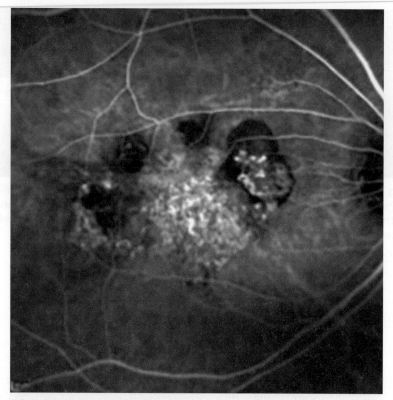

Fig. 16.9: Case 2: A case with multifocal polyps around macula. Repeat ICG angiogram shows occlusion of temporal and superior polyps but persistence of nasal polyps and BVN.

3. The subretinal hemorrhage can potentially be shifted away from the posterior pole using a combination of gas tamponade and tissue plasminogen activator (TPA).
4. Large subretinal hemorrhages tend to break through into vitreous cavity at some stage or the other, more so after the injection of gas.
5. Most often pars plana vitrectomy is performed to remove the vitreous component of the hemorrhage, and sometimes to remove the subfoveal portion of the subretinal hemorrhage.
6. Small sub-RPE hemorrhages can sometimes resolve without affecting the overlying retinal function significantly.
7. Heroic surgeries with 360-degree retinotomy and removal of extensive hemorrhages are rarely associated with acceptable functional results, mostly due to extensive damage to the RPE as well risk of PVR.

END POINT OF TREATMENT

Ideally one would like to have no secondary effects in the form of retinal/subretinal/sub-RPE fluid or hemorrhage, and the closure of all polyps and BVN. Such a happy ending is unfortunately not the rule. In general:

- Continued treatment is definitely indicated if the lesions are active and symptomatic.
- Continued treatment is possibly indicated if the lesions are active although not symptomatic.
- No treatment is indicated if polyps are seen clinically and angiographically but have no activity (on OCT and clinically).

RESULTS

The 'EVEREST' clinical trial has shown that polyp regression was greatest with combination of PDT and Ranibizumab injection (77.8%) followed by PDT alone (71.4%) and least with Ranibizumab alone (28.6%).[39] A younger age, better presenting vision, smaller baseline hemorrhage, and a smaller lesion size were independent factors predictive of better visual outcomes after PDT monotherapy. PDT has not been as effective to cause regression of BVN or its exudative activity. Studies which compare visual outcomes between PDT and anti-VEGF therapy have generally reported better results with anti-VEGF therapy. [37] In the EVEREST study, despite higher rate of polypoidal lesion closure, the PDT arm achieved less visual gain.[39] Also, studies have shown that in PCV eyes treated with PDT, visual outcome was stable until 2 years, but worsened at 3 years, especially in eyes with recurrence.[40] Reduced fluence PDT has been proposed to reduce the risk of PDT-related complications.[41]

In LAPTOP study, patients with PCV were randomized to either ranibizumab monotherapy or PDT monotherapy. At month 12, a higher proportion of patients in the ranibizumab arm gained 0.2 log MAR units and visual improvement was maintained to month 24.[42]

Currently ongoing randomized controlled trials for PCV (EVEREST 2 and PLANET) can provide further evidence regarding the benefits of PDT in combination with ranibizumab or Aflibercept. "EVEREST 2" is a 24-month, phase 4, randomized, double masked multicenter study of ranibizumab monotherapy or ranibizumab in combination with verteporfin photodynamic therapy on the visual outcome in patients with symptomatic macular PCV. "PLANET" is a randomized, double-masked, sham-controlled phase 3b/4 study of the efficacy, safety, and tolerability of intravitreal Aflibercept monotherapy compared to Aflibercept with adjunctive photodynamic therapy as indicated in subjects with PCV.[43,44]

Cho HJ et al.[45] in a study compared Ranibizumab and Aflibercept in PCV. They reported a higher rate of polyp regression in eyes treated with Aflibercept (39.5%) than Ranibizumab (21.6%), although the effect on central macular thickness and visual improvement was similar.

Recurrent Polypoidal Choroidal Vasculopathy

Polypoidal choroidal vasculopathy is associated with frequent recurrences (64% at 2 years, 77% at 3 years and 78.6% at 5 years).[40] Hence the long-term results are very often not satisfactory. Recurrences are characterized by hemorrhagic or exudative manifestation, and are due to the appearance of new polyps, polyps that did not close with treatment, or from BVN. Repeated PDT leads to cumulative damage to the normal choroidal vasculature and RPE. Thus, recurrent disease is treated with selective ablation of new or persistent polypoidal lesions with PDT or focal laser, while BVN activity can be managed using anti-VEGF monotherapy.

Treatment of Peripapillary Polypoidal Choroidal Vasculopathy

Currently, there are no optimal guidelines for the management of peripapillary PCV as these cases are generally excluded from randomized clinical trials. Ablative treatment with laser/PDT is associated with risk of damage to the optic nerve and papillomacular bundle, despite some studies suggesting that PDT even involving the disk is safe.[46] Hence, very often these situations are managed with anti-VEGF monotherapy.

PROGNOSTICATING FACTORS

1. Presentation as serous detachments have better prognosis compared to presentation as hemorrhagic detachments of RPE and retina.
2. Multiple polyps have worse prognosis compared to isolated lesions.[47,48]
3. Types of abnormal vascular network, polyps supplied by interconnecting channels were found to have the best visual outcome following treatment, followed by PCV with non-leaking BVN while PCV with leaking BVN had the worst visual outcome.[18]
4. A pulsating PCV on the ICG video angiography had a higher risk of extensive hemorrhagic events.
5. Choroidal vascular hyperpermeability on ICGA and thicker choroid on OCT may be a poor prognostic factor for response to anti-VEGF therapy in PCV.[49]

GENETICS

In a recent meta-analysis of 66 published articles on the association of genetic variants with PCV identified 31 polymorphisms in 10 genes/loci.[50] These genes have been shown to be involved in the complement cascade (e.g. CFH), inflammatory pathway, extracellular matrix/basement membrane regulation pathway (ARMS2, HTRA1) and lipid metabolism (CETP). Several other studies have found CETP genetic variants to be associated with a high risk of PCV,[51-54] suggesting a possible role of the high-density lipoprotein pathway in the pathogenesis of PCV.

Interestingly, some studies have suggested genotypic–phenotypic correlation in PCV. The *ARMS2 LOC387715* rs10490924 variant has been shown to be associated with larger lesion size, higher risk of vitreous hemorrhage, and worse visual outcome after PDT treatment.[55] In addition, the HTRA1-rs 11200638 is associated with poorer visual acuity 12 months after PDT treatment.[56] Certain risk genotypes (TT of rs10490924 and AA of rs11200638 at ARMS2/HTRA1) have been shown to have significantly poorer visual acuity outcome 1 year after combination therapy of PDT and intravitreal bevacizumab injection.[57] However, the limitations of these pharmacogenomics studies include their small sample size and restrospective design, which have limited their clinical applicability. Of note, the *ARMS2 A69S* and *CFH 162V* polymorphisms are associated with increased choroidal thickness and choroidal vascular hyperpermeability, similar to central serous chorioretinopathy.[58]

CHALLENGES AND FUTURE DIRECTION

Substantial uncertainty still remains whether PCV is part of the AMD spectrum, or a completely separate clinical entity. More importantly, the pathogenesis of PCV remains unclear. The exact role of VEGF in PCV is unclear, though it is widely believed that the VEGF is less crucial in PCV than in CNV-AMD. This may partially explain the limited efficacy of anti-VEGF monotherapy in PCV. Also, although multiple pathways have been eluded to play a role in PCV pathogenesis, such as complement activation, extra-cellular regulation, lipid metabolism and angiogenesis, how they contribute exactly to PCV formation remains unclear. Moreover, we still do not know what causes the branching vascular network, and why they do not respond well to either PDT or anti-VEGF agents.

As can be seen, this lack of understanding of the underlying pathogenesis has resulted in unclear treatment strategies for the various components of PCV. Addressing these gaps in our knowledge will allow us to develop targeted and effective treatment for PCV.

REFERENCES

1. Stern RM, Zakov ZN, Zegarra H, et al. Multiple recurrent serosanguineous retinal pigment epithelial detachments in black women. Am J Ophthalmol. 1985;100:560-9.
2. Kleiner RC, Brucker AJ, Johnston RL. The posterior uveal bleeding syndrome. Retina. 1990;10:9-17.
3. SHo K, Takahashi K, Yamada H, et al. Ploypoidal choroidal vasculopathy: incidence, demographic features and clinical characteristics. Arch Ophthalmol. 2003;121:1392-6.
4. Wen F, Chen C, Wu D, et al. Polypoidal choroidal vasculopathy in elderly Chinese patients. Graefes Arch Clin Exp Ophthalmol. 2004;242:625-9.
5. Byeon SH, Lee SC, Oh HS, et al. Incidence and clinical patterns of polypoidal choroidal vasculopathy in Korean patients. Jpn J Ophthalmol. 2008;52:57-62.
6. Scasellat-Sforzolini B, Mariotti C, Bryan R, et al. Polypoidal choroidal vasculopathy in Italy. Retina. 2001;21:121-5.
7. Ladas ID, Rouvas AA, Moschos MM, et al. Polypoidal choroidal vasculopathy and exudative age related macular degeneration in Greek population. Eye. 2004;18:455-9.
8. Lafaut BA, Leys AM, Snyers B et al. Polypoidal choroidal vasculopathy in Caucasians. Greaefes Arch Clin Exp Ophthalmol. 2000;238:752-9.
9. Imaizumi H, Takeday M. Knobby-like choroidal neovascularization accompanied with retinal pigment epithelial detachment. Nippon Ganka Gakkai Zasshi. 1999;103:527-37.

10. Hou J, Tao Y, Li XX, et al. Clinical characteristics of polypoidal choroidal vasculopathy in Chinese patients. Graefes Arch Clin Exp Ophthalmol. 2011;249:975-9.
11. Spaide RF, Yannuzzi LA, Slakter JS. Indocyanine green videoangiography of idiopathic polypoidal choroidal vasculopathy. Retina. 1995;15:100-10.
12. Yannuzzi LA, Sorenson J, Spaide RF, Lipson B: Idiopathic polypoidal choroidal vasculopathy. Retina. 1990;10:1-8.
13. Coscas G, Yamashiro K, Coscas F, et al. Comparison of exudative age-related macular degeneration subtypes in Japanese and French patients: multicenter diagnosis with multimodal imaging. Am J Ophthalmol. 2014;15:309-318.
14. Otsuji T, Tsumura A, Takahashi K, et al. Evaluation of cases of polypoidal choroidal vasculopathy showing classic choroidal neovascularization in their natural course. Nippon. Ganka Gakkai Zasshi. 2006;110:454-461.
15. Maruko I, Iida, T, Saito, M, et al. Combined cases of polypoidal choroidal vasculopathy and typical age-related macular degeneration. Graefe's Arch Clin Exp Ophthalmol. 2010;248:361-8.
16. Desmettre T, Devoisselle JM, Mordon S. Fluorescence properties and metabolic features of indocyanine green (ICG) as related to angiography. Surv Ophthalmol. 2000;45:15-27.
17. Koh AK. On behalf of The expert PCV panel. Polypoidal choroidal vasculopathy-Evidence based guidelines for clinical diagnosis and treatment. Retina. 2013;33:686-716.
18. Tan CSH, Ngo WK, Lim LW, et al. A novel classification of the vascular patterns of polypoidal choroidal vasculopathy and its relation to clinical outcomes. Br J ophthalmol. 2014;98:1528-33.
19. Yuzawa M, Mori R, Kawamura A. The origins of polypoidal choroidal vasculopathy. Br. J. Ophthalmol. 2005;89:602-7.
20. Kang SW, Chung SE, Shin WJ, et al. Polypoidal choroidal vasculopathy and late geographic hyperfluorescence on indocyanine green angiography. Br J Ophthalmol. 2009;93:759-64.
21. Lijima H, Iida T, Imai M, et al. Optical coherence tomography of orange-red subretinal lesions in eyes with idiopathic polypoidal choroidal vasculopathy. Am J Ophthalmol. 2000;129:21-6.
22. Sato T, Kishi S, Watanabe G, et al. Tomographic features of branching vascular networks in polypoidal choroidal vasculopathy. Retina. 2007;27:589-94.
23. Ozawa S, Ishikawa K, Ito Y, et al. Differences in macular morphology between polypoidal choroidal vasculopathy and exudative macular degeneration detected by optical coherence tomography. Retina. 2009;29:793-802.
24. Chung SE, Kang SW, Lee JH, et al. Choroidal thickness in polypoidal choroidal vasculopathy and exudative age related macular degeneration. Ophthalmology. 2011;118:840-5.
25. Jirarattanasopa P, Ooto S, Nakata I, et al. Choroidal thickness, vascular hyperpermeability, and complement factor H in age related macular degeneration and polypoidal choroidal vasculopathy. Invest ophthalmol. 2012;53:3663-72.
26. Agarwal R, Gupta P, Tan KA, et al. Choroidal vascularity index as a measure of vascular status of the choroid: measurements in healthy eyes from a population-based study. Sci Rep. 2016;12:6.
27. Chung SE, Kang SW, Kim JH, et al. Engorgement of vortex vein and polypoidal choroidal vasculopathy. Retina. 2013;33:834-40.
28. Saito M, Iida T, Nagayama D. Cross sectional and enface optical coherence tomographic features of polypoidal choroidal vasculopathy. Retina. 2008;28:459-64.

29. Srour M, Querques G, Semoun O, et al. Optical coherence tomography angiography characteristics of polypoidal choroidal vasculopathy. Br J Ophthalmol. 2016;100:1489-93.

30. Yamagishi T, Koizumi H, Yamazaki T, et al. Changes in fundus autofluorescence after treatments for polypoidal choroidal vasculopathy. Br J Ophthalmol. 2014;98:780-4.

31. Japanese study group of polypoidal choroidal vasculopathy. Criteria for diagnosis of polypoidal choroidal vasculopathy. Nippon Gangka Gakkai Zasshi. 2005;109:417-27.

32. Koh AHC. On behalf of The expert PCV panel. Polypoidal choroidal vasculopathy-Evidence based guidelines for clinical diagnosis and treatment. Retina. 2013;33:686-716.

33. Lee MW, Yeo I, Wong D, et al. Argon laser photocoagulation for the treatment of polypoidal choroidal vasculopathy. Eye. 2009;23(1):145-8.

34. Yuzawa M, Mori R, Haruyama M. A study of laser photocoagulation for polypoidal choroidal vasculopathy. Jpn J Ophthalmol. 2003;47, 379-84.

35. Wong RL, Lai TY. Polypoidal choroidal vasculopathy: an update on therapeutic approaches. J Ophthalmic Vis Res. 2013;8:359-71.

36. Hirami Y, Tsujikawa A, Otani A, et al. Hemorrhagic complications after photodynamic therapy for polypoidal choroidal vasculopathy. Retina. 2007;27:335-41.

37. Fan NW, Lau LI, Chen SJ, et al. Comparison of the effect of reduced-fluence photodynamic therapy with intravitreal bevacizumab and standard-fluence alone for polypoidal choroidal vasculopathy. J Chin Med Assoc JCMA. 2014;77:101-7.

38. Inoue M, Arakawa A, Yamane S, et al. Long term outcome of intra vitreal Ranibizumab treatment compared to photodynamic therapy in eyes with polypoidal choroidal vasculopathy. Eye. 2013;27:1013-20.

39. Koh A, Lee WK, Chen LJ, et al. EVEREST study: efficacy and safety of verteporfin photodynamic therapy in combination with ranibizumab or alone versus ranibizumab monotherapy in patients with symptomatic macular polypoidal choroidal vasculopathy. Retina. 2012;32:1453-64.

40. Wong CW, Cheung CM, Mathur R, et al. Three-year results of polypoidal choroidal vasculopathy treated with photodynamic therapy: retrospective study and systematic review. Retina. 2015;35:1577-93.

41. Yoshida Y, Kohno T, Yamamoto M, et al. Two-year results of reduced-fluence photodynamic therapy combined with intravitreal ranibizumab for typical age-related macular degeneration and polypoidal choroidal vasculopathy. Jpn J Ophthalmol. 2013;57:283-93.

42. Oishi A, Tsujikawa A, Yamashiro K, et al. Comparison of the effect of ranibizumab and verteporfin for polypoidal choroidal vasculopathy: 12-month LAPTOP study results. Am J Ophthalmol. 2013;156:644-51.

43. ClinicalTrials. Visual Outcome in Patients with Symptomatic Macular PCV Treated with Either Ranibizumab as Monotherapy or Combined with Verteporfin Photodynamic Therapy. (EVEREST II). [online] Available from https://clinicaltrials.gov/ct2/show/NCT01846273. [Accessed January, 2018].

44. ClinicalTrials. Aflibercept in Polypoidal Choroidal Vasculopathy (PLANET). [online] Available from https://clinicaltrials.gov/ct2/show/NCT02120950. [Accessed January, 2018].

45. Cho HJ, Kim KM, Kim HS, et al. Intra vitreal Aflibercept and Ranibizumab injections for polypoidal choroidal vasculopathy. Am J Ophthalmol. 2016;165:1-6.

46. Bernstein PS, Horn RS. Verteporfin photodynamic therapy involving the optic nerve for peripapillary choroidal neovascularization. Retina. 2008;28:81-4.

47. Suzuki M, Nagai N, Shinoda H, et al. Distinct responsiveness to intravitreal Ranibizumab therapy in Polypoidal choroidal vasculopathy with single or mutliple polyps. Am J Ophthalmol. 2016;166:52-9.

48. Uyama M, Wada M, Nagai Y, et al. Polypoidal choroidal vasculopathy: natural history. Am J Ophthalmol. 2002;133:639-48.

49. Kim H, Lee SC, Kwon KY, et al. Subfoveal choroidal thickness as a predictor of treatment response to anti vascular endothelial growth factor therapy for polypoidal choroidal vasculopathy. Graefes Arch Clin Exp Ophthalmol. 2015;254:1497-503.

50. Ma L, Li Z, Liu K, et al. Association of genetic variants with polypoidal choroidal vasculopathy: a systemic review and updated meta-analysis. Ophthalmology. 2015;122(9):1854-65.

51. Liu K, Chen LJ, Lai TY, et al. Genes in the high-density lipoprotein metabolic pathway in age-related macular degeneration and polypoidal choroidal vasculopathy. Ophthalmology. 2014;121:911-6.

52. Nakata I, Yamashiro K, Yamada R, et al. Genetic variants in pigment epithelium-derived factor influence response of polypoidal choroidal vasculopathy to photodynamic therapy. Ophthalmology. 2011;118:1408-15.

53. Nakata I, Yamashiro K, Kawaguchi T, et al. Association between the cholesteryl ester transfer protein gene and polypoidal choroidal vasculopathy. Invest Ophthalmol Vis Sci. 2013;54:6068-73.

54. Zhang X, Li M, Wen F, et al. Different impact of high-density lipoprotein-related genetic variants on polypoidal choroidal vasculopathy and neovascular age-related macular degeneration in a Chinese Han population. Exp Eye Res. 2013;108:16-22.

55. Chen H, Liu K, Chen LJ, et al. Genetic associations in polypoidal choroidal vasculopathy: a systematic review and metaanalysis. Mol Vis. 2012;18:816-29.

56. Tsuchihashi T, Mori K, Horie-Inoue K, et al. Prognostic phenotypic and genotypic factors associated with photodynamic therapy response in patients with age-related macular degeneration. Clin Ophthalmol. 2014;8:2471-8.

57. Park DH, Kim IT. LOC387715/HTRA1 variants and the response to combined photodynamic therapy with intravitreal bevacizumab for polypoidal choroidal vasculopathy. Retina. 2012;32:299-307.

58. Yoneyama S, Sakurada Y, Kikushima W, et al. Genetic factors associated with choroidal vascular hyperpermeability and subfoveal choroidal thickness in polypoidal choroidal vasculopathy. Retina. 2016;36:1535-41.

CHAPTER 17

Macular Phototoxicity

Dhananjay Shukla

INTRODUCTION

While the primary function of eyes is to perceive the light produced by or reflected from the material world, we "see," more the light is certainly not the Merrier for the vision. In fact, suboptimal light is way better than supraoptimal light in terms of comfortable visibility and safety. Too bright a light, when seen for too long, can permanently damage the ocular media and retina. "Too bright" is defined by two parameters: intensity of the light and the duration of the ocular exposure.[1] An extremely bright flash of light can vaporize the target ocular tissue in a fraction of a second, and such damage is called *photomechanical injury*, e.g. accidental exposure to industrial or military Q-switched lasers (this effect is also used therapeutically in posterior capsulotomy by the Nd:YAG laser).[1,2] These acute and severe injuries usually have a clear-cut cause, and are fortunately rare. Subacute light injuries occur over a longer exposure, usually in seconds, and cause retinal burn by raising the tissue temperature to about 10–20°C.[1,2] Classic examples of *photothermal injuries* are retinal photocoagulation (intentional or accidental, depending on the target area) or laser pointer injuries, caused by staring into the pointer. Though more common than photomechanical accidents, they are also relatively rare.[1,3] The most common and insidious light injuries are those caused by long-term exposure to light at an intensity considered safe for a brief duration. These are *photochemical injuries* (also called *phototoxic* or simply, *photic* injuries), and cause subtle but cumulative damage, which therefore goes undetected, unreported and underdiagnosed to a large extent.[1-3] Further, while the photic damage to the transmission media is reversible or manageable to a large extent, retinal phototoxicity tends to be permanent and irreversible. This review, therefore focuses on retinal photic injuries, and elaborates on the key offenders in the visible spectrum, the hazardous environmental settings, the risk factors, the early diagnostic signs, and the preventive measures.

PHOTOCHEMICAL INJURIES: PATHOGENETIC MECHANISM

Photochemical toxic reactions occur at temperatures too low to cause thermal burns (so it is technically wrong to call the resultant skin or retinal lesions *sunburns* or *eclipse burns*), at light brightness above the normal physiological levels, and exposure times in seconds to minutes.[1,3] The injury occurs only when the above parameters of light exposure are so excessive that they overwhelm the retinal repair mechanisms. The extent of damage is influenced by coexistent ocular disease, clarity of crystalline lens, the subject's age, diet and body temperature (fever *primes* retina for the low-intensity burns) as well as the systemic intake of certain photosensitizing drugs (see later).[1-3]

Phototoxicity is mediated by free radical release when the energy in the photons of the incident light excites the atoms of the substrate tissue, damaging the cell membranes, proteins, and nucleic acids. The higher the energy in photons, the more is the photochemical damage.[2] As the lower wavelengths of light have greater energy, they are more phototoxic. Very low-to-low wavelengths (UV-A and UV-B, violet) are absorbed to a large extent by the cornea and crystalline lens.[1,4,5] The prominent type of photochemical injury is therefore also referred to as *blue-light hazard*. The substrate for blue light absorption is the retinal pigment epithelium (RPE), specifically, the lipofuscin pigment. The toxicity develops over 1–2 days.[1,2,4] To a lesser extent, a slightly higher wavelength (500 nm, blue-green) can also directly damage the photoreceptors, mainly rods. This type of damage requires repetitive exposure over several days.[2-5]

AGENTS OF PHOTOTOXICITY

Sunlight and Welding Arc

Looking up at the sun momentarily, even on a sunny day, is unlikely to cause retinal damage due to instinctive aversion of gaze and pupillary constriction, which limit both the retinal exposure and heating.[1] However, sun worshippers (a centuries old practice indeed, cutting across religions) who erroneously believed that *sun-gazing* was good for their eyes, and practiced it every day for several years. All these subjects had significant RPE mottling with corresponding visual decline (which they refused to admit). A similar picture has been reported in psychiatric patients and addicts with altered consciousness due to hallucinogenic drugs.[6,7] A more common presentation in the saner general population is observed after watching a solar eclipse, where the damage is enhanced by a greater pupillary dilatation and the ability to watch the darkened sun for a longer period. The typical acute lesion is a subtle yellow-white foveolar spot (Figs. 17.1A to F), which could be missed unless looked for.[8] The lesion may fade away over a few months, generally leaving

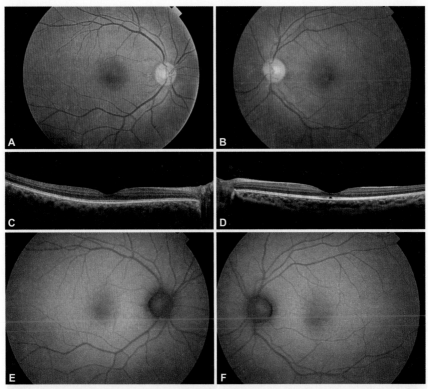

Figs. 17.1A to F: This 62-year-old physician accidentally noted distorted and subnormal vision in his left eye a week back. Best-corrected visual acuity was 6/6 in the right eye and 6/18 in the left. On asking a leading question, he confessed to having seen an eclipse several years back, squinting with his right eye. (A and B) Right fundus showed only a few drusen while the left fovea had a central depigmented spot. (C) Spectral domain optical coherence tomography (SD-OCT, grid view) showed a normal foveal contour in the right eye. (D) SD-OCT of the left eye (cross line) revealed a disruption of the outer retinal lines corresponding to the ellipsoid zone and the interdigitation zones (see text for details); the external limiting membrane was intact. Central foveal thickness was reduced to 143 μm (normal range: 220–260 μm approximately). (E) Fundus autofluorescence imaging was normal in the right eye; (F) left showed a central speck of increased hypoautofluorescence, with hyperautofluorescent parafoveal area.

no clinical traces or subtle RPE mottling. The children are more vulnerable to damage due to their clear lenses (which allow more short wavelengths) and lack of awareness.[8,9] An important aspect in the diagnosis is proactive history-taking about solar exposure, which the patient may dismiss as insignificant, especially in chronic solar retinopathy with mild-moderate visual symptoms (blurred vision, central scotoma).[10] The reflection of bright sunlight from large surfaces such as lakes and snow-covered landscapes can also predispose mountain trekkers and skiers to chronic indirect solar retinopathy.[4,11]

Welders experience both acute painful corneal erosions (photophthalmia) and chronic photic injuries from the occupational exposure to near-UV wavelengths in welding arc light (CJO). Chronic injuries are probably very common, and largely under-reported globally,[12] most pertinently in India, where it is common to see welders not wearing protective glasses (Figs. 17.2A to D). The younger (below 30 years) welding apprentices are more vulnerable due to the clear lens permitting more UV-A light.[4,12] The fundus picture is similar to solar retinopathy in both acute and chronic stages.[1,4,12]

Phototoxicity from Microscope, Endoilluminators and Ambient Light

Improved brighter lighting during intraocular surgery has improved surgical outcomes, but ironically, has also increased the scope of retinal phototoxicity.[1] The spectral components of white light (blue, green, and yellow), which are most helpful for tissue identification by the surgeon are also unfortunately most damaging to the retina of the eye under scalpel.[13] Light injuries have been reported after cataract, glaucoma, corneal and retinal surgeries. The latter two are more vulnerable due to longer duration (more than 30 minutes).[1] Cataract surgery, however, is the one most commonly performed, and when accidentally or inherently complicated and therefore longer (e.g. trans-scleral fixation of PCIOL),

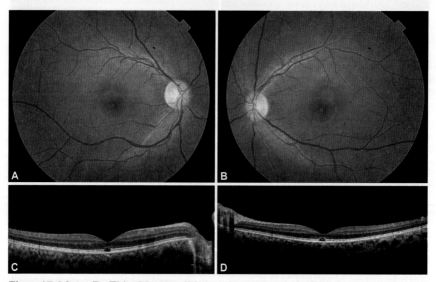

Figs. 17.2A to D: This 30-year-old man has been a welder for more than 10 years, and has been stoically living with a best-corrected Snellen visual acuity of 6/18 in both eyes. (A and B) Fundi revealed a central identical pale spot at the fovea in both eyes. (C and D) SD-OCT revealed a disruption of the outer retinal lines corresponding to the ellipsoid and interdigitation zones; the external limiting membrane was intact in both eyes. Central foveal thickness was subnormal in both right (171 μm) and left eyes (163 μm).

can result in phototoxicity in close to 10% of cases, with adverse visual outcomes in half the subjects.[14] Retinal surgeries are, however, inherently vulnerable due to the use of endoscopic lights. This concern is more relevant now with the use of small-gauge endoilluminators, which require double the power in light source as compared to 20G endo-lights.[13] The risk is further increased in macular surgeries, use of dyes (especially Indocyanine green), immobile chandeliers (which do not allow retinal recovery from constant exposure), surgical video making (which multiply the light requirement) and trainee surgeons taking more time in surgery.[13,15]

Though less common, such damage can also follow prolonged exposure to the fundus camera, the indirect ophthalmoscope, and imaging devices. This should be remembered especially during examination of vulnerable eyes.[1] The light-emitting diodes (LED), which are fast becoming the preferred source of domestic lighting, emit much more blue light than conventional lamps. An experimental study reported photochemical damage from the "white light" LED designs in albino rats and recommended further investigation on pigmented human retina.[16] Cases of macular phototoxicity of macula due to excessive, continued exposure to a video gaming device or computer screen, which are known to emit blue light from LED screens have been documented (unpublished data).

FACTORS AFFECTING VULNERABILITY TO PHOTOTOXICITY

Aging

Ocular media, mainly the cornea and the lens, are the most important protectors against photic injuries. Protection from the cornea against UV light remains uniform throughout life, while the crystalline lens becomes more protective as age advances. We have already seen how welders above the age of 30 years are more protected from the UV light of the welding arc. With further yellowing of the aging lens, it starts blocking the visible blue light too, which remains a threat through life. This protection is partly offset by the accumulation of lipofuscin pigment in the RPE which increases phototoxic vulnerability.[1,3] Cataract surgery therefore has the potential to increase the retinal exposure to blue light, besides the potential for intraoperative phototoxicity. There has been a prolonged debate on the use of UV- or blue-blocking intraocular lenses (IOLs) to mimic the protection of the aging lens.[1,17] On the other hand, blue-blocking IOLs have been accused of disturbing the circadian rhythm and the quality of sleep of the elderly.[18] These fears have been put to rest by recent trials;[19] there are, however, insufficient data to show the tangible benefits of these IOLs as well, particularly in terms of phototoxic damage resulting in age-related macular degeneration (AMD).[20]

Retinal Disease

Like aging, the diseases that result in lipofuscin accumulation in the RPE, such as Best disease and Stargardt's disease, make the retina more susceptible to light damage. Other diseases that affect the photo-pigment regeneration, like retinitis pigmentosa, have also shown the potential for photic damage in animals, though this potential is so far unproven in human subjects.[3] On the other hand, the role of cumulative phototoxic damage by short wavelengths, in the causation of AMD has been discussed and debated for close to a century.[1] Though a large body of experimental evidence is available in favor of this causative link, it remains unproven till date.[1]

Diet, Supplements and Drugs

The retina, being the most metabolically active tissue in the body, is highly vulnerable to oxidative injury.[21] An antioxidant rich diet has been proposed to make the retina resistant to light damage; [22] however, the modern diet is woefully deficient in macular carotenoids lutein and zeaxanthin, which could easily be provided by a diet rich in fruits and vegetables.[21]

Photosensitizing drugs are typically composed of tricyclic, heterocyclic or porphyrin rings, which allow them to bind to the melanin in the RPE, and make ordinarily harmless visible light (400–600 nm) phototoxic.[15] In view of the vast range of pharmacotherapeutic drugs, including antibiotics (e.g. tetracycline), antimalarials (e.g. hydroxychloroquine), psychoactive drugs (benzodiazepines), antiarrhythmic drugs (amiodarone), diuretics (furosemide, hydrochlorothiazide), NSAIDs (indomethacin) and even herbal supplements (St John's wort), the incidence of drug-induced phototoxicity appears to be grossly under-reported.[1,3,15]

DIAGNOSIS OF ACUTE AND CHRONIC MACULAR PHOTOTOXICITY

Irrespective of the cause, the most common retinal lesion is a faint yellow dot at the central macula in most cases of acute phototoxicity (Figs. 17.1B and 17.2A); a more dramatic blanching of the retina has been described, but rare.[1] The most important diagnostic clue is an exposure to a source of bright light immediately preceding the reduction in vision. If the intensity of the exposure does not appear to match the severity of the macular lesion, the it is instructive to look at the systemic status (febrile illness, diabetes, and hypertension), the use of photosensitizing drugs, and associated intraocular disease (heredomacular degenerations).[1,3,15]Associated photokeratitis (as in welding-arc exposure) is a simple giveaway.[1,12] The lesion fades quickly, leaving no footprints or a faint RPE stippling, and partial or complete visual recovery. Subacute and chronic cases are therefore much more difficult to diagnose: the fundus may look normal, the visual complaint vague and non-specific, and the patient may not remember the exposure (e.g. looking at an eclipse).[10,11] In this scenario, leading questions must be asked about the occupation (welder, mountaineer, sun-worshipper) and residence (mountains, cold regions), besides the usual suspects.

The key investigation, especially in the more obscure chronic cases, is spectral domain optical coherence tomography (SD-OCT). Previous versions of OCT are unable to demonstrate the finer details in the outer retina that characterize photic retinopathy.[11] In the acute phase, OCT shows a central triangular or vertical zone of hyperreflectivity in the outer nuclear layer,[23,24] with or without the interruption of the bright lines corresponding to the inner segment-outer segment junction (IS-OS junction, now called *ellipsoid zone*) of the photoreceptors (cones), and their apices (COST line or Verhoeff's line, now called *interdigitation zone*).[23,25] The chronic picture, however, characteristically shows an interruption of the outer retinal lines (the interdigitation and the ellipsoid zones) with an intact external limiting membrane, with or without the central foveal thinning/atrophy (Figs. 17.1C and D and 17.2C and D).[23]

The OCT findings are well supplemented by the fundus autofluorescence (FAF) imaging, which reveals the loss of the characteristic hypo-autofluoroscent signal at the central fovea in the acute phase.[10,23,24] After a few months, the FAF shows recovery of the normal central hyposignal. In some cases with recurrent photic insults (e.g. welders), the spot corresponding to the outer retinal interruption develops an accentuated punctate hypoautofluorescence (typically, but not universally at the central fovea), while the surrounding region shows hyperautofluorescence (Figs. 17.1E and F).[10,11,23] Multiple hyposignals can be found scattered around the fovea in some chronic cases.[11] Fluorescein angiography is a less informative investigation, which reveals nothing in subtle cases; window defects occur only at the stage where clinical RPE stippling is anyway clinically evident.[26]

In conclusion, the SD-OCT is the key investigation in acute and chronic, proven or suspected photic retinopathy, particularly that secondary to chronic recurrent exposure, like solar and welding arc retinopathy. The outer retinal findings, while characteristic, are not pathognomonic of photochemical damage, and could be mimicked by type 2 macular telangiectasia, maculopathy due to tamoxifen (early changes in vitreomacular traction and postoperative images of a closing macular hole[27]). Some of the mimics can be ruled out by history alone (tamoxifen use, macular hole surgery), others by additional OCT findings in the affected and fellow eye (macular telangiectasia and vitreomacular traction), or by additional investigations such as fluorescein angiography and FAF imaging (macular hole and telangiectasia).[27]

The General Assembly of the United Nations proclaimed 2015 as the *International Year of Light and Light-based Technologies*.[28] It is therefore high time for us to review the effect of light on the eyes. In modern times, young women are rightly conscious of sun-tan and sunburn, and often take protective measures. We, however, remain woefully ignorant of the several ways light can damage the eyes, where the most insidious and permanent damage is often at the retinal level. The threat of chronic phototoxicity has ironically become more real and relevant today in spite of reduced outdoor activities, due to the increasing exposure of children and young adults (with clear lenses, and therefore more vulnerable retina) to the LED light of electronic media, as well as domestic bulbs, the duration of exposure further increased by our greater life expectancy.[16,28] Marshall has poetically labeled the global light levels as approaching what could be described as *light pollution*.[28] While waiting for technological improvements in these devices to make them safer, it is wise to recognize and limit exposure to blue-light sources; even though a recent review absolves the current electronic media (TV, computers, tablets and smartphones) and LED lights of the blame for phototoxicity.[29] On the other hand, outdoor workers in general, and mountain trekkers and welders in particular, need to be educated about the hazards of chronic and repetitive exposure to reflected sunlight and the welding arc, and the imperative need for protective eye gear in hazardous occupations.[1-4,11,12,16] Acceptable levels of light exposure need to be defined by regulatory authorities, especially in India, where laborers toil away in environments that are largely unprotected both physically and legally.[3,11] UV-protecting sunglasses especially for individuals with fever, diabetes, and hypertension, on photosensitizing drugs, and after a cataract surgery offer reasonable protection.[1] As eye surgeons, we ourselves should exercise precautions such as minimal lighting compatible with comfortable intraocular surgery, avoiding routine oxygen intubation, checking out sensitizing drugs, etc. preoperatively.[1,13,15,20] While we march towards a digital age in a technology-savvy India, prudent use of safety measures and precautions inside and outside our homes shall allow us to enjoy the comforts of modern life without getting burnt by the very light that illuminates and nurtures our lives.

REFERENCES

1. Mainster MA, Turner PL. Photic retinal injuries: Mechanisms, Hazards, and Prevention. In: Ryan SJ (Ed). Retina, 5th edition. St Louis: Elsevier; 2013. pp. 1551-63.
2. Wu J, Seregard S, Algvere PV. Photochemical damage of the retina. Surv Ophthalmol. 2006;51:461-81.
3. Hunter JJ, Morgan JI, Merigan WH, et al. The susceptibility of the retina to photochemical damage from visible light. Prog Retin Eye Res. 2012;31:28-42.
4. Söderberg PG. Optical radiation and the eyes with special emphasis on children. Prog Biophys Mol Biol. 2011;107:389-92.
5. Youssef PN, Sheibani N, Albert DM. Retinal light toxicity. Eye. 2011;25:1-14.
6. Kamp PS, Dietrich AM, Rosse RB. Sun gazing by psychiatric patients. Am J Psychiatry. 1990;147:810-1.
7. Schatz H, Mendelblatt F. Solar retinopathy from sun-gazing under the influence of LSD. Br J Ophthalmol. 1973;57:270-3.
8. Khatib N, Knyazer B, Lifshitz T, et al. Acute eclipse retinopathy: a small case series. J Optom. 2014;7:225-8.
9. Gregory-Roberts E, Chen Y, Harper CA, et al. Solar retinopathy in children. J AAPOS. 2015;19:349-51.
10. dell'Omo R, Konstantopoulou K, Wong R, et al. Presumed idiopathic outer lamellar defects of the fovea and chronic solar retinopathy: an OCT and fundus autofluorescence study. Br J Ophthalmol. 2009;93:1483-7.
11. Shukla D. Optical coherence tomography and autofluorescence findings in chronic phototoxic maculopathy secondary to snow-reflected solar radiation. Indian J Ophthalmol. 2015;63:455-7.
12. Yang X, Shao D, Ding X, et al. Chronic phototoxic maculopathy caused by welding arc in occupational welders. Can J Ophthalmol. 2012;47:45-50.

13. Charles S. Illumination and phototoxicity issues in vitreoretinal surgery. Retina. 2008;28:1-4.

14. Kweon EY, Ahn M, Lee DW, et al. Operating microscope light-induced phototoxic maculopathy after transscleral sutured posterior chamber intraocular lens implantation. Retina. 2009;29:1491-5.

15. Siu TL, Morley JW, Coroneo MT. Toxicology of the retina: advances in understanding the defence mechanisms and pathogenesis of drug- and light-induced retinopathy. Clin Experiment Ophthalmol. 2008;36:176-85.

16. Shang YM, Wang GS, Sliney D, et al. 2014. White light-emitting diodes (LEDs) at domestic lighting levels and retinal injury in a rat model. Environ Health Perspect. 2014;122:269-76.

17. Mainster MA. Violet and blue light blocking intraocular lenses: photoprotection versus photoreception. Br J Ophthalmol. 2006;90:784-92.

18. Henderson BA, Grimes KJ. Blue-blocking IOLs: a complete review of the literature. Surv Ophthalmol. 2010;55:284-9.

19. Brøndsted AE, Sander B, Haargaard B, et al. The effect of cataract surgery on circadian photoentrainment: a randomized trial of blue-blocking versus neutral intraocular lenses. Ophthalmology. 2015;122:2115-24.

20. Yang H, Afshari NA. The yellow intraocular lens and the natural ageing lens. Curr Opin Ophthalmol. 2014;25:40-3.

21. Hammond BR, Johnson BA, George ER. Oxidative photodegradation of ocular tissues: beneficial effects of filtering and exogenous antioxidants. Exp Eye Res. 2014;129:135-50.

22. Vaughan DK, Nemke JL, Fliesler SJ, et al. Evidence for a circadian rhythm of susceptibility to retinal light damage. Photochem Photobiol. 2002;75:547-53.

23. Shukla D, Sharan A, Venkatesh R. Optical coherence tomography and autofluorescence findings in photic maculopathy secondary to distant lightning strike. Arch Ophthalmol. 2012;130:656-8.

24. Bruè C, Mariotti C, De Franco E, et al. Solar retinopathy: a multimodal analysis. Case Rep Ophthalmol Med. 2013;2013:906-20.

25. Staurenghi G, Sadda S, Chakravarthy U, et al. International Nomenclature for Optical Coherence Tomography (IN•OCT) Panel. Proposed lexicon for anatomic landmarks in normal posterior segment spectral-domain optical coherence tomography: the IN•OCT consensus. Ophthalmology. 2014;121:1572-8.

26. Jain A, Desai RU, Charalel RA, et al. Solarretinopathy: comparison of optical coherence tomography (OCT) and fluorescein angiography (FA). Retina. 2009;29:1340-5.

27. Comander J, Gardiner M, Loewenstein J. High-resolution optical coherence tomography findings in solar maculopathy and the differential diagnosis of outer retinal holes. Am J Ophthalmol. 2011;152:413-9.

28. Marshall J. Light in man's environment. Eye. 2016;30:211-4.

29. O'Hagan JB, Khazova M, Price LL. Low-energy light bulbs, computers, tablets and the blue light hazard. Eye. 2016;30:230-3.

CHAPTER 18

Chloroquine Retinopathy: Diagnosis

Aljoscha Steffen Neubauer

INTRODUCTION

Screening strategies for antimalarial retinal toxicity are still controversial, mainly because there is a difficulty in defining the early stages of retinopathy. Additionally, in well-monitored and dosed patients, the incidence of retinopathy is low. It is, therefore, important to first define chloroquine-associated toxicity. Most ophthalmic textbooks divide retinopathy into five stages.[1]

PREMACULOPATHY

The earliest fundus findings are usually some irregularity of the macular pigmentation and loss of the foveal reflex.[2,3] Subtle retinal changes such as pigmentary stippling or granular appearance of the macula with the patient still being asymptomatic (and not exhibiting defects in visual field testing) may be the first signs of retinopathy.[4,5] The presence of mild macular abnormalities without significant functional abnormalities has been termed as *premaculopathy* or *preretinopathy* by some authors.[6,7] However, the early stages of maculopathy are nearly indistinguishable from changes frequently occurring with aging. These changes are believed to be mostly reversible.

EARLY MACULOPATHY

Early maculopathy is defined by visual impairment (including some reduction in visual acuity). On ophthalmoscopy, the typical "Bull's eye" maculopathy can be seen associated with impaired visual acuity and central visual field defects.[8,9] Changes are believed to be irreversible in this stage.

ESTABLISHED MACULOPATHY

The maculopathy becomes more and more evident on funduscopy. Visual acuity is reduced to approximately 20/60.

ADVANCED MACULOPATHY

Advanced maculopathy is characterized by marked atrophy of retinal pigment epithelium (RPE) and a visual acuity of or less than 20/200.

FINAL-STAGE MACULOPATHY

This stage is characterized by RPE atrophy and visibility of the choroidal vasculature. Retinal arteries may be narrowed and pigment changes are observed in the retinal periphery.

The above definition illustrates the course of fundus changes with increasing toxicity. However, as the higher stages are rare and have not much relevance for screening, a simpler definition appears appropriate for screening and other purposes.[8,10]

1. "Mild form" of retinopathy corresponds to stage 1 "premaculopathy." Some pigmentary macular changes are observed, which are suspected to be drug associated, and not age-related. No reproducible defects on Amsler and static macular visual field testing (10–2 program) exist and visual acuity is not significantly impaired. Changes are most likely reversible.

2. In a more advanced, established maculopathy (corresponding to stages 2–4 of the definition given above), typical pigmentary macular changes are observed on funduscopy ("Bull's eye appearance"). Visual acuity is affected to a variable degree and may be nearly normal in earlier stages. Visual field testing shows reproducible, bilateral paracentral field defects.[9] Changes are more likely irreversible. An early example of this stage is shown in Figure 18.1.

Ocular toxicity caused by antimalarials[11,12] was first described in as early as 1957. As antimalarials are effective not only for the treatment and prophylaxis of malaria but also for many rheumatoid diseases, they are used ever more frequently nowadays and are administered as a long-term medication. The risk of ocular toxicity is, therefore, considerable. The incidence of early retinopathy in ophthalmologically unmonitored patients was estimated in an early review by Bernstein[6] to be 10% for chloroquine and 3–4% for hydroxychloroquine. In contrast, newer studies found much lower rates of toxicity. For example, in 1,207 patients taking hydroxychloroquine, only one definite and five patients with indeterminate but probable toxicity were identified.[13] While part of the lower incidence of retinopathy may be attributed to ophthalmologic screening, it should be stressed that adequate dose refinements are vital for avoiding toxicity. Reports in older literature on retinopathy suggested that cumulative dose was the critical factor. However, when considering the reports of toxicity, it becomes evident that rather daily dose is important. As body fat is irrelevant for the distribution of the drug,[14] the ideal body weight is the basis to refer to. Care

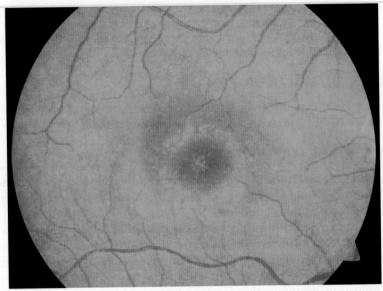

Fig. 18.1: Typical paracentral pigment changes in early chloroquine retinopathy (visual acuity 20/25).

must be, therefore, especially exercised when relatively small patients are given the standard daily dose of 250 mg of chloroquine.[9] Applying this concept of using a dosage of less than 4 mg/kg/day of chloroquine or less than 6.5 mg/kg/day of hydroxychloroquine, a study had showed no toxicity over a mean follow-up of 7 years in over 900 patients.[15] A review of published literature showed that less than 20 cases of toxicity in well over 1 million individuals using the drug have been reported despite not exceeding a daily dose of 3 mg/kg chloroquine and 6.5 mg/kg hydroxychloroquine.[16] All cases occurred after more than 5 years usage of the drugs. Those numbers make toxicity a very unlikely event if the recommended daily dosage is not exceeded.

MECHANISM OF CHLOROQUINE TOXICITY

Over the last decades, several experimental studies on animals and cell cultures have improved our knowledge on toxicity and caused a change in the considerations for clinical screening. Most early studies and occasionally some recent literature[16,17] assumed that a binding of chloroquine to melanin was responsible for retinal toxicity.[18,19] While this might be suspected from the ophthalmoscopic picture of Bull's eye maculopathy, there is a strong proof that melanin is not at all involved in ocular toxicity.[14] This is supported by the fact that retinopathy can be reproduced equally both in albino and in pigmented rabbits, rats, and cats.[20-24]

Early histopathologic reports of retinal changes showed membranous cytoplasmic bodies predominantly in the ganglion cells of the retina in both man[25] and monkey,[26] and rodents,[27] whereas the pigment epithelium showed changes only in more advanced retinopathy. This mechanism of initial ganglion cell function impairment proposes that the strategy for a clinical screening should focus on those cells and, to a lesser extent, on RPE.

The underlying cell-biologic mechanism involves lipid complex accumulation containing lysosomes within the ganglion cells, Müeller cells, and bipolar cells.[21] It appears that changes of the RPE occur only in the later stages as a secondary effect,[14] whereas another study[28] showed a lysosomal dysfunction in both the neural retina and the RPE. As far as it is known, chloroquine forms complexes with gangliosides imparting further degradation,[29] finally leading to an accumulation of lipid complexes in the neuroretina.[30,31] Ultimately, this may cause irreversible damage to cones and, to a lesser extent to rods.[28] The damage may progress even after cessation of the drug.[32,33] Perhaps the interference of chloroquine with deoxyribonucleic acid plays a role.[9,30,31]

CORNEAL DEPOSITS

Some degree of corneal deposits (verticillata) can be demonstrated in most patients taking chloroquine (Fig. 18.2), but these changes rarely impair vision.[34] Corneal deposits occur more frequently with chloroquine than with hydroxychloroquine.[35] The deposits are located in the epithelium and subepithelial stroma[36,37] and are mostly reversible.[37] In experiments with albino rats, a more peripheral localization and a dose-dependent effect were found.[38] The dose-dependent corneal changes in corneal epithelium and anterior stroma could be confirmed on patients in vivo by confocal microscopy.[37] It is also known that up to 95% of patients on chloroquine (in contrast to

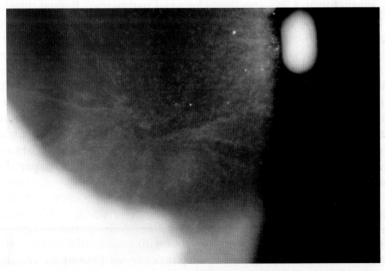

Fig. 18.2: Typical corneal deposits (verticillata) intraepithelial, whorl-like deposits in the cornea appear frequently but do not impair vision.

approximately 10% of patients taking hydroxychloroquine) exhibit corneal deposits.[35] A correlation with overdosage, especially in hydroxychloroquine, has been discussed,[35] but unfortunately most reports do not even mention corneal status.[39-42] Still it seems important to carefully examine the cornea for verticillata[17,34,35] as this may hint toward retinopathy, although the diagnostic significance is limited.[10,35]

Screening strategies include visual acuity testing and a dilated fundus examination. Subtle macular changes and transient defects in visual field and color vision may be symptoms of "preretinopathy," but are difficult to differentiate from other causes such as age-related changes. Therefore, to facilitate follow-up, especially when already some age-related changes are present at the time of initiation of therapy, fundus photography is recommended. Fluorescein angiography is not routinely applied for screening purpose.[43]

VISUAL FIELD TESTING

Visual field testing is frequently performed for monitoring ocular toxicity of the drug.[44,45] Its importance derives from the definition of definitive retinopathy by reproducible bilateral visual field defects,[9,46] while early maculopathy does not show such defects.[7] The use of Amsler grid for testing is inexpensive and fast and, therefore, is frequently recommended.[5,16,17,44,47] However, it is very dependent on the compliance of the patient and nonspecific as approximately 6% of the normal population has defects.[48] Amsler grid testing may still give hints and allow a less frequent use of automated static perimetry.[17]

Although routinely many centers use static 10-2 automated perimetry, only few reports exist regarding its suitability for screening. Easterbrook found 91% sensitivity and 58% specificity for a red perimetry.[34] Retinal threshold profile, a technique related to visual field testing, has been shown to be a very sensitive test.[49] A typical early visual field defect is an arcuate paracentral scotoma.[50] The early defects appear more commonly superior to the fixation.[45] In more advanced cases, a typical ring-like scotoma is found at the area of highest ganglion cell density corresponding to secondary changes of the RPE. Peripheral changes in visual fields such as constriction may also occur but are nonspecific. Using red test objects seems to improve the sensitivity.[7] A case example for a developing retinopathy is given in Figures 18.3 and 18.4. It also shows that 10-2 perimetry better defines the defects (refer Fig. 14.4), although screening by 30-2 testing (Fig. 18.3) was sufficient to detect retinopathy at a relatively early stage with good visual acuity.

COLOR VISION

Defects in color vision are known to occur with antimalarial treatment that causes retinal toxic changes[3] and may precede visible fundus changes.[5] However, these early changes may be subtle and often are not detected by conventional color testing.[2,9,48,49,51,52] Moreover, it is assumed that the earliest

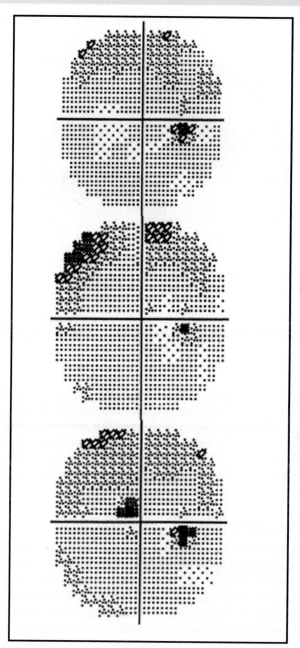

Fig. 18.3: Developing chloroquine retinopathy on 30-2 Swedish interactive threshold algorithm (SITA) visual field testing (6-months follow-up intervals from top to bottom; the same patient as in Figure 18.1).

changes resulting from retinal toxicity occur with blue–yellow (i.e. tritan) colors, while protan defects occur in more advanced cases.[53,54] This explains why every color test is not equally applicable. The usual color-plate test such

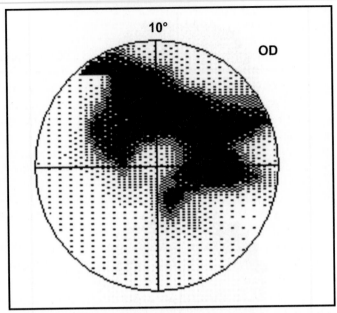

Fig. 18.4: Typical central visual field defect on 10-2 testing in the same patient at the same time-point.

as Ishihara plates is not optimal for testing. Better test is Farnsworth panel test. Computerized quantitative color tests become more and more widespread and have the advantage of being performed fast and easily (less than 5 min for both eyes). They offer high sensitivity and specificity for chloroquine-induced maculopathy.[10,50] When applying large optotypes, there is only a trivial disturbance in color perception due to age,[55,56] which might even help distinguish toxic from age-related changes.[50,56]

ELECTROOCULOGRAM

Testing of patients taking chloroquine with the electrooculogram (EOG) was introduced early and showed promising results.[2,57] EOG is believed to show the interaction between RPE and rods of the human eye[58] and was, therefore, considered to be valid diagnostic tool.[57,59] However, it was soon noticed that screening for antimalarial toxicity by EOG requires a baseline testing due to high interindividual variations.[57] It also became obvious that an Arden quotient (AQ) of 180% is not an appropriate cut-off for diagnostic testing.[60,61] Because of 10% intraindividual variance, a cut-off of 20% reduction of AQ was proposed.[62,63] Furthermore, it was noted that a reduction in EOG occurred frequently not only due to chloroquine medication but also by the course of the rheumatic disease itself.[64-67] Due to a very limited diagnostic value of EOG even when optimizing cut-offs, it is nowadays only rarely indicated for detecting chloroquine retinopathy.

ELECTRORETINOGRAM AND MULTIFOCAL ELECTRORETINOGRAM

The full-field electroretinogram (EOG) was evaluated as a screening tool for chloroquine toxicity.[57,68] but never showed any advantage over EOG.[57,63,65,67,69,70] It is, therefore, performed rarely for this indication.[44] Only a few data exist on pattern ERG.[71] This technique focuses on the neuroretinal response and is especially performed as a multifocal technique, a promising new approach for detecting chloroquine retinopathy.[50,72]

The photopic multifocal ERC (mfERC) is gaining increasing importance in clinical routine diagnosis. It has also been applied successfully for screening in chloroquine retinopathy.[73-77] Changes in mfERC responses appear to be present even in mild (pre) retinopathies,[75,78] which makes the mfERC a very promising diagnostic tool. However, further studies are needed before this technique can be validly assessed.

Ophthalmologic screening for retinal toxicity of chloroquine is performed quite differently, which shows very inhomogeneous results.[44] In general, over the last few years, the proposed screening requirements have become more and more limited to clinical tests,[16,17] especially when considering the low incident of retinopathy in patients with lower dosage. Screening intervals derived from the literature usually recommend 6-12 months follow-up visits. For the safer hydroxychloroquine, even no specific toxicity screening is at all recommended by the Royal College of Ophthalmologists.[8]

The American Academy of Ophthalmology[16,17] recommends screening after a mandatory baseline examination for both the antimalarials based on the anticipated risk for the patient. The proposed routine screening includes an ophthalmologic examination and visual field testing by an Amsler grid or Humphrey 10-2. Optional tests recommended include color testing, fundus photography, fluorescein angiography, and multifocal ERG. Patients are classified low-risk[16,79] if they do not exceed 6.5 mg/kg hydroxychloroquine or 3 mg chloroquine, they are using the medication for less than 5 years, have normal habitus, no renal or retinal diseases, and are less than 60 years old. The low-risk patients are recommended a baseline examination and follow-up examinations based on their age: 20-29 years once, 30-39 years twice during treatment period, 40-64 years every 2-4 years, and over 65 years every 1-2 years. For high-risk patients (including >5 years of medication) annual screening is recommended. In case of doubtful findings, a re-evaluation after 3 months should be performed.

In case of established diagnosis of (hydroxy) chloroquine retinopathy, the drug should be immediately stopped. This may mean worsening of the underlying systemic disease with the need for different medications with serious side effects. On the other hand, severe visual loss must be prevented. It is known that patients with early toxic changes may improve in visual acuity and lose their scotoma if the drug is discontinued early enough.[4] Usually after the cessation of chloroquine or hydroxychloroquine therapy, in long-term follow-up, the retinopathy tends to remain stable after the drug is discontinued.[42]

Rarely, there may be regression in early (pre) retinopathy, and on occasion, further deterioration may occur.[4]

When the recommended 3 mg chloroquine and 6.5 mg hydroxychloroquine per kilogram body weight are not exceeded, the risk for retinopathy can be considered very low. Hydroxychloroquine appears to be safe, meaning that less frequent or even no monitoring is necessary for this drug. Still a baseline examination appears wise. Regular screening is, however, indicated for patients taking chloroquine and should consist of vision testing, corneal and fundus examination, Amsler, and if possible, 10-2 perimetry. Further tests such as fundus photography, appropriate color vision testing, and fluorescein angiography or electrophysiological testing may be required in some to differentiate other retinal changes. A baseline examination, when retinopathy can still be excluded due to a low total chloroquine dose, say within the first 6 months, is recommended. The minimal effective dose should be used or less than the recommended daily milligrams per kilogram ideal body weight dose. Follow-up examinations for chloroquine medication appear useful one to two times per year in cases with some risk. For patients with low risk, screening intervals may be extended.

REFERENCES

1. Kanski JJ. Clinical Ophthalmology: A Systematic Approach, 5th edition. Oxford: Butterworth-Heinemann; 2003. pp. 928.
2. Henkind P, Carr RE, Siegel IM, Early chloroquine retinopathy: Clinical and functional findings. Arch Ophthalmol. 1964;71:157-65.
3. Okun E, Gouras P, Bernstein H, et al. Chloroquine retinopathy: a report of eight cases with ERG and dark adaptation findings. Arch Ophthalmol. 1963;58:774-8.
4. Nozik RA, Weinstock FJ, Vignos PJ. Ocular complications of chloroquine. A series and case presentation with a simple method for early detection of retinopathy. Am J Ophthalmol. 1964;58 774-8.
5. Niemeyer G, Fruh B. Examination strategies in the diagnosis of drug-induced retinal damage. Klin Monatsbl Augenheilkd. 1989;194(5):355-8.
6. Bernsten HN. Ophthalmologic considerations and testing in patients receiving long-term antimalarial therapy. Am J Med. 1983;75(1A):25-34.
7. Percival SP, Behraman J. Ophthalmological safety of chloroquine. Br J Ophthalmol. 1969;53(2):101-9.
8. Fielder A, Graham E, Jones S, et al. Royal college of ophthalmologists guidelines: ocular toxicity and hydroxychloroquine. Eye. 1998;12(Pt 6):907-9.
9. Easterbrook M. Ocular effects and safety of antimalarial agents. Am J Med. 1988;85(4A):23-9.
10. Neubauer AS, Samari-Kermani K, Schaller U, et al. Detecting chloroquine retinopathy: Electro-oculogram versus colour vision. Br J Ophthalmol. 2003;87(7):902-8.
11. Cambioggi A. Unusual ocular lesions in a case of systemic lupus erythematosus. Arch Ophthalmol. 1957;57:451-3.
12. Hobbs H, Sorsby A, Freedman A. Retinopathy following chloroquine therapy. Lancet. 1959;2:478.
13. Levy GD, Munz SJ, Paschal J et al. Incidence of hydroxychloroquine retinopathy in 1,207 patients in a large multicenter outpatient practice. Arthritis Rheum. 1997;40(8):1482-6.

14. Leblanc B, Jezequel S, Davies T, et al. Binding of drugs to eye melanin is not predictive of ocular toxicity. Regul Toxicol Pharmacol. 1998;28(2):124-32.
15. Mackenzie AH. Dose refinements in long-term therapy of rheumatoid arthritis with antimalarials. Am J Med. 1983;75(1A):40-5.
16. Marmor MF, Carr RE, Easterbrook M, et al. Recommendations on screening for chloroquine and hydroxychloroquine retinopathy: a report by the American Academy of Ophthalmology. Ophthalmology 2002;109(7)1377-82.
17. Easterbrook M. Current concepts in monitoring patients on antimalarials. Aust NZJ Ophthalmol. 1998;26(2):101-3.
18. Potts AM. Further studies concerning the accumulation of polycyclic compounds on uveal melanin. Invest Ophthalmol. 1964;3:399.
19. Gonasun LM, Potts AM. In vitro inhibition of protein synthesis in the retinal pigment epithelium by chloroquine. Invest Ophthalmol. 1974;13(2):107-15.
20. Francois J, Maudgal MC. Experimental chloroquine retinopathy. Ophthalmologica. 1964;148:442-52.
21. Gregory MG, Rutty DA, Wood RD. Differences in the retinotoxic action of chloroquine and phenothiazine derivatives. J Pathol. 1970;102(3):139-50.
22. Legros J, Rosner I. Electroretinographic modifications in albino rats after chronic administration of toxic doses of hydroxychloroquine and desethyl hydroxy-chloroquine. Arch Ophthalmol Rev Gen Ophthalmol. 1971;31(2):165-80.
23. Kuhn H, Keller P, Kovács E, et al. Lack of correlation between melanin affinity and retinopathy in mice and cats treated with chloroquine or flunitrazepam. Albrecht Von Graefes Arch Klin Exp Ophthalmol. 1981;216(3):177-90.
24. Ivanina TA, et al. Ultrastructural alterations in rat and cat retina and pigment epithelium induced by chloroquine. Graefes Arch Clin Exp Ophthalmol. 1983;220(1):32-8.
25. Ramsey MS, Fine BS. Chloroquine toxicity in the human eye. Histopathologic observations by electron microscopy. Am J Ophthalmol. 1972;73(2):229-35.
26. Rosenthal AR, Kolb H, Bergsma D, et al. Chloroquine retinopathy in the rhesus monkey. Invest Ophthalmol Vis Sci. 1978;17(12):1158-75.
27. Hodgkinson BJ, Kolb H. A preliminary study of the effect of chloroquine on the rat retina. Arch Ophthalmol. 1970;84(4):509-15.
28. Mahon GJ, Anderson HR, Gardiner TA, et al. Chloroquine causes lysosomal dysfunction in neural retina and RPE: Implications for retinopathy. Curr Eye Res. 2004;28(4):277-84.
29. Lüllmann-Rauch R. Lipoidosis of the retina due to cationic amphiphilic drugs. In: Jones TC, Mohr U, Hunt RD (Eds). Eye and Ear Monography on Pathology of Laboratory Animals. Berlin: Springer-Verlag; 1991. pp. 87-92.
30. Meier-Ruge W, Cerletti A. Zur experimentellen Pathologie der Phenothiazin Retinopathie. Ophthalmologica. 1966;151:512-33.
31. Tanenbaum L, Tuffanelli DL. Antimalarial agents. Chloroquine, hydroxy-chloroquine, and quinacrine. Arch Dermatol. 1980;116(5)587-91.
32. Duncker G, Bredehorn T. Chloroquine-induced lipidosis in the rat retina: functional and morphological changes after withdrawal of the drug. Graefes Arch Clin Exp Ophthalmol. 1996;234(6):378-81.
33. Duncker G, Schmiederer M, Bredehorn T. Chloroquine-induced lipidosis in the rat retina: A functional and morphological study. Ophthalmologica. 1995;209(2):79-83.
34. Easterbrook M. Detection and prevention of maculopathy associated with antimalarial agents. Int Ophthalmol Clin. 1999;39(2):49-57.
35. Easterbrook M. Is corneal deposition of antimalarial any indication of retinal toxicity? Can J Ophthalmol. 1990;25(5):249-51.

36. Francois K, Maudgal MC. Experimentally induced chloroquine retinopathy in rabbits. Am J Ophthalmol. 1967;64(5):886-93.
37. Slowik C, Somodi S, von Gruben C, et al. Detection of morphological corneal changes caused by chloroquine therapy using confocal in vivo microscopy. Ophthalmology. 1997;94(2):147-51.
38. Francois J, Maudgal MC. Experimental chloroquine keratopathy. Am J Ophthalmol. 1965;60(3):459-64.
39. Mavrikakis M, Papazoglou S, Sfikakis PP, et al. Retinal toxicity in long-term hydroxychloroquine treatment. Ann Rheum Dis. 1996;55(3):187-9.
40. Tobin DR, Krohel G, Rynes RI. Hydroxychloroquine. Seven-year experience. Arch Ophthalmol. 1982;100(1):81-3.
41. Mills PV, Beck M, Power BJ. Assessment of the retinal toxicity of hydroxy-chloroquine. Trans Ophthalmol Soc UK. 1981;101(1):109-13.
42. Brinkley JR Jr, Dubois EL, Ryan SJ. Long-term course of chloroquine retinopathy after cessation of medication. Am J Ophthalmol. 1979;88(1):1-11.
43. Cruess AF, Schachat AP, Nicholl J, et al. Chloroquine retinopathy. Is fluorescein angiography necessary? Ophthalmology. 1985;92(8):1127-9.
44. Mazzuca SA, Yung R, Brandt KD, et al. Current practices for monitoring ocular toxicity related to hydroxychloroquine (Plaquenil) therapy. J Rheumatol. 1994;21(1):59-63.
45. Hart WM Jr, Burde RM, Johnston GP, et al. Static perimetry in chloroquine retinopathy. Perifoveal patterns of visual field depression. Arch Ophthalmol 1984;102(3)377-80.
46. Easterbrook M. The ocular safety of hydroxychloroquine. Semin Arthritis Rheum. 1993;23(2 Suppl 1):62-7.
47. Easterbrook M. The use of Amsler grids in early chloroquine retinopathy. Ophthalmology. 1984;91(11):1368-72.
48. Percival SP, Meanock I. Chloroquine: Ophthalmological safety, and clinical assessment in rheumatoid arthritis. Br Med J. 1968;3(618):579-84.
49. Carr RE, Gouras P, Gunkel RD. Chloroquine retinopathy. Early detection by retinal threshold test. Arch Ophthalmol. 1966;75(2):171-8.
50. Neubauer AS, Stiefelmeyer S, Berninger T, et al. The multifocal pattern electroretinogram in chloroquine retinopathy. Ophthalmic Res. 2004;36(2):106-13.
51. Nylander U. Ocular damage in chloroquine therapy. Acta Ophthalmol. (Copenh) 1966;44(3):335-48.
52. Bartel PR, Roux P, Robinson E, et al. Visual function and long-term chloroquine treatment. S Afr Med J. 1994;84(1):32-4.
53. Jaeger W. Acquired colour-vision deficiencies caused by side effects of pharmacotherapy (author's transl). Klin Monbl Augenheilkd. 1977;170(3):453-60.
54. Grutzner P. Acquired color vision defects secondary to retinal drug toxicity. Ophthalmologica. 1969;158(Suppl):592-604.
55. Berninger T, Drobner B, Hogg C, et al. Color vision in relation to age: a study of normal values. Klin Monbl Augenheilkd. 1999;215(1) 37-42.
56. Arden GB, Wolf JE. Colour vision testing as an aid to diagnosis and management of age-related maculopathy. Br J Ophthalmol. 2004;88(9):1180-5.
57. Kolb H. Electro-oculogram findings in patients treated with antimalarial drugs. Br J Ophthalmol. 1965;49(11):573-89.
58. Arden GB, Kelsey JH. Changes produced by light in the standing potential of the human eye. J Physiol. 1962;161:189-205.
59. Arden GB, Friedmann AI, Kolb H. Anticipation of chloroquine retinopathy. Lancet. 1962;1:1164-5.

60. Graniewski-Wijnands HS, van Lith GH, Vijfvinkel-Bruinenga S. Ophthal-mological examinaiton of patients taking chloroquine. Doc Ophthalmol. 1979;48(2):231-4.
61. Percival SP. The ocular toxicity of chloroquine. Trans Ophthalmol Soc UK. 1967;87:355-7.
62. van Lith GH, Mak GT, Wijnands H. Clinical importance of the electrooculogram with special reference to the chloroquine retinopathy. Bibl Ophthalmol. 1976;(85):2-9.
63. van Lith GH. Electro-ophthalmology and side effects of drugs. Doc Ophthalmol. 1977;44(1):19-21.
64. Reijmer CN, Tijssen JG, Kok GA, et al. Interpretation of the electrooculogram of patients taking chloroquine. Doc Ophthalmol. 1979;48(2):273-6.
65. Pinckers A, Broekhuyse RM. The EOG in rheumatoid arthritis. Acta Ophthalmol (Copenh). 1983;61(5):831-7.
66. Bishara SA, Matamoros N. Evaluation of several tests in screening for chloroquine maculopathy. Eye 1989;3(Pt 6):777-82.
67. Gouras P, Gunkel R. The EOG in Chloroquine and other retinopathies. Arch Ophthalmol. 1963;70:91-100.
68. Sverak J, Erbenová Z, Peregrin J, et al. The ERG and EOG potentials after a long-term Resochin therapy. Klin Monbl Augenheilkd. 1970;157(3):389-92.
69. Bernstein HN. Chloroquine ocular toxicity. Surv Ophthalmol. 1967;12(5):415-47.
70. Infante R, Martin DA, Heckenlively JR. Hydroxychloroquine and retinal toxicity. Doc Ophthalmol Proc Ser. 1983;37:121-6.
71. Cursiefen CU, Grunert A Junemann. Chloroquine-induced bull's eye maculopathy without electrophysiologic changes. Klin Monbl Augenheilkd. 1997;210(6):400-1.
72. Wolfelschneider P, Kohen L, Wiedemann P. Maculopathy in long-term chloroquine therapy. Ophthalmology. 1998;95(3):186-7.
73. Kellner U, Kraus H, Foerster MH. Multifocal ERG in chloroquine retinopathy: regional variance of retinal dysfunction. Graefes Arch Clin Exp Ophthalmol. 2000;228(1):94-7.
74. So SC, Hedges TR, Schuman JS, et al. Evaluation of hydroxychloroquine retinopathy with multifocal electroretinography. Ophthalmic Surg Lasers Imaging. 2003;34(3):251-8.
75. Maturi RK, Yu M, Weleber RG. Multifocal electroretinographic evaluation of long-term hydroxychloroquine users. Arch Ophthalmol. 2004;122(7):973-81.
76. Tzekov RT, Serrato A, Marmor MF. ERG findings in patients using hydroxy-chloroquine. Doc Ophthalmol. 2004;108(1):87-97.
77. Moschos MN, Moschos MM, Apostolopoulos M, et al. Assessing hydroxychloroquine toxicity by the multifocal ERG. Doc Ophthalmol. 2004;108(1):47-53.
78. Penrose PJ, Tzekov RT, Sutter EE, et al. Multifocal electroretinography evaluation for early detection of retinal dysfunction in patients taking hydroxychloroquine. Retina. 2003;23(4):503-12.
79. Marmor MF. New American Academy of Ophthalmology recommendations on screening for hydroxychloroquine retinopathy. Arthritis Rheum. 2003;48(6):1764.

CHAPTER 19

Macular Hole

Meena Chakrabarti, Arup Chakrabarti, Sonia S John

INTRODUCTION

A macular hole is a defect of the foveal retina involving its full thickness from the internal limiting membrane (ILM) to the outer segment of the photoreceptor layer. The condition was first described by Knapp[1] in 1869 in a patient who sustained blunt trauma to the eye. Subsequent case reports and series pointed to antecedent episodes of ocular trauma such that the two were customarily linked to each other. In the present century, ophthalmologists have increasingly recognized that the condition occurs more commonly in atraumatic settings and have differentiated these macular holes from trauma-induced holes by describing them as idiopathic full-thickness macular holes. In fact, case series as far back as the 1970s reported that more than 80% of macular holes are idiopathic and that only less than 10% are associated with the history of trauma to the eye.

The overall prevalence macular hole is approximately 3.3 cases in 1,000, in persons older than 55 years. Peak incidence of idiopathic macular hole is found in the seventh decade of life, and women typically are affected more than men. Reasons for sex difference are not known. Cardiovascular disease, hypertension, and a history of hysterectomy have been reported as risk factors. However, none of these has been proven to have any significant effect on macular hole formation. The prevalence rate of hole in India is reported to be 0.17%, with a mean age 67 years.[2] The Beijing Eye Study[3] found the rate of macular holes to be 1.6 out of 1,000 elderly Chinese with a strong female predilection.

The natural history of a macular hole varies because of its current clinical stage. It has been reported that around 50% of stage 0 and stage 1 macular hole (Fig. 19.1A) may resolve both in the anatomic changes and in the symptoms. Stage 2 holes progress in most cases to stage 3 or stage 4 (Fig. 19.1B), resulting

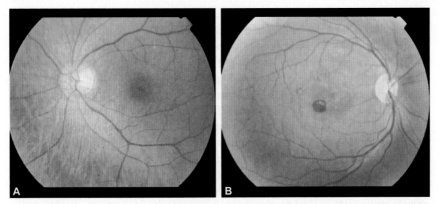

Figs. 19.1A and B: Fundus photographs of stage 1 (A) and stage 4 (B) macular holes. Note the presence of localized subretinal fluid around (B).

BOX 19.1: Natural course of idiopathic macular holes.

- Nearly 50% of holes undergo spontaneous vitreofoveal separation, relief of retinal traction, and show no further progression.
- About 8–10% holes show spontaneous resolution and one-third of these cases have visual improvement.
- About 40% progress to early small macular hole within several months. Most stage 2 holes progress to larger stage 3 holes.

---

in worsening vision (Box 19.1). Occasionally, a full-thickness macular hole may spontaneously close with resultant good vision.[4]

An estimate for the incidence of development of an idiopathic full-thickness macular hole in the fellow eye is approximately 12%.[5,6]

The figures in Box 19.1 suggest that the natural history of macular hole is that of deterioration over a few years with subsequent stabilization of both visual acuity and size of the hole.

PATHOGENESIS OF MACULAR HOLES

The exact pathogenesis of macular holes remains unknown. The first reported macular holes in the late 19th century were believed to result from trauma that caused cystoid changes in the macula. Concurrent with the discovery around 1970 that the majority of macular holes were not associated with trauma, the predominant thought was that macular hole etiology was related to the presence of cystoid macular edema (CME), including any condition which may lead to CME.

The vitreomacular traction theory of pathogenesis of macular hole gained in popularity with the recognition that peripheral retinal breaks occur secondary to vitreoretinal traction and that strong adhesion exists between the vitreous and fovea. The recognition of a temporal association between posterior vitreous detachment (PVD) and full-thickness macular hole assisted Gass[7] in the development of the grading scheme. Optical coherence tomography has enhanced our understanding of the orientation of this traction, which is now thought to be predominantly anteroposterior (AP) in direction.

There is also mounting evidence that A-P traction may not be the only factor in macular hole formation. Researchers have documented macular hole formation after complete PVD/vitrectomy as well as spontaneous closure of macular hole in eyes without PVD [documented by ocular coherence tomography (OCT)]. Such observations led to the development of other theories of macular hole pathogenesis, such as the hydrodynamic model, in which the macular hole is formed or maintained by fluid flow caused by the macular retinal pigment epithelium (RPE) pump.

The hydration theory of pathogenesis of macular holes was put forward in 2003 by Tornambe et al.[8] In this theory, posterior hyaloidal traction on fovea resulting in a tear in inner fovea was the first step in the genesis of macular holes. Seepage of fluid vitreous into the spongy layers of the macula through this defect resulted in the creation of a cavity in inner retina, enlargement of hole, and spread of fluid to the outer retina. Resistance is offered by RPE and Bruch's membrane to the seepage of fluid vitreous. Therefore, the swollen retina remains elevated and retracted.

In reality, the etiology of macular hole is probably multifactorial, and determining the primary event may be less important than the recognition that vitreomacular traction, foveolar dehiscence, and other factors are likely to play a role.

Macular hole has long been recognized as a female-predominant disease, yet despite extensive research, the reason for such a gender predilection is unclear, and there is no strong evidence to support an association between estrogen replacement[9] and macular hole.

STAGING OF MACULAR HOLES

Gass classified macular hole in the following stages:

- *Stage 1a:* Tangential vitreous traction results in the elevation of the fovea marked by presence of foveal detachment and increased clinical prominence of xanthophyll pigment. This stage is occasionally referred to as the *yellow dot stage* and can also be seen in cases of central serous chorioretinopathy, CME, and solar retinopathy. Fundus photograph of a stage 1a macular hole presents characteristic yellow spot at the center of the fovea.
- *Stage 1b:* As the foveal retina elevates to the level of the perifovea, the yellow dot of xanthophyll pigment changes to a donut-shaped yellow ring. Persistent traction on the fovea leads to dehiscence of deeper retinal layers at the umbo.
- *Stage 2:* This is the first stage when a full-thickness break in the retina exists. It is defined as a full-thickness macular hole less than 400 μm in size. The full-thickness defect may appear eccentric, and there may be a pseudo-operculum at this stage if there has been spontaneous vitreofoveolar

separation. These opercula have been examined and found to be vitreous condensation and glial proliferation without harboring any retinal tissue.

- *Stage 3:*A full-thickness macular hole in the retina exists. It is greater than 400 μm in size and is still with partial vitreomacular adhesion/traction.
- *Stage 4:* A full-thickness macular hole exists inthepresence of a complete separation of the vitreous from the macula and the optic disk. There is recent evidence, however, that, even in the presence of an apparent PVD, a thin shell of residual may still remain and contribute to the macular hole.

The advent of OCT has provided in vivo structural support to the hypotheses focused on vitreous traction underlying idiopathic macular holes. Both biomicroscopic examination and OCT can evaluate the various stages of the macular holes (Fig.19.2). The OCT has allowed careful evaluation of the vitreoretinal interface demonstrating persistent adhesion on the fovea resulting in oblique traction on the fovea even with a partial PVD. The persistent traction

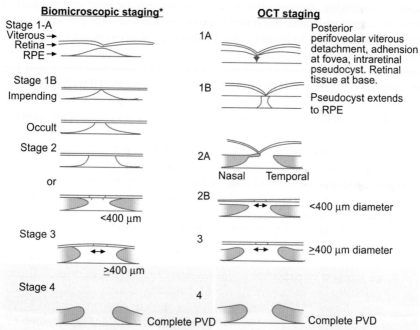

Fig. 19.2: Comparison between the biomicroscopic and OCT staging of macular holes.
Source: Ryan SJ (Ed). Retina. 1994;1169-85.
(PVD: posteriorvitreous detachment; OCT: ocular coherence tomography; RPE: retinal pigment epithelium)
Stage 1A: Perifoveal PVD with central adherence. Intraretinal pseudocysts with retinal tissue at the base.
Stage 1B: Impending hole with pseudocyst extending to RPE.
Stage 2A: Full thickness with partial opening of roof. And focal vitreous adhesion to flap of less than 400 μm size.
Stage 2B: Full thickness operculated MH less than 400 μm with traction on fovea released.
Stage 3: Full thickness operculated greater than 400 μm with vitreous traction released.
Stage 4: Full thickness MH with complete PVD.

on the fovea prior to anatomic changes to the fovea has been referred to as stage 0.[10] The clinical appearance may resolve without progression in 40–50% of patients.

Screening of eye[11,12] at regular intervals can document progression macular hole in the eye (Figs.19.3A to D). In eyes without preexisting PVD, the cumulative risk of developing macular hole is 4.6% in 3 years, 6.5% in 5 years, and 7.1% in 6 years. In eyes with PVD, the risk is negligible.

Visual dysfunction in patients with macular hole[13] is directly related to the absence of retinal tissue in the fovea. However, visual dysfunction may seem out of proportion to the size of the macular hole and potentially may also be related to the presence of a cuff of subretinal fluid with associated photoreceptor atrophy.

Patients with idiopathic macular holes present with a variety of symptoms. Initial symptoms include blurred central vision or metamorphopsia. Patients may characterize these symptoms as being mild and only apparent when reading or driving. Because the initial changes may be mild and gradual, it may be sometime before the patient discovers that something is wrong with their vision. Macular holes may only be discovered when patients cover one eye and notice blurred vision and metamorphopsia in the opposite eye. Rarely, some patients may describe the exact moment at which the hole developed, but more commonly, they describe the onset as slow and gradual if at all noticeable. Later, a larger macular hole may produce a central defect, or scotoma, in the central vision of the patient.[14] Some patients may be a symptomatic, and the hole is diagnosed only on routine ophthalmologic examination. The visual acuity of the patient varies according to the size, location, and the stage of the macular hole. Patients with small, eccentric holes may retain excellent visual acuity in the range of 6/9–6/12. In addition, a macular hole that is not full thickness can have very good visual acuity in the range of 6/18–5/60. However, once a macular hole is well developed or full thickness, the usual range of visual acuity is from 6/24 to 2/60, averaging at 6/60 (Table 19.1).[15]

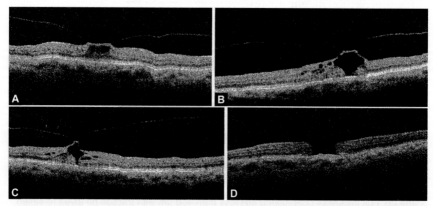

Figs. 19.3A to D: Serial OCT follow-up of a 60-year-old female patient. During 9 months, the hole progressed to full thickness.

TABLE 19.1: Clinical features of various stages of macular holes.

Clinical features	Stage 1A and 1B	Stage 2	Stage 3	Stage 4
Initial symptoms	Metamorphopsia mild loss	>6/12	6/12–6/60	>1/60
Microscopy/OCT	VMT/prefoveolar detachment	VMTTR on flap pseudo-operculum	Pseudo-operculum	PVD
Fundus	Foveolar depression yellow spot/ring (100–300)	Central/eccentric small, 400 µm full thickness	>400 µm neurosensory RD	400–1500 µm neurosensory RD
FFA	Hyperfluorescence	Hyperfluorescence	Hyperfluorescence	Hyperfluorescence

A full-thickness macular hole visualized with direct ophthalmoscope[16] is characterized by a well-defined round or oval lesion in the macula with yellow-white deposits at the base. These yellow dots probably represent lipofuscin-laden macrophages or nodular proliferations of the underlying pigment epithelium with associated eosinophilic material. With biomicroscopic (slit-lamp) examination,[17] around excavation with well-defined borders interrupting the beam of the slit-lamp can be observed.

In most patients, an overlying semitranslucent tissue, representing the pseudo-operculum, can be seen suspended over the hole. There is often a surrounding cuff of subretinal fluid. Cystic changes of the retina may also be evident at the margins of the hole. The RPE is usually intact and normal in acute stages but may undergo chronic changes, such as atrophy and hyperplasia, with time. Fine crinkling of the inner retinal surface caused by an epiretinal membrane (ERM) may be present and sometimes may even distort the appearance of the hole.

The most useful diagnostic tests for ophthalmologists to distinguish full-thickness macular holes from other lesions are the Watzke–Allen and the laser aiming beam tests. The Watzke–Allen test[18] is performed at the slit-lamp using a macular lens and placing a narrow vertical slit-beam through the fovea. A positive test is elicited when patients detect a break in the bar of light that they perceive. This reaction is due to the fact that there is a lack of retinal element in the area of the hole, thus producing a central defector scotoma. Narrowing or distortion of the bar of light is not diagnostic of full-thickness macular holes and should be interpreted with caution. The laser aiming beam test also is performed similarly, but this time a small 50 µm spot size laser aiming beam is placed within the lesion. A positive test is obtained when the patient fails to detect the aiming beam when it is placed within the lesion but is able to detect it once it is placed onto a normal retina. In addition, some slit-lamps are equipped with a setting to project a small test object, often a star, onto the fovea. Again, the patient is asked whether they perceive the test object.

ETIOLOGY OF MACULAR HOLES

Trauma

Approximately 6% of patients experiencing a contusion injury of the eye develop a macular hole following the trauma. Trauma[19-22] is also commonly associated with commotio retinae involving the macula, subretinal hemorrhage, and intraretinal hemorrhage.

Progressive High Myopia (Foveal Schisis)

Patients with high myopia[23-26] may develop foveal schisis, which can progress to a full-thickness macular hole. Of those patients in whom foveal schisis identified, 31% developed macular holes. Risk factors include axial eye length, macular chorioretinal atrophy, and vitreoretinal interface factors.

Preceding Rhegmatogenous Retinal Detachment Repair

Less than 1% of patients with a successfully repaired rhegmatogenous retinal detachment[27] will present with macular holes several years later.

Differential Diagnosis

The macular hole must be differentiated from the following conditions:
1. Pseudohole due to epimacular membrane[28]
2. Cystoid macular edema[29]
3. Lamellar macular hole.[30,31]

Primary consideration should be given to conditions that may mimic the appearance of a macular hole. While most of these conditions are readily apparent clinically, subtle presentations may present as a macular hole. These conditions include any disease that can cause the development of CME[e.g. choroidal neovascularization (CNVM), retinal vein occlusions, and retinitis pigmentosa]. An appropriate work-up and examination should identify these conditions. OCT allows high-resolution cross-sectional imaging of the retina. OCT allows the physician to detect the presence of a macular hole as well as changes in the surrounding retina. OCT can distinguish lamellar holes and cystic lesions of the macula from macular holes. Also, the status of the vitreomacular interface can be evaluated. This allows the clinician to evaluate the earliest of the stages of a macular hole as well as evaluate for other vision-limiting conditions associated with macular holes, such as a surrounding cuff of subretinal fluid and ERMs. Fluorescein angiography may be a useful test in differentiating macular holes from masquerading lesions, such as CME and CNVM. Full-thickness stage 3 holes typically produce a window defect early in the angiogram. The arteriovenous phase of the angiogram best demonstrates a granular hyperfluorescent window associated with the overlying pigment layer changes. No leakage or accumulation of dye is observed as opposed to other lesions. In CME, a gradual accumulation of dye occurs in the cystoids spaces, eventually demonstrating a petaloid appearance late in the angiogram. B-scan ultrasonography may be helpful in elucidating the relationship of the macula to the vitreous; therefore, it may be helpful in staging the disease but is not sensitive to distinguish a true macular hole from masquerading lesions.

INVESTIGATIONS

- *Amsler grid abnormalities,*[32] although sensitive for macular lesions, are not specific for macular holes. Plotting of small central scotomas caused by full-thickness macular holes using the Amsler grid is difficult, because of the poor fixation in the affected eye. However, bowing of the lines and micropsia frequently are appreciated. This could be attributable to the surrounding area of retinal edema and intraretinal cysts, which can be seen in macular holes as well as other lesions like CNV.
- *Microperimetry*[33] and *multifocal electroretinography*[34] have also been used to evaluate patients with idiopathic macular holes. These studies show loss of retinal function corresponding to the macular hole with subsequent recovery of function following surgical repair of the hole.

Medical Care

No current medical treatment exists for macular holes. Historically, therapy for macular holes has evolved from pharmacologic interventions, such as anxiolytics and vasodilators, to an assortment of surgical techniques, such as cerclage, scleral buckles, direct photocoagulation of the hole edges, and intraocular gas tamponade without the aid of vitrectomy. In 1982, Gonvers and Machemer[35] were the first to recommend vitrectomy, intravitreal gas, and prone positioning for retinal detachments secondary to macular holes. Kelly and Wendel[36] reported that vision might be stabilized or even improved if it were possible to surgically relieve tangential traction on the macula, reduce the cystic changes, and reattach the cuff of detached retina surrounding the macular hole. They proposed that by performing this surgery, they could flatten the retina and possibly reduce the adjacent cystic retinal changes and neurosensory macular detachment.

In 1991, Kelly and Wendel[36] demonstrated that vitrectomy, removal of cortical vitreous and ERMs, and strict face-down gas tamponade could successfully treat full-thickness macular holes. The overall results of their initial report were a 58% anatomic success rate and visual improvement of two or more lines in 42% of eyes. A succeeding report showed a 73% anatomic success rate and 55% of patients improving two or more lines of visual acuity. Present anatomic success rates range from 82% to 100% depending on the series.[37-41] Possible mechanisms to explain why vitrectomy and fluid–gas exchange can close a macular hole include relief of traction (tangential and AP) and stimulation of fibroglial proliferation to plug the hole. Histopathological evidence has revealed hyperplastic RPE and fibroglial cells associated with spontaneously closed macular holes. A variety of adjuvant therapies have been used at the time of surgery in an effort to enhance glial proliferation. Prospective, randomized studies of transforming growth factor beta (TGF-β)[42] and autologous platelets[43] have, however, shown little benefit in terms of anatomic closure or final visual acuity. Case reports exist that describe the use of autologous plasmin for idiopathic and traumatic macular holes. Ongoing clinical trials are evaluating the role of plasmin[44] as a means of "chemovitrectomy." In these studies, case illustrations have demonstrated resolution of idiopathic macular holes following intravitreal injection of plasmin and no surgical intervention.

There are several controversies regarding the surgical management of macular holes.

1. How soon to advice surgical intervention?

OCT will help to detect stage 1 and stage 2 macular holes. It is best to observe eyes with VA 6/6 and monitor progression (<6/12).

Some stage 2A holes can be closed without surgical intervention by inducing vitreofoveolar separation by air injection and maneuvering the air bubble under the flap to detach the posterior hyaloid phase adherent to the flap. This was demonstrated by Ruiz-Moreno[45] with OCT demonstration of vitreofoveolar separation. Surgical results are best for macular holes less than a year duration. But some chronic holes do well as demonstrated by Steele et al. who achieved a closure rate of 83% in holes of greater than 4.2 years duration; and 39% of these eyes achieved a final vision of greater than 20/70.

Thus, it is reasonable to offer surgery for macular holes of 1–5 years duration, especially if the fellow eye has a visually debilitating and progressive macular or optic nerve pathology. The potential for better vision, as well as the 12% chance that the fellow eye will develop another macular hole has prompted ophthalmologists to seek for a viable treatment of this condition.

Indications for consideration in the surgical management of macular holes are based on the presence of a full-thickness defect. Once this defect has developed, the potential for spontaneous resolution is low. Thus, surgical management is recommended with documentation of a stage 2 or higher, full-thickness macular hole. Stage 1 holes and lamellar holes are managed conservatively with observation at this time.

Lamellar holes cause symptoms but minimal loss of central visual acuity. Management has historically been conservative. Garretson et al.[30] reported a series of successfully repaired lamellar macular holes, wherein 93% eyes demonstrated improved visual acuity. The mean improvement was 3.2 Snellen lines.

Some aspects of the surgery may vary, but the basic technique is the same. The anterior and middle vitreous is removed via a standard three-port pars plana vitrectomy. Patients with macular hole frequently undergo vitrectomy using smaller gauge vitrectomy systems (i.e. 25 gauge or the 23 gauge). The critical step appears to be the removal of the perimacular traction. Factors contributing to this traction, such as the posterior hyaloid, the ILM, and coexisting epimacular membranes, need to be addressed. The traction exerted by the posterior hyaloid on the macula should be relieved by either removing just the perimacular vitreous or combining it with the induction of a complete

PVD. Various surgical techniques have been described to accomplish this task, including the use of a soft-tipped silicon cannula or the vitrectomy cutter using suction alone. A "fish-strike sign"[46] or bending of the silicon cannula has been described as a sign that the posterior hyaloid has been engaged. Then, it may be released from the underlying retina and removed with the vitrectomy cutter.

2. To peel or not to peel ILM?

The removal of ILM is considered to be a contributing factor in the success of macular hole surgeries. ILM peeling may be accomplished via a"rhexis" not unlike that of a capsulorrhexis in lens surgeries.[47] Very fine forceps maybe used to peel the ILM from the underlying retina. Careshould be taken not to include the deeper layers in the forceps' grasp, which may further damage the surrounding retinal tissues. Many surgeons use vital dyes to stain the ILM making it easier to visualize and manipulate. Peeling of ERM or ILMD, through the release of cytokines, is thought to induce a similar fibroglial proliferation in order to facilitate macular hole closure.[48] ILM peeling may also remove any contractile ERM formed above it, thereby relieving tangential traction. In addition, membrane removal can enhance the mobility of the hole edges, thereby facilitating reapproximation. Data on whether the benefit of ILM peeling is translated into improved anatomical and functional results are not available. Several retrospective studies suggest that ILM peeling is beneficial[49-52] in attaining improved visual acuity and anatomic closure in macular holes of less than 6 months duration. A multicenter controlled randomized trial[53] showed a significant increase in closure rates with ERM peeling, but no effect on visual acuity. Accordingly, there has been some concern regarding damage to the retina secondary to membrane peeling. Another study showed that ILM peeling at the time of macular hole surgery significantly improves the closure rate of macular holes larger than 400 μm in diameter but has no effect on the closure rate of smaller macular holes. Based on an association between ERM formation and late hole reopening, some have postulated that ILM peeling may prevent macularhole recurrence. Indocyanine green (ICG) dye[54] has been successfully used to facilitate visualization during ILM peeling; however, several studies have demonstrated significant retinal toxicity and decreased visual acuity results associated with this technique. A recent review[55] showed that the use of ICG during macular hole surgery is not associated with worse visual outcome, suggesting that retinal toxicity may not be clinically significant.

One study using scanning laser ophthalmoscopy[56] revealed paracentral scotomas in more than half of patients after ILM peeling. However, a prospective study[57] with a 5-year follow-up revealed that macular hole surgery with ILM peeling is a safe and effective procedure with 95% of patients achieving anatomic closure and 92% achieving improvement in visual acuity. In that study, the majority of patients (97%) were pseudophakic at 5 years, but there were no cases of late hole reopening or ERM formation after successful hole closure. The absence of a large randomized clinical trial likely accounts for the lack of consensus regarding the efficacy of and indications for ILM peeling.

TABLE 19.2: Comparative analysis of the efficacy and toxicity of ICG used for ILM staining in MHS and ERM peels.

S.No	Authors	Year	Procedure	ICG effect	Complication
1.	Sheidow et al.[58]	2003	MHS	Worse visual acuity when ICG used as adjuvant	
2.	Gass et al.[59]	2003	MHS	Worse visual acuity when ICG used as adjuvant	
3.	Ando et al.[60]	2004	MHS	Worse visual acuity when ICG used as adjuvant	Optic atrophy
4.	Hillenkampet al.[61]	2006	ERM	No difference with and without ICG	Optic atrophy
5.	Lochead et al.[62]	2004	MHS	No adverse effects	
6.	Slaughter and Lee[63]	2004	MHS	No adverse effects	
7.	Rodrigues and Meyer[64]	2007	MHS	No difference in anatomic outcome	Worse functional outcome

Use of vital dyes for ILM peeling

ICG dye was the first vital dye used for macular surgery. There is considerable literature questioning the toxicity of ICG dye to the retina and RPE. Despite the laboratory and literature cautioning the use of ICG dye, an equal amount of literature documented good surgical and visual results. ICG dye is still used by surgeons with care taken to limit the exposure of the retina and, potentially more importantly, the RPE to the dye (Table 19.2).

Trypan blue has also been used to stain the ILM without the literature suggesting toxicity. On the other hand, trypan blue does not appear to stain the ILM as effectively as ICG dye. Triamcinolone acetonide has also been used to facilitate peeling of the ILM.

Brilliant blue G is less toxic to the RPE and stains both ERM and ILM well.

Majority of studies used ICG in higher concentration and this factor could be responsible for the toxicity. We suggest following safety measures when using ICG for ILM peeling.

- Perform a fast surgical procedure in order to minimize the duration of contact with RPE cells and to minimize the ICG exposure to light from endoilluminator.
- Use ICG concentrations lower than 0.5 mg/mL to minimize the risk of RPE damage and possible retinal toxicity.
- Avoid ICG injection direct through the macular hole by any method to control ILM staining (slow injection, use of the 20 gauge, prototype painting brush called vitreoretinal ILM color enhancer[65] or by the use of perfluorocarbons over the macular hole, etc.).
- ERMs, if present, should also be removed. Techniques in completing this procedure vary from surgeon to surgeon.

3. Are adjuvants necessary to optimize surgical outcome?

Bovine TGF-β,[66] recombinant TGFβ[67] platelets,[68] autologous serum,[69] and plasmin[70,71] are adjuvants commonly used in macular hole surgery. Which one is effective? Does it have effect on late reopening? Does ILM peeling create adjuvants?—are all partially answered questions with various studies demonstrating a positive outcome or no added effect following the use of adjuvant. The use of adjuvant[71] may be necessary in recurrent holes, myopic holes, ruptured cyst, traumatic holes, chronic holes, and pediatric holes . The use of pharmacologic adjuncts, such as a TGF-beta and autologous serum, to facilitate hole closure has not been proven to have any added benefit compared with controls and hence their use has not gained much popularity.[72]

4. Which gas to be used intraocular for temponade?

After careful indirect ophthalmoscopic examination of the peripheral retina for tears, a total air–fluid exchange is performed to desiccate the vitreous cavity. A nonexpansile concentration of a long-acting gas is exchanged for air. Studies have shown that a longer period of internal tamponade equated to a higher success rate.[73]

Sterile air and varying concentrations of either perfluoropropane or sulfur hexafluoride have been used based on surgeon preference for internal tamponade. The primary difference achieved using different gases is the duration of action of the gas bubble and, consequently, the amount of internal tamponade achieved within the first several days after surgery.

The rate of hole closure of idiopathic macular holes is based on many important factors mentioned below:
1. Size of the hole
2. Duration of symptoms
3. Whether ILM peeling has been performed or not
4. Type of tamponade (air/C3F8, SF6, or silicone oil)
5. Length of face-down position.

The mechanism by which the gas bubble closes the hole is not really known. It was initially thought that the buoyancy of the gas was what reattached the retina. Berger et al.[74] successfully proved that the buoyancy exerted by the intraocular gas bubble is small. It was later postulated that it was the interfacial tension rather than the buoyancy that reattached the retina. Therefore, if surface tension is all that is important, the gas must be in contact with the hole all the time.

Longer-acting gas like C3F8 allows for 2–3 weeks of contact between the hole and gas if supine position is avoided. Hence, there is more leeway in positioning. Shorter acting gas therefore requires more rigorous positioning to achieve hole/gas contact as bubble dissipates. Positioning may actually be more critical as the bubble dissipates. Majority of surgeons use C3F8 (64% C3F8 versus 33% SF6). Intraocular tamponade with C3F8 gas produces 6 weeks of visual debility which is as cumbersome to the patient as the prone positioning. Ulnar neuropathy has also been reported in patients on prolonged face down positioning.

The duration for which face-down prone positioning is advocated is also variable. Majority of surgeons[75-83] advocated at least 2 weeks of face down positioning (63%) while 25% advised only 1 week of prone positioning (Tables 19.3 and 19.4).

Historically, strict face-down positioning had been recommended for patients for up to 4 weeks, with consequent difficulties of compliance and patient's quality of life during that period. Traditionally, it has been believed that the shorter the period of face-down positioning, the lower the rate of successful hole closure. In 1997, Tournambe et al. described a pilot study of patients without face-down positioning. They reported a success rate with one surgery of 79% and suggested that pseudophakia was necessary for consideration of liberalization of positioning requirements. The advent of ILM peeling has encouraged a second look at minimal to no face-down positioning. Rubinstein et al.[84] described a case series of 24 eyes of patients who underwent ILM peeling and then did not position postoperatively. In this case series, 22 eyes were successfully closed and had visual improvement. Both eyes that failed were stage 4 large holes. Others have reported comparable, if not better, results in patients with only 1 day of positioning.

Dhawahir-Scala et al.[85] suggest that a critical factor is the size of the gas bubble on postoperative day 1 being greater than 70%. Tranos et al.[78] showed, however, that there may be more rapid progression of cataract formation with less face-down positioning. Tranos et al. were among several authors who recommended combined phacovitrectomy for phakic patients to allow less stringent positioning requirements.

Macular hole surgery is generally associated with good anatomical success. Various periods of face down positioning have been suggested to allow for

TABLE 19.3: Duration of face-down prone position reported by various authors.

Author	Patients	Size/duration	ILM	Gas	Position	Closure
Park et al.[80] 1999	58	All	+	Air	4 days	91%
Isomae et al.[81] 2002	21	Recent	–	C3F8	1 day	91%
Sato et al.[82] 2003	23	Small	+	Air	1 day	91%
Krohn et al.[77] 2005	24	All	–	C3F8	3 days	87.5%
Wickens et al.[83] 2006	21	All	+	Mostly C3F8	3 days	95%

TABLE 19.4: Meta-analysis of available literature on results of macular hole surgery sans positioning.

Author	Patients	Size/duration	ILM	Gas	Position	Closure
Tornambe et al.[76] 1997	33	21% Chronic	–	C3F8		79%
Simcock et al. 2001	20	Stages 2 and 3	–	C2F6		90%
Tranos et al.[78] 2007	16	All	+	C3F8		88%
Merkur et al.[79] 2007	72	Recent	+	C3F8		92%

anatomical closure. The addition of ILM peeling has been reported to increase the rate of anatomical hole closure.

Histologic analysis of ILM specimens removed during macular hole surgery indicated that with higher stages of macular holes there was an increased amount of myofibroblasts. ILM peeling may reduce the tangential tractional forces by assuring that any remaining cortical vitreous or surface myofibroblasts are removed. As the edges of the hole become more mobile, the hole closes in a shorter period, allowing for a reduced period of face down positioning. In addition to reducing tangential traction, other investigators have suggested that ILM removal may increase cytokine release and thus enhance glial proliferation that leads to hole closure. Previous reports have evaluated the necessity of extended periods of face down positioning. Krohn et al.[77] found similar hole closure rates for 3-day and 1-week face down positioning with vitrectomy, gas tamponade, and no ILM peeling. Macular holes closed when surgery was performed with vitrectomy, ILM peeling, intravitreous air, and face down positioning for 4 days. Tornambe et al.[76] described macular hole surgery without any face down positioning. In a series of 33 macular holes, 79% closed when surgery was performed with 15% C3F8, no ILM peeling, and no face down requirements. In a single case observation, Sato et al. reported with optical coherence tomographic images that a full thickness macular hole closed completely within 3 days after ILM peeling and gas tamponade. These studies support a shortened period of face down positioning. A difficulty with macular hole surgery is often motivating the patient to accept face down positioning. Extended periods of face down positioning often produce neck or back pain. There have been reports of complications, including ulnar nerve neuropathy and pressure sores. In addition to these medical complications, there are the financial costs of lost time from work, caregiver requirements, and expensive medical equipment. These associated costs of macular hole surgery may be reduced if a shorter period of for postoperative positioning of patient, such as the retina recovery system face-down positioning was required.

A shortened prone positioning period offers patients decreased risk of medical complication, increases patient convenience, and lowers the indirect costs of macular hole surgery.

In the surgical management, we often use air or gas bubble, long-acting gas, ILM peeling, and vitrectomy depending on the stage and duration of macular hole. Old patients seldom follow instructions regarding facedown positioning. Our results in terms of anatomical closure of the hole and visual improvement are encouraging (Figs. 19.4A to D).

Long-acting gas with face down positioning for up to 3 weeks was used earlier in the development of surgery for macular hole. There is evidence, however, that macular holes can be effectively closed without strict positioning regimens. One study of stage 3 and 4 macular holes revealed a 90% closure rate with significant improvement in visual acuity 1 year after vitrectomy combined with ILM peeling, instillation of C3F8 gas, and 15 days postoperative period avoiding the supine position. OCT has demonstrated anatomic resolution

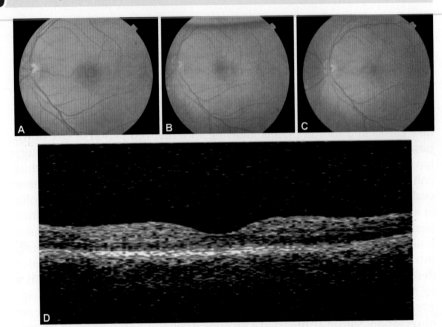

Figs. 19.4A to D: (A) Preoperative stage 3 macular hole; (B) Postoperative appearance on day 20; (C) At 1 month; (D) OCT after surgery.

beginning as soon as 1 day after surgery. Infusion of silicone oil or a gas bubble theoretically provides a scaffolding or template for fibroglial proliferation. Face-down positioning is commonly used to facilitate macular hole tamponade and closure postoperatively.

Silicone oil has also been used as an internal tamponade for patients with difficulty positioning or altitude restrictions. However, the use of silicone oil necessitates a second subsequent surgery to remove the oil. Furthermore, the visual results are not comparable to the use of gas tamponade, possibly as a result of silicone oil toxicity at the level of the photoreceptors and RPE.

Tafoya et al.[86] showed, at 1 year, a final postoperative visual acuity difference of 20/96 (LogMAR 0.208) for silicone oil eyes versus 20/44 (LogMAR 0.453) for gas treated eyes. Lai et al.[87] also showed the visual acuity advantage of gas tamponade with a smaller difference (20/70 versus 20/50). However, Lai et al.[87] also showed the rate of single operation closure being only 65% for silicone oil and 91% for gas tamponade. Thus, unless limited by patient circumstances, gas tamponade for macular hole repair is preferable to silicone oil tamponade. It has been suggested that silicone oil may improve the tamponade effect and decrease the need for face-down positioning; however, there is evidence that success rates with gas are superior. One study[88] demonstrated greater one-surgery anatomic success and superior visual acuity with gas tamponade compared to silicone oil.

20-Gauge versus 23-Gauge versus 25-Gauge Vitrectomy Systems

While no one system poses a significant long-term advantage, smaller gauge vitrectomy systems, with frequently self-sealing wounds, avoid induced astigmatism from suturing sclerotomies, resulting in a more rapid recovery of vision. An initial increase in endophthalmitis[89,90] appears to have been addressed by changing the means of wound construction but may still be considered a disadvantage to small gauge vitrectomy systems. Smaller gauge vitrectomy systems, especially 25-gauge systems, lack shaft stiffness because of the smaller barrel and also complicate the actual vitrectomy surgery for surgeons trained using 20-gauge systems.

Important Predictor of Postoperative Vision

- Preoperative visual acuity and duration of the macular hole.
- Preoperative minimum hole diameter and base diameter (Fig. 19.5) are prognostic factors.
- The larger the size of the macular hole and the longer its duration, the final anatomic as well as functional outcome is adversely affected.

Surgical Complications

With improving surgical techniques, we have seen a decline in complication rates of the macular hole surgery. A review of three multicenter[91-93] randomized, controlled trials found the following complications to be most prevalent: cataract (>75%), late macular hole reopening (2–10%), retinal detachment (3%), and endophthalmitis (<1%). Because the rate of cataract formation is so high, some surgeons remove the lens prior to or simultaneous with the macular hole surgery. A study[94] of 631 eyes revealed a high rate of peripheral retinal tears, but a significantly lower rate of retinal detachment (2%), less

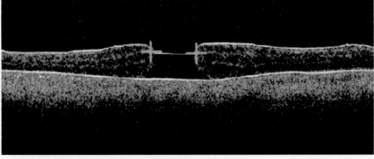

a = Base diameter of hole   = 932 microns
b = Minimum hole diameter = 449 microns
c = Length of left arm   = 280 microns
d = Length of right arm   = 333 microns
HFF = c+d/a   = 280 + 333 / 613   = 0.65

Fig. 19.5: Measurement of the macular hole.

than reported in previous studies. Visual field defects are another reported complication of macular hole surgery. These deficits have been hypothesized to occur secondary to mechanical injury and/or dehydration of the nerve fiber layer during intraoperative air–fluid exchange.

Reoperation

Reoperations are considered for failed primary surgery and reopened macular hole.[95,96] Failed primary surgery is seen in 1–15% of cases.[97] The incidence of primary failures decreases with increasing experience, use of adjuvants and ILM peel. Reopened macular holes have an incidence of 4–9%[98] operated cases. Increase in axial length, pseudophakia and the presence of ERM[99] are the risk factors for late reopening of operated macular holes that may respond to the same surgery with visual improvement.

The various combinations of procedures which can be carried out to improve the anatomical success rate in reoperations are given in Box 19.2.

The pattern of hole closure and foveal contour has a definite relation to the visual prognosis. The patterns of hole closure that are commonly seen are:[106]

- U-pattern: Normal foveal contour
- V-pattern: Steep fovealcontour
- W-pattern: Foveal defect of neurosensory retina

The visual prognosis is best with a U-pattern of closure.It progressively worsens with V- and W-patterns of closure (U < V <W).

SUMMARY

A summary of current management strategies of macular holes is presented in Box 19.3.

BOX 19.2: Procedure for reoperations.

- Repeat standard PPV
- PPV + ILM peel
- PPV + ILM peel + DYE
- Operate FAE with laser to retinal pigment epithelium
- Use longer-acting gas as tamponade
- Stress on face-down positioning
- Silicone oil tamponade

BOX 19.3: Current treatment strategies.

- Almost all macular holes can achieve success
- Internal limiting membrane peel improves hole closure rate (85–90 to 95%)
- Internal limiting membrane peel slows visual recovery
- Use of dye staining facilitates complete peel
- Prone positioning: Duration decreased with ILM peel
- 1 week gas adequate in most eyes
- Long-term (5+ years) results excellent: 60% >6/12

Since macular holes were first recognized in the 19th century, there have been many developments in our understanding and treatment of the condition. This evolution has been facilitated by advancing theories of pathogenesis, improved imaging modalities, including OCT, as well as refinement of surgical technique. Accordingly, outcomes for patients with macular hole have improved dramatically since surgical results were initially reported in 1991. However, many questions remain unanswered and are currently being investigated regarding the pathogenesis and optimal surgical techniques for macular holes.

REFERENCES

1. Aaberg TM. Macular holes: a review. Survey Ophthalmol.1970;15:139-62.
2. Sen P, Bhargava A, Vijaya L, et al. Prevalence of idiopathic macular hole in adult rural and urban south Indian population.Clin Experiment Ophthalmol.2008;36:257-60.
3. Wang S, Xu L, Jonas JB. Prevalence of full-thickness macular holes in urban and rural adult Chinese: the Beijing Eye Study. Am J Ophthalmol. 2006;141(3):589-91.
4. Freund KB, Ciardella AP, Shah V, et al. Optical coherence tomography documentation of spontaneous macular hole closure without posterior vitreous detachment. Retina. 2002;22:506-9.
5. Spaide R. Measurement of the posterior precortical vitreous pocket in fellow eyes with posterior vitreous detachment and macular holes.Retina. 2003;23:481-5.
6. Casuso LA, Scott IU, Flynn HW, et al. Long-term follow-up of unoperated macular holes. Ophthalmology. 2001;108:1150-5.
7. Johnson RN, Gass JD. Idiopathic macular holes.Observations, stages of formation, and implications for surgical intervention.Ophthalmology. 1988;95(7):91724.
8. Tornambe PE. Macular hole genesis (the hydration theory). Retina. 2003;23:421-4.
9. The Eye Disease Case-Control Group. Risk factors for idiopathic macular holes. Am J Ophthalmol. 1994;118:754-61.
10. Azzolini C, Patelli F, Brancato R. Correlation between optical coherence tomography data and biomicroscopic interpretation of idiopathic macular hole. Am J Ophthalmol. 2001;132:348-55.
11. Ezra E, Wells JA, Gray RH, et al. Incidence of idiopathic full-thickness macular holes in fellow eyes (a 5-year prospective natural history study). Ophthalmology. 1998;105:353-9.
12. Lewis ML, Cohen SM, Smiddy WE, et al.Bilaterality of idiopathic macular holes. Grafes Arch ClinExpOphthalmol. 1996;234:241-5.
13. Madreperla SA, Geiger GL, Funata M, et al. Clinicopathologic correlation of a macular hole treated by cortical vitreous peeling and gas tamponade. Ophthalmology.1994;101(4):682-6.
14. Judson PH, Yannuzzi LA.Macular hole.Retina.1994;2:1169-85.
15. Chew EY, Sperduto RD, Hiller R, et al. Clinical course of macular holes (the eye disease case-control study). Arch Ophthalmol. 1999;117:242-6.
16. Krzystolik M, Ciulla TA, Frederick AR. Evolution of a full-thickness macular hole. Am J Ophthalmol. 1998;125:245-7.
17. Ho AC. Macular hole. Retina Vitreous Macula.1999;2:217-29.
18. Ho AC, Guyer DR, Fine SL. Macular hole. SurvOphthalmol. 1998;42(5):393-416.
19. Cox MS, Schepens CL, Freeman HM. Retinal detachment due to ocular trauma. Arch Ophthalmol. 1966;76(5):678–85.

20. Rubin JS,Glaser BM, Thomson JT, et al. Vitrectomy, fluid-gas exchange and transforming growth factor â for the treatment of traumatic macular holes. Ophthalmology. 1995;102:1840-5.
21. Margheria RR,Schepens CL: Macular breaks: diagnosis,etiology and observation. Am J Ophthalmol. 74:219;1972.
22. Wilkinson CP,Rice TA,Michels retinal detachment, St Louis, MO: Mosby; 1997. pp. 1163.
23. Gaucher D, Haouchine B, Tadayoni R, et al. Long-term follow-up of high myopic foveoschisis: natural course and surgical outcome. Am J Ophthalmol. 2007;143(3):455-62.
24. Blakenship GW,Ibanez-Langlois S,Treatment of myopic macular hole and detachment: intravitreal gas exchange. Ophyhalmology. 1987;94:333-6.
25. Croll U,Croll M. Hole in the macula.Am J Ophthalmol. 1950;33:249-52.
26. Campo RV, Lewis RS. Lightning induced macular holes. Am J Ophthalmology.1984;97:792-4.
27. Benzerroug M, Genevois O, Siahmed K, et al. Results of surgery on macular holes that develop after rhegmatogenous retinal detachment. Br J Ophthalmol.2008;92(2):217-9.
28. Gass JDM, JoondephBC. Observations concerning patients with suspected impending macular holes. Am J Ophthalmol. 1990;109:638-46.
29. Rao PK, Shah G, Blinder KJ. Bilateral macular hole formation in a patient with retinitis pigmentosa. Ophthalmic Surg Lasers. 2002;33:152-4.
30. Garretson BR, Pollack JS, Ruby AJ, et al. Vitrectomy for a symptomatic lamellar macular hole. Ophthalmology. 2008;115(5):884-6.
31. Smiddy WE, Michels RG, Glaser BM, et al. Vitrectomy for impending idiopathic macular holes. Am J Ophthalmol.1988;105:371-6.
32. Guyer DR, Fine SL, Ho AC. Macular holes—major review. SurvOphthalmol. 1998;42;393-416.
33. Sjaarda RN. Macular hole.IntOphthalmolClin. 1995;35:105-22.
34. Smiddy WE, Gass JDM. Masquerades of macular holes.Ophthalmic Surg. 1995;26:1624.
35. GonversM, Machemer R.Anew approach to treating retinal detachment with macular holes.Am J Ophthalmol. 1982;94:468-72.
36. Kelly NE, Wendel RT. Vitreous surgery for idiopathic macular holes. Results of a pilot study. Arch Ophthalmol. 1991;109(5):654-9.
37. De Bustro S. Vitrectomy for prevention of macular holes: results of a randomized multicentre clinical trial.Vitrectomy for prevention of macular holes study group. Ophthalmology. 1994;101:1055-9.
38. James M,Feeman SS, Macular holes. Graefes Arch Clin Exp Ophthalmol. 1980;215:59-63.
39. Morgan CM,Schatz H. Idiopathic macular holes. Am J Ophthalmol. 1985;99:437-44.
40. Gass JDM. Stereoscopic Atlas of Macular Diseases: Diagnosis and Treatment,4th edition.St Louis, MO: Mosby; 1996.pp. 1080.
41. Freeman WR. Vitrectomy surgery for full-thickness macular holes.Am J Ophthalmol.1992;2:233-5.
42. Thompson JT, Glasser BM, Sjaarda RN, et al. Progression of nuclear sclerosis and long-term visual results of vitrectomy with transforming growth factor beta-2 for macular holes. Am J Ophthalmol.1995;119:48-54.
43. Faude F, Edel E, Dannhauer M, et al. Autologous thrombocyte administration in treatment of idiopathic macular foramen. Ophthalmologe. 1997;94:877-81.

44. Sakuma T, Tanaka M, Inoue M, et al. Efficacy of autologous plasmin for idiopathic macular hole surgery. Eur J Ophthalmol. 2005;15(6):787-94.

45. Ruiz-Moreno JM, Staicu C, Pinero DP, et al. Optical coherence tomography predictive factors for macular hole surgery outcome. Br J Ophthalmol. 2008;92(5):640-4.

46. Wendel RT, PatelNC, Kelly NE.Vitreous surgery for macular holes. Ophthalmology. 1993;100:1671-6.

47. MeenaChakrabarti, Arup Chakrabarti et al. Macular hole surgery in the young. KJO. 2007;17:23-6.

48. Smiddy WE, Feuer W, Cordahi G. Internal limiting membrane peeling in macular hole surgery. Ophthalmology. 2001;108:1471-8.

49. Kumagai K, Furukawa M, Ogino N, et al. Vitreous surgery with and without internal limiting membrane peeling for macular hole repair. Retina. 2004;24:721-7.

50. Brooks HL Jr. Macular hole surgery with and without internal limiting membrane peeling. Ophthalmology. 2000;107(10):1939-48. Discussion 1948-9.

51. Rodriguez EB, Meyer CH, Farah ME, et al. Intravitreal staining of ILM using ICG in the treatment of macular holes. Ophthalmologica. 2005;219:251-62.

52. Nakamura.T, Murata T et al. Ultrastructure of the vitreoretinal interface following the removal of ILM using ICG. CurrEye Res. 2004;27:395-9.

53. Hillenkamp J, Saikia P, Herrmann WA, et al. Surgical removal of idiopathic ERM with or without the assistance of ICG: a randomised controlled clinical trial.Graefes Arch ClinExpOphthalmol. 2006;21.

54. Maia.M, Haller JA, Pieramici DJ et al. Retinal pigment epithelial abnormalities after internal limiting membrane peeling guided by ICG staining. Retina. 2004;24:157-60.

55. Guo S, Tutela AC, Wagner R, et al. A comparison of the effectiveness of four biostains in enhancing visualization of the vitreous.J PediatrOphthalmol Strabismus. 2006;43:281-4.

56. Haritoglou C, GassCA, Schaumberger M, et al. Macular changes after peeling of the internal limiting membrane in macular hole surgery. Am J Ophthalmol. 2001;132:363-8.

57. Kim JW, Freeman WR, Azen SP, et al. Prospective randomized trial of vitrectomy or observation for stage 2 macular holes. Am J Ophthalmol. 1996;121:605-14.

58. Sheidow TG, Blinder KJ, Holekamp N, et al. Outcome results of macular hole surgery: an evaluation of internal limiting membrane peeling with and without indocyanine green. Ophthalmology.2003;110:1697-1701.

59. Gass CA, Haritoglou C, Schaumberger M, et al. Functional outcome of macular surgery with and without indocyanine green assisted peeling of the ILM. GraefesArch clinExpOphthalmol. 2003;241:716-20.

60. AndoF, Sasano K, Ohba N, et al. Anatomic and visual outcomes after ICG assisted peeling of the retinal ILM in Indiopathic macular hole surgery. Am JOphthalmol. 2004;137:744-6.

61. Hillenkamp J, Saikia P, HerrmannWA et al. Surgical removal of idiopathic ERM with or without the assistance of ICG: a randomised controlled clinical trial. Ophthalmology. 2005;146:432-5.

62. Lochhead J, Jones E, Chui D et al. Outcome of ICG assisted ILM peel in macular hole surgery. Eye. 2004;18:804-8.

63. Slaughter K, Lee IL. Macular hole surgery with and without ICG assistance. Eye. 2004;8:376-8.

64. Rodrigues EB, Meyer CH. Meta-analysis of chromovitrectomy with ICG in macular hole surgery. Ophthalmologica. 2007;114:587-90.

65. Meyer CH, Rodrigues EB. A novel applicator for the selective painting of pre-retinal structures during vitreo retinal surgery.Graefes Arch ClinExpOphthalmol. 2005;243:487-9.

66. Thompson JT, Smiddy WE, Williams GA, et al. Comparison of recombinant transforming growth factor-beta-2 and placebo as an adjunctive agent for macular hole surgery. Ophthalmology. 1998;105:700-6.

67. Minihan M, Goggin M, Cleary PE. Surgical management of macular holes: results using gas tamponade alone, or in combination with autologous platelet concentrate, or transforming growth factor beta 2. Br J Ophthalmol. 1997;81:1073-9.

68. Dosquet C,Chastang C, Mathis A, et al. Effect of autologous platelet concentrate in surgery for idiopathic macular hole: results of a multicenter, double-masked, randomized trial. Platelets in Macular Hole Surgery Group. Ophthalmology.1999;106:932-8.

69. Blumenkraz MS Use of autologous plasmathrombin mixture as adjuvant therapy for macular holes. Ophthalmology. 1994;101(suppl):69.

70. Liggett PE. Human autologous serum in the treatment of idiopathic macular holes. Ophthalmology. 1993;102:1071-6.

71. LansingMB, Glaser BM. The effect of transforming growth factor beta 2 without epiretinal membrane peeling in full-thickness macular holes.Ophthalmology. 1993;100:868-72.

72. Kotobelnik, Hannouche D, Belayachi N, et al. Autologous platelet concentrate as an adjunct in macular hole healing: a pilot study. Ophthalmology.1996;103:590-4.

73. Thompson JT, Smiddy WE, Glaser BM. Intraocular tamponade duration and success of macular hole surgery. Retina. 1996;16:373-82.

74. Berger JW. Buoyancy of gas bubble in macular hole surgery. Ophthalmology. 1997;113:390-4.

75. Benson WE, Cruickshank KC, Fong DS. Surgical management of macular holes; a report by the American academy of Ophthalmology. Ophthalmology.2001;108:1328-35.

76. Tornambe PE, Poliner LS, Grote K. Macular hole surgery without face-down positioning. A pilot study.Retina. 1997;17:179-85.

77. Krohn AD. Macular hole surgery with shortened face down positioning. Am J Ophthalmol. 2005;146:285-7.

78. Tranos PG, Peter NM, Nath R, et al. Macular hole surgery without prone positioning. Eye. 2007;21(6):802-6.

79. Merkur AB, Tuli R. Macular hole repair with limited nonsupine positioning. Retina. 2007;27(3):365-9.

80. Park DW, Sipperley JO, Sneed SR, et al. Macular hole surgery with internal-limiting membrane peeling and intravitreous air. Ophthalmology. 1999;106:1392-8.

81. Merkur AB, Tuli R. Macular hole repair with ILM peeling and limited positioning. Am J Ophthalmol. 2002;136:185-7.

82. Sato H, Kawasaki R, Yamashita H. Observation of idiopathic full-thickness macular hole closure in early postoperative period as evaluated by optical coherence tomography. Am J Ophthalmol. 2003;136:185-7.

83. Soiberman U, Shai D, Loewenstein A,et al. Macular hole surgery with internal-limiting membrane peeling and Intravitreous C3F8 and shortened 3 day positioning; 2005.

84. Rubinstein A, Ang A, Patel CK. Vitrectomy without postoperative posturing for idiopathic macular holes. Clin Experiment Ophthalmol. 2007;35(5):458-61.

85. Dhawahir-Scala FE, Maino A, Saha K, et al. To posture or not to posture after macular hole surgery. Retina. 2008;28(1):60-5.

86. Tafoya ME, Lambert HM, Vu L, et al. Visual outcome of silicone oil versus gas tamponade for macular hole surgery. Semin. 2003;18(3):127-31.
87. Lai JC, Stinnett SS, McCuen BW.Comparison of silicone oil versus gas tamponade in the treatment of idiopathic full-thickness macular hole.Ophthalmology. 2003;110:1170-4.
88. Goldbaum MH, McCuen BW, Hanneken AM, et al. Silicone oil tamponade to seal macular holes without position restrictions. Ophthalmology.1998;105(11):2140-8.
89. Park SS, Marcus DM, Duker JS, et al. Posterior segment complications after vitrectomy for macular hole. Ophthalmology. 1995;102(5):775-81.
90. Kusuhara S, TeraokaEscano MF, Fujii S, et al. Prediction of postoperative visual outcome based on hole configuration by optical coherence tomography in eyes with idiopathic macular holes. Am J Ophthalmol.2004;138(5):709-16.
91. Chen CJ. Glaucoma after macular hole surgery. Ophthalmology. 1998;105:94-100.
92. Poliner LS, TornambePE. Retinal pigment epitheliopathy after macular hole surgery. Ophthalmology. 1992;99:1671-7.
93. Sjaarda RN, Glaser BM, Thompson JT, et al. Distribution of iatrogenic retinal breaks in macular hole surgery. Ophthalmology. 1995;102:1387-92.
94. Hutchins RK.Complications of macular hole surgery.Ophthalmology.1998;105:762.
95. Pasques S, Passin P Visual field loss after vitrectomy for full thickness macular holes. Am J Ophthalmol. 1997;124:88-94.
96. Pendergast SD, McCuen BW. Visual field loss after vitrectomy for full thickness macular holes.Ophthalmology. 1996;103:1069-71.
97. Johnson RN, McDonald HR, Schatz H, et al. Outpatient postoperative fluid-gas exchange after early failed vitrectomy surgery for macular hole. Ophthalmology. 1997;104:2009-13.
98. Ohana E, Blumenkranz MS. Treatment of reopened macular hole after vitrectomy by laser and outpatient fluid-gas exchange. Ophthalmology. 1998;105:1398-403.
99. Baba T, Yamamoto S, Arai M, et al. Correlation of visual recovery and presence of photoreceptor inner/outer segment junction in optical coherence images after successful macular hole repair. Retina. 2008;28(3):453-8.

CHAPTER 20

Macular Hole Surgery

Abhinav Dhami, Dhanashree Ratra, Tarun Sharma

INTRODUCTION

A macular hole is a tear or a defect of the foveal retina involving its full-thickness from the internal limiting membrane (ILM) to the outer segment (OS) of the photoreceptor layer. Until recently, it was thought to be an infrequent ocular condition that was invariably untreatable. Advances in the field of vitreoretinal surgery, especially in the last decade, have sparked renewed interest in this disease paving the way for an increased awareness and understanding of its pathogenesis, natural course, and, more importantly, management.

In 1869, Knapp first reported the case of a macular hole in a patient who sustained blunt trauma to the eye. Subsequent case reports and series pointed to antecedent episodes of ocular trauma such that the two were customarily linked to each other.[1] However, throughout this century, ophthalmologists have increasingly recognized this condition in atraumatic settings such that it has now come to be known as full-thickness idiopathic macular hole (IMH). In fact, case series as far back as 1982 reported that 83% of macular holes were idiopathic and that only 17% have associated history of trauma to the eye.[2]

EPIDEMIOLOGY

The prevalence of IMH has been estimated at around 0.1–0.8% of adults older than 40 years, while the reported age-adjusted incidence is 7.8 per 100,000 of the general population per year.[3] The peak incidence is seen in the seventh decade. The condition is unilateral in around 80% of cases and approximately two-thirds are women. Reasons for this, at best, are speculative at this point. Some epidemiological risk factors have been reported such as cardiovascular disease, hypertension, elevated plasma fibrinogen, and a history of hysterectomy. A number of factors have been suggested to increase the risk of

IMH development, such as, while in women, the use of estrogen-replacement therapy is associated with a reduced risk of IMH. In individuals with severe myopia (−14 to −32 diopters), the prevalence of IMH has been reported to be as high as 6%.[4] Notably, the risk of IMH development in fellow eyes without manifest vitreous separation has been estimated at around 7–12% after 5 years and 17% at 10 years.[5,6]

PATHOPHYSIOLOGY

Our current understanding of the pathogenesis of IMH is based on the correlation between clinical observations with known histopathology of the condition. Several theories exist about how an IMH is produced.

Trauma

In the latter part of the 19th century and early 20th century after the first description by Knapps, several other investigators believed trauma to be the primary cause of macular hole formation.[2,7] One mechanism that was proposed was that contrecoup forces from the trauma led to an immediate rupture or laceration of the macular retina.[7-9] Another theory was that post-traumatic cystic degeneration from reactive vasoconstriction and vasodilation in time led to macular hole formation.[10] Interestingly, the latter served as the basis for the atraumatic theories that were subsequently proposed.

Vascular/Cystoid Degeneration Theory

The early part of the last century saw the first histopathologic description of macular holes by Coats, Fuchs, and Kuhnt. Based on findings of intraretinal cystic changes adjacent to the holes, Coats suggested that macular holes could likewise be caused by atraumatic mechanisms.[11]

The most popular of these theories was the vascular-cystoid theory wherein it was proposed that aging changes in the retinal vasculature led to cystoid degeneration of the macular retina. Coalescence of these cysts along with the progressive thinning of the retina eventually leads to macular hole formation. This theory was the basis for a myriad of interesting pharmacologic therapies including anxiolytics, vasodilating agents, hormones, nicotinic acid, and even retrobulbar atropine injections.[7]

Vitreous Traction Theory

More recently, great emphasis has been placed on the role of the vitreous in the pathogenesis of macular holes. In 1924, Lister[9] described anteroposterior vitreous traction bands originating from the vitreous base, which he believed to cause macular distortion, traction retinal detachments, macular cystoid degeneration, and subsequently, macular hole formation. Later, histological findings of vitreomacular attachment (VMA) plaques,[12] attachments of vitreous traction fibers on macular hole opercula, and direct attachments of vitreous fibers to the macula from the base[13] appear to support this theory. Indirect support also came from the clinical finding that eyes with posterior vitreous detachment were relatively protected against macular hole formation. McDonell et al.[2] thought vitreous separation to be critical in the pathogenesis of macular holes. However, Ho et al.[6] and Akiba et al.[14] observed progression to full-thickness macular hole without the occurrence of a posterior vitreous detachment. Several investigators could not reconcile with this theory of contracting vitreous bands with clinical observations of relatively clear vitreous in the majority of cases.[15]

However, more recent research using ultrasound and optical coherence tomography (OCT) has elucidated that IMHs are initiated during perifoveal peripheral vascular disease as a consequence of anteroposterior and dynamic vitreomacular traction (VMT).

The anterior tractional forces acting at the foveola first produce an intrafoveal split, which evolves into a foveal pseudocyst.

The pseudocyst may then become extended, disrupting and separating the outer retinal layer while raising the inner retinal layer. Degeneration of the retinal tissue secondary to these tractional forces at the foveola may facilitate this process. Dehiscence of the foveal cyst creates a full-thickness defect, including the inner segment (IS)/OS junction of the photoreceptor layer. Complete detachment of the cyst roof appears as an operculum within the vitreous gel, which consists of glial tissue and hyperplastic Müller cells from the inner retinal surface, as well as components of the outer retina including cone cells in up to 65% of cases.[14-16]

CLASSIFICATION OF IDIOPATHIC MACULAR HOLE

In 1988, Gass and Johnson described a classification scheme for IMHs and their precursor lesions incorporating their ideas of the pathogenesis of these lesions.[15] Gass later updated his biomicroscopic classification and anatomic interpretation of macular hole formation (Table 20.1).[15,17]

TABLE 20.1: Staging of macular hole.	
Stages	Gass classification
Stage 0	VMA in the fellow eye of a patient with a known/previous IMH without any change in foveal architecture
Stage 1	Impending macular hole with outer retinal elevation from RPE at foveal center
Stage 2	≤400 µm IMH with VMA
Stage 3	>400 µm IMH without VMA
Stage 4	IMH with complete vitreous separation including from optic disk

(VMA: vitreomacular attachment; IMH: idiopathic macular hole; VMT: vitreomacular traction; OCT: optical coherence tomography)

Stage 1A

In this stage, a yellow spot with 100–200 µm diameter is seen, resulting from a foveolar detachment secondary to spontaneous tangential traction by the prefoveolar vitreous cortex. The yellow spot is presumed to be intraretinal xanthophyll pigment, which becomes more visible due to the foveolar detachment. This is not a pathognomonic sign of a macular hole, as it can also be seen in some cases of central serous chorioretinopathy, cystoid macular edema (CME), and solar maculopathy.

Stage 1B

The foveal retina elevates to the level of the perifovea, elongating the foveal retina around the umbo. The yellow spot is transformed into a doughnut-shaped yellow ring of approximately 200–300 µm in size centered on the foveola. This finding appears to be specific for macular hole formation. Vision in stage 1 lesions typically is in the 20/25 to 20/70 range associated with some degree of metamorphopsia.

Eventually, the centrifugal forces exerted on the fovea lead to the dehiscence of the deeper retinal layers at the umbo. The overlying ILM and prefoveolar vitreous condensation may remain intact and thereby preclude detection. The center of the yellow ring may appear reddish, and the yellow ring itself develops serrated or irregular edges.[17]

Stage 2

This stage is the first evidence of a full-thickness macular hole (<400 µm). At this stage, the hole may become evident in two ways. More often, it appears as an eccentric hole caused by the separation of the prefoveolar cortex from one edge of the occult hole. Rarely, the prefoveolar cortex separates from the center of the macular hole. Spontaneous vitreofoveal separation occurs creating a semitransparent opacity, the pseudo-operculum, which often is larger than the underlying occult macular hole. Pseudo-opercula have been found not to harbor any retinal receptors and mainly are made up of vitreous condensation and reactive glial proliferation. At this stage, the yellow ring disappears because of the relief of prefoveolar traction on the edge of the occult macular hole.[17]

Stage 3

Stage 2 macular hole generally progresses to stage 3 hole, which is defined as hole larger than 400 µm associated with partial vitreomacular separation.

Stage 4

This stage has a complete separation of the vitreous from the entire macular hole and the optic disc.

One would think that the visual decline caused by macular holes would be related to the size of the retinal defect. Although this might be true to some extent, other factors are also involved in the causation of poor vision in these cases. IMH may range in size from as small as 100 μm to more than 800 μm, averaging at around 500 μm in diameter. Based on optical and physical principles alone, the size of these full-thickness defects is not enough to produce the drop in visual acuity experienced by patients.

Studies have shown that a full-thickness macular hole one-half disc diameter in size (750 μm) centered on foveal fixation would produce a visual acuity of 20/60. In order for a macular hole alone to produce the 20/200 vision experienced by the majority of patients, a 3,000-μm full-thickness defect should be present. This discrepancy could be explained by the fact that these holes have been found to be surrounded by a cuff of subretinal fluid and underlying photoreceptor atrophy. This localized detachment and associated receptor atrophy occupy a much larger area than the hole itself, thereby explaining the heightened visual decline, which is usually found.[6]

A variety of traumatic events including blunt trauma, phototoxicity, spontaneously resolved VMT, and other unrecognized causes can cause localized outer retinal defects, which appear as tiny (50–100 μm) apparent foveal micro holes. The inner retina remains intact and the condition is nonprogressive, occurring in patients of all ages. The visual acuity is good but the patient may be aware of a central scotoma.[16]

OCULAR MANIFESTATIONS

Symptomatic patients with macular holes usually complain of blurred central vision and metamorphopsia. Particularly when the condition is mono-ocular, it may be some time before they discover that something is wrong with their vision. The defect is discovered when they cover one eye and notice blurred vision and metamorphopsia in the opposite eye. Usually, patients characterize these symptoms as being mild and only apparent when reading or driving. Impairments in physical activity, engaging in close activities, and decreased social interaction, as well as emotional effects have been reported. Vision-dependent activities such as reading small print, reading road signs, and driving at night can all be affected.[16]

CLINICAL EVALUATION

Visual acuity in patients with macular holes may vary depending, for the most part, on their size and location. Patients with small, eccentric holes may retain excellent visual acuity in the range of 20/25 to 20/40. However, most series report that the usual range of visual acuity is from 20/80 to 20/400 averaging at 20/200.[6] A well-defined round or oval lesion in the macula characterizes a full-thickness macular hole visualized with direct ophthalmoscopy, with yellow-white deposits at the base. These yellow dots probably represent lipofuscin-laden macrophages or nodular proliferations of the underlying pigment epithelium with associated eosinophilic material.

With slit-lamp biomicroscopic examination preferably with a contact lens, a round excavation with well-defined borders interrupting the beam of the slit lamp can be observed. In the majority of patients, an overlying semitranslucent tissue, representing the pseudooperculum, can be seen suspended over the hole. The macular hole is typically surrounded by a gray halo of detachment of the retina. Cystic changes of the retina may also be evident at the margins of the hole. The retinal pigment epithelium (RPE) is usually intact and normal in acute stages but may undergo chronic changes, such as atrophy and hyperplasia, with time. Fine crinkling of the inner retinal surface caused by an epiretinal membrane (ERM) may be present and sometimes may even distort the appearance of the hole.

The most useful diagnostic tests for ophthalmologists to distinguish full-thickness macular holes from other lesions are the Watzke–Allen and the laser aiming beam tests.

The Watzke–Allen's test is performed at the slit lamp using a macular lens and placing a narrow vertical slit beam through the fovea. A positive test is elicited when patients detect a break in the bar of light that they perceive and not the narrowing or distortion of the bar.[6]

The laser aiming beam test is also performed similarly, but this time a small 50 μm spot size laser aiming beam is placed within the lesion. A positive test is obtained when the patient fails to detect the aiming beam when it is placed within the lesion, but is able to detect it once it is placed onto the normal retina.[16]

Optical coherence tomography remains the most accurate method for visualizing and identifying IMH. Within the last couple of years, spectral domain OCT has become more widely available, providing even higher resolution images (axial resolution of as little as 5 μm) and reducing artifacts produced by the moving parts of conventional OCT. This improved technology can therefore provide detailed visualization of VMT, ERM, retinal distortion, and macular detachment.

Apart from the detailed evaluation of the morphology of the macular hole, the OCT also provides the most accurate and noninvasive way of measuring the defect. Over the past few years, various researchers have devised certain indices and OCT parameters, which can be used for calculating the prognosis.[18] They are listed in Table 20.2. Figure 20.1 shows the calculation of one such index called the hole form factor.

Ancillary Investigations

Fluorescein angiography may be a useful test in differentiating macular holes from masquerading lesions such as CME and choroidal neovascularization.[16]

B-scan ultrasonography may be helpful in elucidating the relationship of the macula to the vitreous; therefore, it may be helpful in staging the disease but is not sensitive to distinguish a true macular hole from masquerading lesions.[16]

Amsler grid abnormalities, although sensitive for macular lesions, are not specific for macular holes. Plotting of small central scotomas caused by full-thickness macular holes using the Amsler grid is difficult because of the

TABLE 20.2: Optical coherence tomography (OCT) parameters for calculating prognosis of macular hole surgery.

Optical coherence tomography parameters	Relation
Minimum hole diameter	Minimum linear dimension Eyes with MHs smaller than 400 µm tend to have greater visual acuity improvement
Basal hole diameter	Linear dimension of MH at the level of the RPE layer The smaller the basal hole diameter better postoperative visual acuity
Hole height	The greatest distance between the RPE layer and the vitreoretinal interface A negative correlation was seen between the final visual acuity and the hole height
IS/OS junction defect length	Neither best postoperative visual acuity nor postoperative visual improvement was correlated with preoperative IS/OS junction defect length
Indices	
Hole form factor (HFF)	The HFF is the quotient of the summation of the left and right arm lengths divided by the basal hole diameter The HFF was positively correlated with postoperative visual acuity
Macular hole index (MHI)	The ratio of the hole height to the basal hole diameter The MHI had a positive correlation with postoperative visual acuity

(RPE: retinal pigment epithelium; OS: outer segment; IS: inner segment)

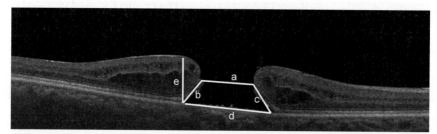

Fig. 20.1: Macular hole indices measured on optical coherence tomography image. [a: Minimum hole diameter; b: left arm length; c: right arm length; d: basal hole diameter; e: hole height; Hole form factor is calculated using the equation, HFF = (b + c)/d].

poor fixation in the affected eye. However, bowing of the lines and micropsia is appreciated. This could be attributable to the surrounding area of retinal edema and intraretinal cysts.[16]

DIFFERENTIAL DIAGNOSIS

Although the diagnosis of a macular hole is quite obvious, it must be differentiated from conditions such as lamellar macular hole, CME, central serous retinopathy, solar retinopathy, ERM, foveal drusen, choroiditis, VMT syndrome, central areolar pigment epitheliopathy, pattern dystrophy, and choroidal neovascular membrane.

NATURAL COURSE

The Vitrectomy for Prevention of Macular Hole Study Group reported that around 40% of stage 1 holes progressed to full-thickness macular hole over a period of 2 years (range 1–13 months from diagnosis).[19] Sixty percent of stage 1 lesions abort and do not progress to later stages. Lamellar holes do not progress to full-thickness holes.[15] Posterior vitreous detachment is believed to confer protection from macular hole.[14] With time, stage 2 holes progress to stage 3 or 4 in the majority of cases (34–96%)[9] associated with a subsequent decline of vision. In rare instances (0–10%), a full-thickness macular hole may spontaneously close with resultant good vision.[20] The estimated incidence for the development of an IMH in the fellow eye is approximately 12%.[21]

TREATMENT OPTIONS

Observation

In the Eye Disease Case–Control Study, after 3 years of follow-up in patients with preexisting IMH, 21.7% demonstrated an enlargement and this rose to 37.1% after 6 years.[16] Spontaneous regression or resolution of IMH was observed in 9% of patients after 6 years of follow-up. Over a period of at least 1 year, deterioration in vision of two Snellen lines or more has been reported for 30% of patients with stage 1, 68% with stage 2, 29% with stage 3, and 13% with stage 4 IMH.[20] However, central retinal detachment secondary to IMH appears to be limited to patients with high myopia.

Surgical Management of Macular Hole

Idiopathic macular holes were considered untreatable until 1991, when Kelly and Wendel[22] reported the first successful closure of a macular hole in 30 out of 52 (58%) patients using vitrectomy and gas tamponade. The success rates in terms of closure of IMH with vitrectomy are in the range of 85–100%, depending on a number of variable prognostic predictors. Figures 20.2A and B show successful closure of a macular hole after surgery on OCT.

Kelly and Wendel[22] based the rationale for their surgery on Gass' observation of macular hole formation and postulated that vitrectomy would remove traction around the hole and combined with gas tamponade would result in the flattening of the ring of perifoveal detachment with some

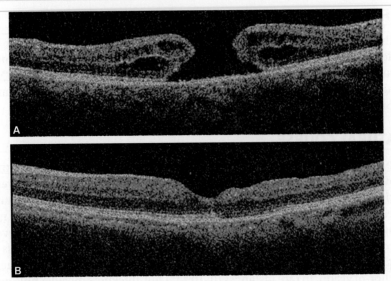

Figs. 20.2A and B: (A) The preoperative full thickness macular hole. (B) The postoperative closure of macular hole following vitrectomy, internal limiting membrane peeling (inverted flap) and gas tamponade.

improvement in vision. Their technique fortunately resulted in hole apposition and closure in many patients with significantly improved vision.

Several variations and additions to the initial technique have been introduced with the aim of improving outcomes and safety. These include the following.

1. *Tamponade type and posturing requirements:* Gas tamponade is believed to additionally aid hole closure by bridging the hole thereby preventing trans-hole fluid flow from the vitreous cavity, allowing the RPE pump to remove the subretinal fluid. It also reduces trans-retinal uveal–scleral outflow with the resultant reduction in the retinal edema. It creates interfacial surface tension forces between the gas bubble and the retina thus acting to pull the edges of the hole together. It also acts as a surface for glial cell migration to bridge the gap across the retinal edges.[16]

    Although Kelly and Wendel[22] used sulfur hexafluoride (SF6) gas as a tamponade agent, in the recent years, there has been a gradual change in practice to increasing use of medium- (C2F6) and short-acting gases (SF6 or air) and a reduction in the duration and strictness of postoperative posturing requirements. It is postulated that the "buoyant force" of a gas bubble on a macular hole in the face-down position is thought to be less important (if all tangential force has been removed) than the bridging of the gap. The gas can still bridge the defect of a macular hole without face-down positioning if the gas fill exceeds 50%. The choice of gas tamponade to be used can be individual surgeon's preference.

2. *Role of ILM peeling:* The removal of the ILM during IMH surgery as a means to improve both anatomical and functional success was first described by Eckardt et al.[23] in 1997 and reported an anatomical success rate of 92% with an equally good functional success rate of 77%.

Internal limiting membrane peeling is believed to improve hole closure by increasing retinal compliance as the ILM, despite being only a few microns thick, contributes very significantly to retinal rigidity. Also, it has a higher rigidity on the retinal side, accounting for its tendency to scroll upward when peeled. Its removal results in increased retinal compliance that aids closure. It also helps in removing residual adherent vitreous cortex remnants on the ILM could exert persistent traction and prevent hole closure.[22,24]

Internal limiting membrane peeling can be surgically challenging, and to facilitate its execution, various dyes have been introduced to help visualize this colorless thin membrane (Table 20.3).[25,26] The technique for peeling ILM is assisted with forceps such as diamond-dusted membrane scraper (DDMS) or end gripping forceps or a Finesse flex loop. DDMS has been shown to be associated with a greater degree of appearance of a dissociated optic nerve fiber layer. The amount of ILM to be peeled does not have a fixed consensus but a radius of peel of between 1.5- and 3-disc diameters has been described in the literature.[23]

Reports of autologous ILM folded into the hole improve closure rates in cases of large primary or persistent macular holes, termed the inverted ILM flap technique and peeling is generally carried out using a pinch-peel technique with fine-tipped forceps (Figs. 20.3A to E). The peeled ILM is used to fill the hole, which acts as a scaffold for the cells to grow and thus aids in hole closure.[27]

TABLE 20.3: Vital dyes for staining internal limiting membrane (ILM).

Dye	Percentage to be used	Property	Toxicity
Indocyanine green (ICG)	0.125–0.5%	Adheres to ILM (collagen type 4, laminin, and fibronectin)	RPE changes Visual field defects Optic atrophy Phototoxicity
Infracyanine green	0.5 mg/mL	High affinity for ILM	Retinal alterations Visual field defects RPE toxicity
Brilliant blue G	Iso-osmolar solution of 0.25 mg/mL	Stains ILM	None reported
Trypan blue	1 mg/mL (0.1%) solution (osmolarity = 300 mOsml)	Recommended mainly for ERM-staining	High osmolar concentration produces retinal toxicity
Bromophenol blue	Concentrations of 0.2% and 0.02%	Stains ERM and ILM	Under study

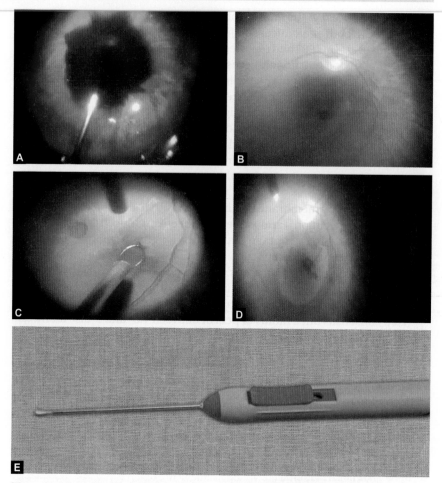

Figs. 20.3A to E: (A) A fundus photo while injecting Brilliant blue G dye under air to stain the internal limiting membrane (ILM) and is kept for 45–120 seconds. (B) The stained ILM along the posterior pole. (C) The scraping of the ILM done around the macular hole with the help of Finesse™ Flex Loop. (D) The peeled ILM with an ILM scaffold filling the macular hole (inverted flap technique). (E) The image of the Finesse™ Flex Loop.

3. *Combined lens surgery with vitrectomy:* Combined lens surgery with vitrectomy has been widely adopted during macular hole surgery to avoid the need for subsequent cataract surgery. With clear corneal phacoemulsification, foldable intraocular lens, and a small gauge minimally invasive vitrectomy, a combined surgery has become a safe and an attractive option. However, potential adverse effects of the procedure can be a higher incidence of posterior synechiae formation, posterior capsule opacity, intraocular lens-related complications, and a small (~0.5 diopter) myopic shift in refraction.[24]

4. *Surgical adjuncts:* The use of a variety of agents at the time of surgery has been described to improve closure rate, namely, transforming growth factor beta 2,[28] autologous serum, and platelets.[29,30] A wide variety of other techniques have been reported, including ILM and capsular flaps,[31] ILM or full thickness retinal transplant,[32] retinal relieving incisions, laser to the base of the hole, mobilization of the edges of the hole,[24] and drainage of chronic fluid from the center of the hole in cases of refractory holes.[31] But by far a simple ILM peeling with gas tamponade or silicone oil is the most common technique followed in routine cases.[24] The earlier described variations are generally reserved for failed macular holes or large primary holes.

Ocriplasmin (Jetrea, ThromboGenics, Inc., Iselin, NJ, United States) has been recently approved for the nonsurgical treatment of symptomatic VMA, including when associated with IMH of less than 400 μm in minimum linear diameter. It is administered by a single 0.1 mL containing 125 μg intravitreal injection. It is a recombinant truncated form of human plasmin and has proteolytic activity against fibronectin and laminin, two major components of the vitreoretinal interface. This action coupled with the activation of endogenous matrix metalloprotease-2 is believed to result in its ability to precipitate vitreoretinal separation. Release of the VMA can result in hole closure in some patients with early IMH. The various side effects as observed in clinical trials are macular hole nonclosure/enlargement, floaters, photopsia, transiently blurred vision, and a variety of outer retinal changes including the development of subretinal fluid, ellipsoid zone changes, electroretinographic changes, dyschromatopsia, impaired pupillary reflex, and lens subluxation/phacodonesis.[16,24]

COMPLICATIONS

- Macular hole surgery shares the same kinds of complications as any other vitreoretinal surgery. The specific complications commonly seen in macular hole surgery include retinal detachment and iatrogenic retinal tears commonly seen inferiorly or temporally (5.5%).[33]
- Enlargement of the hole, macular light toxicity, postoperative pressure spikes, and cataractogenesis may occur. The almost universal development of nuclear sclerotic cataracts (81% in 2 years) may preclude visual improvement seemingly defeating the purpose of the original surgery. At least 25% will require postoperative cataract surgery. Postoperative pressure spikes usually can be managed pharmacologically but may sometimes require an anterior chamber or vitreous tap.[24]
- Some studies have reported wedge-shaped field defects[34] in the temporal field, which may be related to mechanical trauma during posterior hyaloid separation or fluid-gas exchange. Failure of the hole to close after the primary surgery as well as late reopening of the macular hole has been noted. These may respond to a repeat vitrectomy with gas tamponade.[35]

- Internal limiting membrane peeling often results in temporary swelling of the arcuate nerve fiber layer which may be the earliest manifestation of dissociated nerve fiber layer that occurs later in the postoperative period. However, it is probably a transient feature that does not affect visual recovery.[16]
- Late reopening of the macular hole can be seen to occur from less than a year to more than two years after surgery.[36] A significant number of patients were associated with reopening after cataract surgery. Others had an ERM formation or CME. Some patients were found to have multiple recurrences and 75% of these patients showed closure after the third surgery. Visual improvement was noted in 56% of patients. It was concluded that patients who had the macular hole closure for some period of time in any of the first two surgeries showed significant visual improvement.[37]

PROGNOSIS

The limited natural history data available indicate that in a small percentage of cases, IMHs, especially small ones and those with VMT, may close spontaneously. The reported incidence of such spontaneously closing IMHs in the literature is 2.7–8.6%.[16] However, holes usually progress, with size reaching up to 600 µm or larger, over 6 years.[18] The reported rate of development of macular holes in fellow eyes is variable, with an overall risk of 5–10% over 5 years.[21]

Traumatic Macular Holes

Trauma is the second most common cause of macular hole formation. A traumatic macular hole (TMH) can occur in 1.4% of closed globe injuries and to a lesser extent (0.15%) among open globe injury cases. It may lead to permanent significant vision loss due to accompanying retinal pathologies, including commotio retinae, diffuse retinal edema, retinal hemorrhage, vitreous hemorrhage, choroidal rupture, photoreceptor and RPE damage, and retinal tears and dialysis. It is more commonly encountered in younger population, usually associated with sports, recreational work, and transportation.[38]

Multiple hypotheses exist regarding the cause for a TMH. In 2001, Johnson et al.[39] proposed contrecoup mechanism in which a sudden decrease in the globe's anterior–posterior diameter causes a compensatory equatorial expansion. Such a dynamic change within the volume-fixed globe can lead to horizontal forces and splitting of the retinal layers at the fovea.

Traumatic macular holes have been shown to close without any treatment. There are many case reports showing that the spontaneous closures usually took place between 2 weeks and 12 months after the trauma.[40] The proposed mechanism of spontaneous closure of TMH encompasses the proliferation of glial cells or retinal pigment epithelial (RPE) cells from bank of the hole's edge to fill the hole bottom and stimulation of astrocyte migration to heal the TMH. Due to the relatively high rate of spontaneous closure of TMH, it has been suggested that adult patients may be observed for 3–6 months after the hole formation, especially young patients with small holes, good visual acuity, and posterior vitreous adhesion to the hole edges. But surgery may be recommended earlier for pediatric patients to prevent amblyopia. The current surgical technique is similar to that of the IMH which includes removal of the posterior hyaloid, ERMs, with or without ILM peeling, and intraocular gas or silicone oil tamponade.[38]

Myopic Macular Holes

Secondary macular holes can occur in eyes with high myopia and the characteristics and demographics of these MHs differ from those of most IMH. Myopic MHs tend to develop in younger subjects and may be associated with a rhegmatogenous retinal detachment surrounding the hole. The mean age of patients in most myopic MH series is mid-1950s. Very high rates of associated retinal detachment ranging from 9% to 21% have been reported in the Japanese and Chinese literature, respectively.[41]

Although its pathophysiology is not fully understood, it is postulated that anteroposterior vitreous traction on the posterior pole due to a posterior staphyloma, tangential traction on the macula from contraction of the cortical vitreous and ERMs, and reduced retinal adherence to the choroid due to RPE atrophy contribute to the higher incidence of MH in myopic eyes.[42]

Although macular buckling was performed routinely prior to the advent of vitrectomy surgery, vitrectomy combined with peeling of the ILM and gas tamponade has become the most commonly chosen primary procedure even for myopic macular holes. Better understanding of the tractional forces and advances in surgical techniques has increased reattachment rates. Silicone oil as a tamponade instead of gas is favored by some for myopic MH. However, failure of macular hole closure and recurrent detachment remain challenging surgical problems, and visual outcomes are variable. Anteroposterior scleral shortening has been accomplished by scleral infolding with or without scleral resection. Scleral resection has been combined with vitrectomy and gas tamponade for MHRD repair.[43] Macular buckle using the Ando's T-shaped and Morin–Devin "T"-shaped macular wedge buckle has shown encouraging results in the closure of myopic macular holes.

CONCLUSION

With advances in the imaging and surgical techniques, macular holes can be easily detected and treated with good surgical results and improved visual outcomes. Various indices measured on the OCT images give a fairly good estimate of the surgical outcome. The surgical technique of ILM peeling is almost universally employed by surgeons to close the macular defect. Vital dyes such as brilliant blue and trypan blue have been shown to be safe for use for a short duration during the surgery. Their use has greatly facilitated ILM peeling by increasing its visibility. Numerous modifications have been employed including inverted flap or autologous, free ILM transplant. Ocriplasmin has shown the way for a nonsurgical closure of the macular hole. Despite these advances, a myopic macular hole still poses a challenge to the surgeon. More work needs to be done in this area. Even though there are certain areas in macular hole management that remain unanswered, the present treatment has established itself as a highly successful treatment option. It is one of the very successful surgical modalities in terms of surgeon and patient satisfaction.

REFERENCES

1. Kipp CJ. Macular holes: a clinical contribution. Trans Am Ophthalmol Soc. 1908;11:518-28.
2. McDonell PJ, Fine SL, Hillis Al. Clinical features of idiopathic macular cysts and holes. Am J Ophthalmol. 1982;93(6):777-86.
3. McCannel CA, Ensminger JL, Diehl NN, et al. Population-based incidence of macular holes. Ophthalmology. 2009;116(7):1366-9.
4. Coppe AM, Ripandelli G, Parisi V, et al. Prevalence of asymptomatic macular holes in highly myopic eyes. Ophthalmology. 2005;112(12):2103-9.
5. Chew EY, Sperduto RD, Hiller R, et al. Clinical course of macular holes. the eye disease case-control study. Arch Ophthalmol. 1999;117(2):242-6.
6. Ho AC, Guyer DR, Fine SL, et al. Macular hole. Surv Ophthalmol. 1998;42(5):393-416.
7. Croll LJ, Croll M. Hole in the macula. Am J Ophthalmol. 1950;33:248-52.
8. Duke-Elder WS. System of Ophthalmology, St. Louis: CV Mosby; 1967.
9. Lister W. Holes in the retina and their clinical significance. Br J Ophthalmol. 1924;8(1):1-20.
10. Samuels B. Cystic degeneration of the retina. Arch Ophthalmol. 1930;4:476-86.
11. Coats G. The pathology of macular holes. Roy London Hosp Rep 1907;17:69-96.
12. Foos RY. Vitreoretinal junctions: Topographical variations. Invest Ophthalmol Vis Sci 1972;11(10):801-8.
13. Avila MP, Jalkh AE, Murakami K. Biomicroscopic study of the vitreous in macular breaks. Ophthalmology. 1983;90(11):1277-83.
14. Akiba J, Quiroz MA, Trempe CL. Role of posterior vitreous detachment in idiopathic macular holes. Ophthalmology 1990;97:1610-13.
15. Johnson RN, Gass JD. Idiopathic macular holes: Observations, stages of formation, and implications for surgical intervention. Ophthalmology. 1988;95(7):917-24.
16. Steel DH, Lotery AJ. Idiopathic vitreomacular traction and macular hole: a comprehensive review of pathophysiology, diagnosis, and treatment. Eye. 2013;27:S1-21
17. Gass JD. Reappraisal of biomicroscopic classification of stages of development of a macular hole. Am J Ophthalmol. 1995;119:752-9.
18. Kusuhara S, Negi A. Predicting visual outcome following surgery for idiopathic macular holes. Ophthalmologica. 2014;231(3):125-32.
19. deBustros S. Vitrectomy for prevention of macular holes: Results of a randomized multicentre clinical trial. Vitrectomy for Prevention of Macular Hole Study Group. Ophthalmology. 1994;101:1055-9.
20. Kim JW, Freeman WR, Azen SP, et al. Prospective randomised trial of vitrectomy or observation for stage 2 macular holes. Am J Ophthalmol. 1996;121:605-14.
21. Akiba J, Kakehashi A, Arbaze CW, et al. Fellow eyes in idiopathic macular hole cases. Ophthalmic Surg. 1992;23:594-97.
22. Kelly NE, Wendel RT. Vitreous surgery for idiopathic macular holes: Results of a pilot study. Arch Ophthalmol. 1991;109:654-9.

23. Eckardt C, Eckardt U, Groos S, et al. Entfernung der Membranalimitansinternabei Makulalöchern Klinische und morphologischeBefunde. Der Ophthalmologe. 1997;94(8):545-51.

24. Madi HA, Masri I, Steel DH. Optimal management of idiopathic macular holes. Clin Ophthalmol. 2016;10:97.

25. Rodrigues EB, Costa EF, Penha FM, et al. The use of vital dyes in ocular surgery. Survey of Ophthalmology. 2009;54(5):576-617.

26. Kumar A, Thirumalesh MB. Use of dyes in ophthalmology. J Clin Ophthalmol Res. 2013;1(1):55.

27. Michalewska Z, Michalewski J, Nawrocki J. Macular hole closure after vitrectomy: the inverted flap technique. Br J Ophthalmol. 2003;87:1015-9.

28. Glaser BM, Michels RG, Kuppermen BD, et al. Transforming growth factor-beta 2 for the treatment of full thickness macular holes: A prospective randomised study. Ophthalmology. 1992;99:1162-72.

29. Ligget PE, Skolik SA, Horio B, et al. Human autologous serum for the treatment of macular holes. Ophthalmology. 1993;102:1071-6.

30. Takano A, Hirata A, Inomata Y, et al. Intravitreal plasmin injection activates endogenous matrix metalloproteinase-2 in rabbit and human vitreous. American Journal of Ophthalmology. 2005;140(4):654-60.

31. Gonvers M, Machemer R. A new approach to treating retinal detachment with macular hole. Am J Ophthalmol. 1982;94:468-72.

32. Grewal DS, Mahmoud TH. Autologous neurosensory retinal free flap for closure of refractory myopic macular holes. JAMA Ophthalmol. 2016;134(2):229-30.

33. Sjaarda RN, Glaser BM, Thompson JT, et al. Distribution of iatrogenic retinal breaks in macular hole surgery. Ophthalmology. 1995;102:1387-92.

34. Haritoglou C, Ehrt O, Gass CA, et al. Paracentral scotomata: A new finding after vitrectomy for idiopathic macular hole. Br J Ophthalmol. 2001;85:231-3.

35. Duker JS, Wendel RT, Patel RC, et al. Late reopening of macular holes following initial successful vitreous surgery. Ophthalmology. 1994;101:1373-8.

36. Pacques M, Massin P, Blain P, et al. Long-term incidence of reopening of macular holes. Ophthalmology. 2000;107:760-5.

37. Thompson JT, Sjaarda RN. Surgical treatment of macular holes with multiple recurrences. Ophthalmology. 2000;107:1073-7.

38. Liu W, Grzybowski A. Current management of traumatic macular holes. J Ophthalmol. 2017;2017:1748135.

39. Johnson RN, McDonald HR, Lewis H, et al. Traumatic macular hole: observations, pathogenesis, and results of vitrectomy surgery. Ophthalmology. 2001;108(5):853-7.

40. Nunode M, Nakajima C, Watanabe CA. Case of traumatic macular hole with interesting course. Jpn J Clin Ophthalmol. 1983;77:922-4.

41. Zhang CF, Hu C. High incidence of retinal detachment secondary to macular hole in a Chinese population. Am J Ophthalmol. 1982;94:817-9.

42. Morita H, Ideta H, Ito K, et al. Causative factors of retinal detachment in macular holes. Retina. 1991;11:281-4.

43. Kono T, Takesue Y, Shiga S. Scleral resection technique combined with vitrectomy for a macular hole retinal detachment in highly myopic eyes. Ophthalmologica. 2006;220(3):159-63.

CHAPTER 21

Giant Retinal Tears

Lingam Gopal

INTRODUCTION

Giant retinal tear (GRT) is defined as a retinal tear with a circumferential extent of more than 90°. The success rate of reattachment of retina was about 30% in the era before vitrectomy and perfluorocarbon liquids (PFCLs).[1] Several important contributions have made it possible to improve the success rate to very high levels as of today. Notable among them are the introduction of vitrectomy by Machemer et al.,[2] prolonged internal tamponade with perfluorocarbon gases by Lincoff,[3] concept of prone fluid–air exchange by Michels et al.,[4] use of silicone oil by Scott[5] and Zivojnovic,[6] and the most important of all the introduction of PFCLs by Chang.[7] The use of PFCLs has enabled the surgery to be performed in supine position and has almost eliminated the problems of slippage of the retina posteriorly, thus improving the success rate of reattachment of fresh GRTs to nearly 90–95%.

ETIOLOGY

Giant retinal tears are common in diseases such as Marfan's syndrome,[8] Ehlers–Danlos syndrome, and Wagener–Stickler's syndrome,[9] but most GRTs are idiopathic in origin. Myopia is a significant association of GRT with nearly 40% of patients with GRT having myopia of more than 8 Diopters.[10] The idiopathic and traumatic varieties are seen more commonly in males. Nasal GRT is known to be associated with nasal coloboma of the lens.[11] Bilaterality is reported in 13% of cases.

Both penetrating and blunt injuries can be associated with GRT. Pars plana vitrectomy can be rarely complicated by postoperative occurrence of GRT.[12] This complication is fortunately rare in this era of wide-angle visualization and microincisional vitrectomy. Attempted removal of dislocated lens fragments by the limbal approach during cataract surgery could be complicated by the occurrence of GRT, especially inferiorly.[13] At least one report exists of GRT occurring following laser-assisted in situ keratomileusis.[14] GRT may be the result of planned retinotomies and retinectomies while operating on eyes with proliferative vitreoretinopathy (PVR).

GIANT RETINAL TEAR VERSUS GIANT DIALYSIS

Giant retinal dialysis is an intrabasal split at ora serrata—mostly caused by trauma—although familial dialysis has been described.[15] Very often the vitreous is not liquefied and the fluid collects slowly leading to relatively chronic detachments, sometimes, with subretinal bands. In contrast, a GRT has vitreous detachment with vitreous adherent to the anterior flap but not the posterior retina. The gel can, sometimes, be seen behind the detached retina.

VARIABLES IN CLINICAL PRESENTATION

The circumferential extent of the GRT can vary from 90° all the way to 360°, leading to different complexities of the problem from the surgical perspective. The edge of the tears is rolled posteriorly in almost all cases while large tears nearing 180° have usually an inverted flap. Severe hypotony and choroidal detachment are not uncommon associations. GRTs can coexist with macular holes—especially in eyes with high myopia. Considering the large size of retinal dehiscence and the corresponding liberation of retinal pigment epithelial cells, PVR can set in fairly early.[16] PVR is characterized by preretinal and subretinal fibrosis. The rolled edger of the tear often harbors some fibrosis. Pars plana epithelium can be found detached in the area of GRT due to the vitreous traction. The vitreous gel can be seen under the detached retina.

MANAGEMENT

Conservative Management

Retinopexy with photocoagulation/cryopexy in the form of barrage treatment may be possible in selected cases of giant tear/dialysis without clinical retinal detachment. This opportunity is more likely to be present with dialysis rather than with GRT, since retinal detachment tends to set in and progress very rapidly in GRT.

Scleral Buckling

The role of scleral buckling is restricted in the present era to the management of giant retinal dialysis of retina. The procedure of scleral buckling involves the placement of relatively broad and shallow buckle. Additional gas injection may be needed to flatten the retinal tear on the buckle.

Vitreoretinal Surgery

As alluded to above, GRT in the present era is almost always managed through a pars plana approach. The actually surgical steps have evolved with time and newer innovations. The most important contribution has been the introduction of PFCLs by Chang.[7] Prior to this, the problem faced by the surgeon was the slippage of the GRT flap posteriorly leading often to folds across macula. Surgeons tried to overcome the problem by the usage of retinal tacks, retinal screws, prone fluid air exchange, etc.[17–20] These techniques have become obsolete with the advent of PFCL. These heavier than water liquids helped to reattach the retina from posterior pole forward progressively, thus achieving a smoothly attached retina without slippage of the retinal flap.

The use of wide-angle visualization (binocular indirect ophthalmo-microscope of ocular instruments, Resight of Zeiss, etc.) has also improved the surgical results significantly by permitting a panoramic visibility of the fundus—especially during the injection of PFCL, PFCL–silicone oil exchange, PFCL–air exchange, etc. The standard of care in the present-day demands the use of wide-angle visualization system.

A 23-gauge vitrectomy system is most commonly used, although smaller gauge instruments (25-gauge) can also be used. A 23-gauge instrument is likely to withstand the maneuvers required in reaching the periphery better.

Lens Management

In most cases, the lens can be retained. Assisted by scleral indentation, a good vitreous base debulking is possible without removing the lens. If there is significant cataract, one has the option of phacoemulsification with or without intraocular lens (IOL) implantation. "Retaining the lens in the first surgery and removing the same along with silicone oil" is obviously a better option since the placement of IOL is in a more controlled situation with better accuracy in calculation of IOL power. The only issue with retained crystalline lens during the surgery to reattach RD with GRT would be in the access to ora serrata if one believes in the treatment of the circumference beyond the limits of the GRT with retinopexy. Endolaser so far into the periphery could be difficult in the presence of crystalline lens and one may use cryopexy or indirect delivery of laser photocoagulation.

Intraocular Lens Management

The IOL, if present, in most cases does not present special problems. Issues such as capsular opacification, pigment, and deposits on the surface of the IOL can be easily managed to facilitate adequate visualization. A grossly subluxated or dislocated IOL would, however, need to be explanted.

Additional Encirclage

There is considerable controversy on the role of the placement of the encircling element to support the vitreous base. In the milieu of a 360° GRT, there is definitely no purpose served by the encirclage. However, in eyes with predominantly superior tear, if the vitreous debulking is limited (as in a phakic eye), there is a theoretical safety in the placement of encirclage in reducing the risk of recurrent retinal detachment. While Kreiger and Lewis[21] reported good results without encirclage; Verstraeten et al.[22] have shown the benefit of additional encirclage (14% reoperation rate with encirclage versus 45% without).

Surgery for Proliferative Vitreoretinopathy

Fresh GRTs are relatively simple to manage, since most of the vitreous is lying in the anterior vitreous cavity and is easy to remove. However, eyes with PVR could be a challenge. The gross mobility of the retina makes it difficult to get a purchase for membrane peeling. On occasion, one may have to resort to bimanual surgery to adequately remove the preretinal and subretinal traction. GRT secondary to penetrating trauma is associated with more severe PVR, which could be in the form of extensive subretinal and preretinal fibrosis. The presence of GRT gives easy access to the subretinal space for meticulous dissection of the membranes.

Role of Retinectomy

The edge of the GRT often is rolled but this does not always indicate the presence of underlying fibrosis. Under PFCL, the edge can often be stroked into position using a silicone brush needle. Obviously, stiff and contracted GRT edge may need to be excised after diathermization. A conversion to 360° GRT may be needed in eyes with severe PVR.

The anterior flap of the GRT is to be excised to the extent possible.

Use of Perfluorocarbon Liquid

Perfluorocarbon liquid can be used in the initial stages of the surgery to stabilize the posterior retina and permit vitrectomy and vitreous base debulking without the flapping retina coming in the way of the cutter. It also permits membrane dissection to some extent—especially anteriorly. Once all traction is relieved, PFCL is used to reattach the retina. It is preferable to fill the PFCL till at least the edge of the GRT. PFCL should be injected slowly into the bubble to avoid fragmentation. Small bubbles can enter subretinal space easily. Failure to relieve traction would also lead to subretinal migration of the PFCL.

A dual-bore cannula is a good tool to inject PFCL.[23] This permits the egress of balanced salt solution (BSS) simultaneously, and hence a more controlled injection is possible without wide fluctuations in intraocular pressure—especially when valved cannulas are used.

Retinopexy

Endolaser is possible fairly easily along the posterior edge of the GRT. Where the PFCL was filled up to the edge of GRT only, the peripheral retina beyond the PFCL bubble will be still detached and not amenable for laser until it is also reattached during air or silicone oil exchange with the PFCL. In phakic eyes with difficulty in reaching the ora serrata, peripheral cryopexy or indirect delivery of laser photocoagulation can be used to complete the treatment.

Internal Tamponade

In most cases of GRT, silicone oil tamponade is chosen. However, long-acting gas such as C_3F_8 can be used in selected cases when the circumferential extent is about 90°.

Most surgeons would choose to directly exchange the PFCL with silicone oil. This avoids the possibility of slippage of the retina. The oil enters slowly permitting the complete evacuation of the fluid (BSS) trapped anteriorly under the peripheral retina anterior to the PFCL bubble. The drying of this fluid is vital to avoid slippage of the retina once the PFCL is removed.

Some surgeons prefer to perform PFCL–air exchange first before injecting silicone oil in the air-filled eye. However, the chances of slippage of retina posteriorly are greater with this technique.

Some surgeons leave the PFCL in the eye for a period of 10 days and then exchange the PFCL with gas by another surgical procedure.[24,25]

Additional Procedure

Inferior iridectomy would be needed in aphakic eyes when silicone oil is the chosen tamponading agent.

Postoperative Management

Prone posturing is needed for GRT of greater than 180° extent. For GRT smaller than 180°, lateral posture to the direction opposite that of the GRT is preferred.

Recurrent Fibrosis

Proliferative vitreoretinopathy remains the most important cause of recurrent retinal detachment after the repair of GRT. Minimal recurrent fibrosis may manifest as macular pucker or some fibrosis near the edge of the tear but not actually creating an open break situation. Such cases can be managed by membrane peeling at the time of silicone oil removal. However, fibrosis can create new breaks or lift up the GRT edge leading to open break situation. One would need to reoperate under these circumstances. Where extensive membrane peeling is required, one would need to remove the oil and redo the surgery. A few cases can be managed under silicone oil with silicone oil being used as infusion to top up the eye from time to time.

Silicone Oil Removal

In general, silicone oil removal is planned after 3–4 months. In case of eyes with penetrating injury-related GRTs, one tends to leave the oil in the eye longer—beyond 6 months.

Silicone oil removal should not be taken lightly. One should evaluate the retina critically before oil removal. Shallow retinal detachments and small macular puckers can be missed unless they are looked for. Following the oil removal, the retina is carefully inspected with endoillumination and wide-angle visualization. Any fibrosis in the posterior pole is definitely removed. Minimal fibrosis in the periphery not threatening the GRT edge can probably be left behind. In a few cases, one may identify shallow recurrent retinal detachment only after oil removal. In these circumstances, one has to clean the retina and put back silicone oil with the hope of a future opportunity to achieve the endpoint of oil-free eye with attached retina.

RESULTS

Chang et al.[26] reported 94% success in retinal reattachment in a series of GRTs using perfluorodecalin, perfluorooctane, or perfluorotributylamine. A similar success was seen in a series by Schulzman and Peyman[27] using vitrectomy. Berrocal et al.[28] in a review of article have quoted a reattachment rate after one procedure of 80–90% and a final reattachment rate of 94–100% in fresh detachments secondary to GRT. This improved success is directly attributable both to the vitreoretinal surgical techniques and to the use of PFCLs.

Fellow Eye with Giant Retinal Tear

Freeman[29] reported 51% incidence of retinal breaks in the fellow eye of nontraumatic GRT. Sixteen percent of fellow eyes developed retinal detachment. Retinal breaks without detachment consisted of GRT in 13% eyes, retinal tears in 12%, holes in 10%, and dialysis in 0.4%. In general, the fellow eye involvement with GRT was seen within 30 years of the first eye treatment for GRT. Freeman identified high myopia (>10 D) and increasing white-without-pressure as risk factors for GRT in fellow eyes. Fellow eyes are recommended for prophylactic treatment for retinal holes and tears. However, the role of prophylactic scleral buckling in eyes with progressive white-without-pressure is controversial.

REFERENCES

1. Freeman HM, Schepens CL, Cervillion GC. Current management of giant retinal breaks. Trans Am Acad Ophthalmol Otolaryngyol. 1970;74:59-74.
2. Machemer R, Buettner H, Norton EWD. Vitrectomy—a pars plana approach. Trans Am Acad Ophthalmol Otolaryngyol. 1971;75:813-20.
3. Lincoff H. A small bubble technique for manipulating giant retinal tears. Ann Ophthalmol. 1981;3:241-3.
4. Michels RG, Rice TA, Blankenship G. Surgical techniques for selected giant retinal tears. Retina. 1983;3:139-53.
5. Scott JD. Silicone oil as an instrument. In: Ryan SJ (Ed). Retina. St. Louis: Mosby Year Book; 1994. pp. 2181.

6. Zivojnovic R. Silicone Oil in Vitreoretinal Surgery. Dodrecht: Martinus Nijhoff/Dr W Junk; 1987. pp. 61.

7. Chang S. Low viscosity liquid perfluorocarbon chemicals in vitreous surgery. Am J Ophthalmol. 1987;103:38-43.

8. Sharma T, Gopal L, Shanmugam MP, et al. Retinal detachment in Marfan's syndrome: clinical characteristics and outcome. Retina. 2002;22:423-8.

9. Ang A, Poulson AV, Goodburn SF, et al. Retinal detachment and prophylaxis in Type 1 Stickler syndrome. Ophthalmology. 2008;115:164-8.

10. Schepens CL, Dobbie JG, Mcmeel JW. Retinal detachments with Giant retinal breaks—preliminary report. Trans Am Acad Ophthalmol Otolaryngol. 1962;66:471-8.

11. Hovland KR, Schepens CL, Freeman HM. Developmental giant retinal tears associated with lens coloboma. Arch Ophthalmol. 1968;80:325-31.

12. Banker AS, Freeman WR, Kim JW, et al. Vision threatening complications of surgery for full thickness macular hole—vitrectomy for macular hole study group. Ophthalmology. 1997;104:1442-52.

13. Aaberg TM, Rubsamen PE, Flynn HW, et al. Giant retinal tear as a complication of attempted removal of intravitreal lens fragments. Am J Ophthalmol. 1997;124:227-9.

14. Ozodamar A, Aras C, Sener B, et al. Bilateral retinal detachment associated with giant retinal tear after laser-assisted in situ keratomileusis. Retina. 1998;18:176-7.

15. Brown GC, Tasman WS. Familial retinal dialysis. Can J Ophthalmol. 1980;15:193-5.

16. Girard P, Mimoun G, Karpouzas I, et al. Clinical risk factors for proliferative vitreoretinopathy after retinal detachment surgery. Retina. 1994;14:417-24.

17. Usui M, Hamazaki S, Takano S, et al. A new surgical technique for the treatment of giant retinal tears with transscleral retinal sutures. Jpn J Ophthalmol. 1979;23:206-15.

18. Federman JL, Shakin JL, Lanning RC. The microsurgical management of giant retinal tears with transscleral retinal sutures. Ophthalmology. 1982;89:832-8.

19. Freeman HM, Castillejos ME. Current management of giant retinal breaks—results with vitrectomy and total air exchange in 95 cases. Trans Am Ophthalmol Soc. 1981;79:89-100.

20. Ando P, Kanoo J. A plastic tack for the treatment of retinal detachment with giant tear. Ann J Ophthalmol. 1983;90:260-1.

21. Kreiger AE, Lewis H. Management of giant retinal tears without scleral buckling—use of radical dissection of vitreous base and perfluorooctane and intraocular tamponade. Ophthalmology. 1992;99:491-7.

22. Verstraeten T, William GA, Chang S, et al. Lens-sparing vitrectomy with perfluorocarbon liquid for primary management of giant retinal tears. Ophthalmology. 1995;102:17-20.

23. Narendran V, Kothari A, Charles S, et al. Principles and Practices of Vitreoretinal Surgery. New Dehli: Jaypee Brothers Medical Publishers (P) Ltd.; 2014. pp. 84.

24. Ventrua MC, Melo C, Diniz JR, et al. Perfluorooctane liquid as a short-term vitreous–retinal tamponade in the postoperative period in patients with retinal detachment due to giant tears. Arq Bras Oftalmol. 2007;70:495-500.

25. Sirmaharaj M, Balachnadran C, Chan WC, et al. Vitrectomy with short-term postoperative tamponade using perfluorocarbon liquid for giant retinal tears. Br J Ophthalmol. 2005;89:1176-9.

26. Chang S, Lincoff H, Zimmerman J, et al. Giant retinal tears—surgical technique and results using perfluorocarbon liquids. Arch Ophthalmol. 1989; 107:761-6.
27. Schulzman JA, Peyman GA. The Vitreous Surgery: Principles and Practice. Norwalk: Appleton and Lange; 1994. pp. 573-8.
28. Berrocal MH, Chenworth ML, Acaba LA. Management of giant retinal tear detachments. J Ophthalmic Vis Res. 2017;12:93-7.
29. Freeman HM. Fellow eyes of giant retinal breaks. Trans Am Acad Ophthalmol Soc. 1978;76:343-82.

CHAPTER 22

Management of Rhegmatogenous Retinal Detachment by Vitreoretinal Surgical Techniques

Yog Raj Sharma, Soman Nair

INTRODUCTION

Rhegmatogenous retinal detachment (RRD) is one of the most common indications of vitreoretinal surgery. Although conventionally RRD has been managed by 20-gauge pars plana techniques, in recent times, sutureless 25-gauge, 23-gauge, and even sutureless 20-gauge techniques have been used. Owing to the increasing familiarity and high success rate obtained with vitreoretinal surgical techniques, scleral buckling has been supplanted, but remains an effective alternative. Presently, surgical approach in uncomplicated retinal detachment is largely surgeon-dependent and also depends on the vitreoretinal surgical armamentarium available. Despite increasing complexity involved in these techniques, the basic steps involved in vitreoretinal surgery for the management of RRD remain the same and shall be discussed in this chapter.

TECHNIQUE OF VITREORETINAL SURGERY

The salient steps involved in the management of RRD are:
1. Sclerotomy port creation
2. Buckling
3. Vitreous removal
4. Traction relief (if any)
5. Retinal reattachment
6. Retinopexy
7. Tamponade.

Creating Sclerotomy Ports

Sclerotomies should be made 4 mm posterior to the limbus in phakic eyes, 3.5 mm in pseudophakic eyes, and 3 mm in aphakic eye or if lensectomy is planned. The incisions should be made with a fresh blade (MVR) to penetrate the choroid and nonpigmented ciliary epithelium without any traction at the vitreous base. A 1.4-mm linear incision, which rounds out to 0.89 mm in circumference, is created with an MVR blade. The sclerotomies should be parallel to the limbus. The infusion cannula incision should be made first just below the 3 or 9 O'clock position inferotemporally. This ensures that the external aspect of the cannula dose not impede inferior vitreous base dissection. Preplaced scleral sutures are passed first to hold the base of the infusion cannula. The tip of the cannula should be inspected to prevent inadvertent suprachoroidal or subretinal infusion. The other two sclerotomies are made just above the 180° line and parallel to the limbus.

Buckling-encircling Element

The step of placing an encircling element is highly controversial.[1,2] The rationale behind the buckling is that the peripheral indent supports the vitreous base area reducing the effect of any peripheral retinal contracture due to proliferative vitreoretinopathy (PVR). It may also prevent the posterior migration of fluid from a peripheral break. Because in phakic RRD with clear lens, peripheral vitreous base dissection may not be always achievable, some surgeons combine vitreoretinal procedures with buckling. We never use any buckling element in management of any type of RRD. Wide-angle panoramic view of fundus, with high-speed cutters, and peripheral indentation permit effective vitreous base dissection without any lens damage in all cases of RRD including phakic RRD. Therefore, the placement of a peripheral encircling element is considered unnecessary with improved techniques of vitrectomy. The routine use of 360° peripheral endolaser retinopexy also makes a peripheral encircling element redundant. There is a growing evidence of a decreasing success rate in patients with high indents and use of heavy silicone oil because of higher incidence of severe PVR. Theoretically, it may be advantageous to use a peripheral encircling element in patients with pre-existing PVR, traumatic retinal detachment, giant retinal tears, and inferior retinal detachments with inferior retinal breaks. However, we do not combine buckling with vitreoretinal surgery in any of these conditions. In the absence of clear guidelines, it remains the surgeons' discretion to decide to use or not to use an encircling element.

When an encircling element is used, it is usually placed before creating the ports. An exception to this rule is in cases of undue hypotony and perforation during the passage of the encirclage sutures. Common encircling elements are either a No. 240 or a No. 241 band, and if a higher indent is needed, a No. 276 buckle with or without a band. The encirclage is tied either after partial vitrectomy or later in an air-filled state.

Escoffery et al.[1] initially reported on the use of primary vitrectomy and gas tamponade in the treatment of RRD. The final reattachment rate in their series was 93% while visual acuities of 20/50 or more were achieved in 81% of the cases. However, this procedure may not be suitable in breaks located anteriorly. In spite of encouraging results obtained by Escoffery et al.,[1] the technique of primary vitrectomy did not receive much attention mainly due to nonavailability of adequate peripheral retinal viewing devices and simultaneous advent of the procedure of pneumatic retinopexy. In a prospective, randomized study, Stangos et al.[3] reported that pars plana vitrectomy (PPV) is as effective as PPV with an additional encircling buckle for pseudophakic patients with RRD. PPV has the benefit of fewer intraoperative and postoperative complications.

Sharma et al. reported that successful reattachment of primary RRD with inferior breaks can be achieved with PPV alone, and that a supplementary scleral band is unnecessary.[4-6] No statistically significant differences in either reattachment rates or visual outcomes between a 360° scleral band and a combined procedure of scleral band with PPV have been reported. On the contrary, a few authors have suggested that scleral band alone is an effective technique in the primary management of uncomplicated RRD with unseen retinal breaks especially when media are clear,[7] but what viewing systems were used is not discussed. We consider vitreoretinal surgery as the first preferred approach for the management of all retinal detachments if full components of modern vitreoretinal surgery are available and the surgeon has good vitreous surgery experience.

Vitreous Removal

Complete removal of vitreous remains one of the most crucial steps in vitreoretinal surgery for RRD. This is achieved in three stages:
1. Core vitrectomy
2. Peripheral vitrectomy
3. Inferior vitreous base excision.

Core vitrectomy is performed at high suction and low cutting rates. This ensures high flow rates and rapid removal of the core vitreous. Once the core vitreous is excised, adjuvants such as triamcinolone acetonide (TA) and trypan blue may be injected. Trypan blue stains the residual cortical vitreous, enables induction of posterior vitreous detachment (PVD), and improves visualization of peripheral vitreous fibrils. TA has additional advantages as it stains the epiretinal membrane enabling its easy removal. We prefer the use of TA alone. It also has significant anti-PVR activity.[6]

Following central vitreous debulking, PVD is induced (Fig. 22.1). This step ensures that the posterior vitreous scaffold is removed preventing PVR postoperatively. Stripping of the posterior hyaloid is helpful in the complete removal of vitreous. This may be achieved either by using the vitrectomy probe in the suction mode only or by using a silicone-tipped aspiration cannula. High suctions (>200–250 mm Hg) are used, and PVD induction is initiated from the peripapillary retina. Vitreous staining agents aid in this procedure (TA).

Subsequently, peripheral vitreous removal is performed. This step usually employs low suction (50–80 mm Hg) and high cut rates (>1,200 cpm). On approaching close to the retina, the cutting is increased and suction is decreased mainly to reduce traction on the retina. The peripheral vitreous is

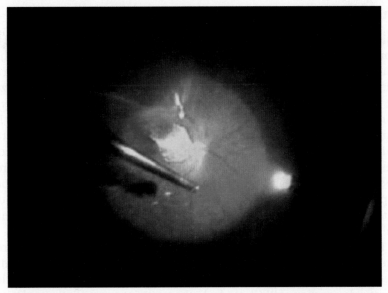

Fig. 22.1: Triamcinolone acetonide-assisted induction of posterior vitreous detachment using vitrectomy probe in the suction mode only.

trimmed all around. One must be especially careful in phakic eyes to prevent lens touch and subsequent cataract formation. Inferior vitreous base shaving may be carried out under indentation. This additional step ensures reduction in the rates of inferior PVR. The use of wide-angle viewing systems (WAVS) is vital.

Management of Proliferative Vitreoretinopathy

The removal of all elements of PVR is extremely essential in achieving retinal reattachment and preventing reproliferation. PVR is commonly associated with traumatic RRDs, recurrent RRDs, pediatric RRDs, and those with large retinal breaks. It commonly takes the form of sheets of contractile membranes either at the posterior pole or in the inferior periphery. This causes fixed retinal folds or large segments of contracted retina. The Silicone Oil Study classifies and quantifies the various types of PVRs.

Following the removal of the vitreous, end gripping or conforming forceps are used to grasp the edges of the membranes and peel them off the retinal surface. Subretinal membranes and bands are removed when possible through retinotomies. If large bands cannot be excised completely, they should be segmented or preferably delaminated, to relieve the traction. Relaxing retinotomies or retinectomies may have to be performed in areas with extremely taut retina or in areas with placoid traction. These maneuvers may be performed under heavy perfluorocarbon liquids (PFCLs) to ensure retinal flattening and achieve hemostasis. It is very important to avoid iatrogenic retinal breaks during these steps.

Retinal Reattachment

Retinal reattachment involves flattening of the retina with displacement of the subretinal fluid. This can be achieved by replacing the vitreous volume with air or heavy liquids. This step must be performed only after all the traction on the retina has been eliminated. If the primary break is inaccessible or not localized, the removal of the subretinal fluid may be achieved through a posterior retinotomy created using endodiathermy probe (Fig. 22.2). Because air has a higher interfacial tension than silicone, fluid–air exchange with internal drainage of subretinal fluid to reattach the retina should precede silicone infusion. A silicone-tipped aspiration cannula is used to aspirate the fluid from the subretinal space (Fig. 22.3). This is achieved either through the retinotomy or preferably through the preexisting break. Thus, a pneumohydraulic reattachment of retina is initiated and completed by simultaneously draining SRF and simultaneously injecting air by an automated air pump.

Pneumohydraulic maneuver is capable of identifying of residual areas of retinal traction. Displacement of the subretinal fluid may be achieved by injecting PFCLs into the intraocular space. In patients with residual traction, subretinal migration of PFCL can be bothersome intraoperative complication and calls for additional traction relief.

Retinopexy

Retinopexy has been used to create permanent adhesion between retina and retinal pigment epithelium. All forms of retinopexy create tissue destruction and have potential to cause reproliferation and should be used as little as

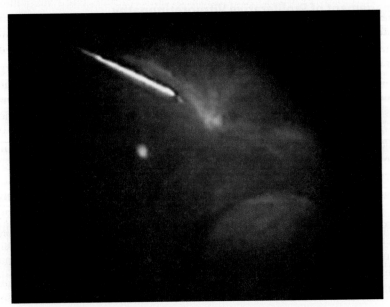

Fig. 22.2: Creation of retinotomy using endodiathermy probe.

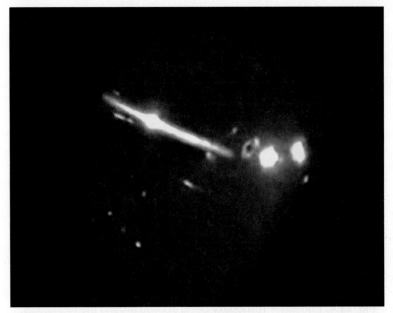

Fig. 22.3: Fluid air exchange through the retinotomy using a silicone-tipped aspiration cannula.

possible. Techniques of retinopexy include endolaser diode photocoagulation or external cryopexy. Retinopexy is classically applied to the edges of retinal breaks (preexisting and iatrogenic) (Figs. 22.4 and 22.5). However, 360° retinopexy with additional rows in the inferior retina is often advocated. This step is believed to reduce the effects of peripheral reproliferation on the posterior pole and prevent redetachment due to a peripheral missed break. The effect of this additional retinopexy on rates of reproliferation is, however, unknown.

Continuous laser endophotocoagulation is preferred to intermittent circular retinopexy because of more uniform tissue destruction and resultant tensile strength. Cryotherapy using external cryoprobe may be performed if larger areas of retinopexy are desired, e.g. giant retinal tears. Cryotherapy overall has become obsolete because of attendant high risk of PVR.

Tamponade

Silicone oil or long-acting gases may be used to tamponade the retina until retinopexy has achieved a permanent effect. Silicone oil should be injected through pressure-controlled power injector, through a short 19-gauge straight cannula or through infusion cannula with very short tubing. The air can be removed by proportional aspiration until the silicone reaches the pupillary plane. An inferior peripheral iridectomy should be created in aphakic patients before fluid–air exchange is performed. This allows aqueous humor to enter the anterior chamber from below and, hopefully, prevents silicone contact

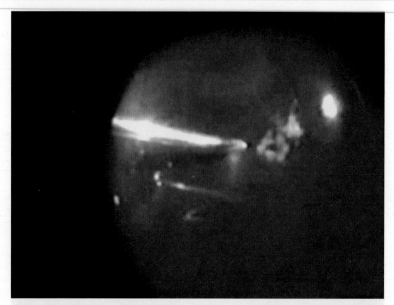

Fig. 22.4: Endolaser retinopexy being applied around the retinotomy.

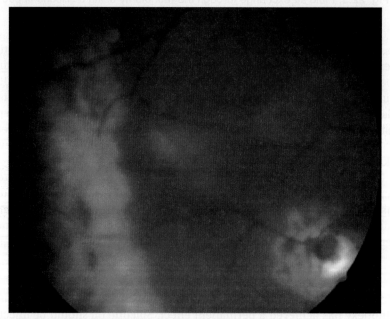

Fig. 22.5: Postoperative view showing prophylactic peripheral retinopexy and laser reaction around the retinotomy.

with cornea. Nonexpansile concentrations of long-acting gases such as perfluoropropane (14–16%) and sulfur hexafluoride (18–20%) are used for tamponade. The duration of tamponade depends upon the gas used (3–6 weeks). The use of silicone oil as a tamponade medium requires a second procedure for its removal, usually after 6 weeks. Longer periods of tamponade may be needed in patients who are one-eyed and have colobomatous retinal detachments or recurrent RRDs. The use of long-lasting gases obviates the need for a second surgical procedure.

Surgical viewing systems ranging from the conventional lenses to the more advanced WAVS are used in the above-mentioned procedures. Viewing through conventional lenses has several disadvantages—chiefly a limited field of view and difficulty in visualizing the fundus in an air-filled eye. Currently available WAVS offer panoramic view of the retina enabling thorough vitreous removal with the availability to perform complex surgical maneuvers. These include the handheld wide-angle viewing lenses (Volk, Ocular), binocular indirect ophthalmo-microscope (BIOM), EIBOS system, and the Peyman–Wessels–Landers (PWL) surgical system. BIOM, EIBOS, and PWL surgical systems are self-retaining and noncontact, and the latter two have integrated reversing optics.[7-11]

The advent of 23- and 25-gauge instrumentations allows for minimally invasive vitreoretinal surgery utilizing smaller sutureless incisions, compared with conventional PPV. Surgically-induced trauma is minimized decreasing the convalescence period, operating time, and postoperative inflammatory response. Lakhanpal et al.[12] reported on a series of 140 nonvitrectomized eyes of 140 patients who underwent 25-gauge transconjunctival posterior segment surgical procedures. Out of 140, 10 patients had RRD. In this retrospective study, the authors reported no intraoperative surgical complications or need to convert to standard 20-gauge system. Shorter surgical time with lesser postoperative inflammation was also observed. However, this study raised several concerns including transient postoperative hypotony, comparable procedural time, cost disadvantages, lesser intraocular illumination, and a longer learning curve. These sutureless surgical techniques are evolving and need to be explored further.

CONCLUSION

Thus, vitreoretinal surgery for the management of RRD represents an exciting aspect of ophthalmic surgical techniques. Despite the increasing complexity of the techniques involved, the basic idea remains simple. The vitreoretinal surgery does indeed make the management of RRD simpler and more successful. The basic steps and the rationale applicable remain the same in all-gauges (20, 23, and 25) vitreoretinal surgeries for RRD, with minor modifications.

REFERENCES

1. Escoffery RF, Olk RJ, Grand MG, et al. Vitrectomy without scleral buckling for primary rhegmatogenous retinal detachment. Am J Ophthalmol. 1985;99(3):275-81.
2. McLeod D. Is it time to call time on scleral buckle? Br J Ophthalmol. 2004;88(11):1357-9.

3. Stangos AN, Petropoulos IK, Brozou CG, et al. Pars-plana vitrectomy alone vs vitrectomy with scleral buckling for primary rhegmatogenous pseudophakic retinal detachment. Am J Ophthalmol. 2004;138(6):952-8.
4. Sharma A, Grigoropoulos V, Williamson TH. Management of primary rhegmatogenous retinal detachment with inferior breaks. Br J Ophthalmol. 2004;88(11):1372-5.
5. Sharma YR, Karunanidhi S, Azad RV, et al. Functional and anatomic outcome of scleral buckling versus primary vitrectomy in pseudophakic retinal detachment. Acta Ophthalmol Scand. 2005;83(3):293-7.
6. Azad RV, Chanana B, SharmaYR, et al. Primary vitrectomy versus conventional retinal detachment surgery in phakic rhegmatogenous retinal detachment. Acta Ophthalmol Scand. 2007;85(5):540-5.
7. Tewari HK, Kedar S, Kumar A, et al. Comparison of scleral buckling with combined scleral buckling and pars plana vitrectomy in the management of rhegmatogenous retinal detachment with unseen retinal breaks. Clin Exp. Ophthalmol. 2003;31(5):403-7.
8. Sunalp M, Wiedemann P, Sorgente N et al. Effects of cytotoxic drugs on PVR in the rabbit cell injection model. Curr Eye Res. 1984;3(4):619-23.
9. Spitznas M. A binocular indirect ophthalmomicroscope (BIOM) for non-contact wide-angle vitreous surgery. Graefes Arch Clin Exp Ophthalmol. 1987;225(1):13-5.
10. Landers B, Peyman GA, Wessels IF, et al. A new, non-contact wide field viewing system for vitreous surgery. Am J Ophthalmol. 2003;136(1):199-201.
11. Sharma YR, Natrajan S, Pal N, et al. Wide-angle vitreous surgery--an indispensable component of modern vitreoretinal surgery. Instruction course: American Academy of Ophthalmology annual meeting, Las Vegas; 2006.
12. Lakhanpal RR, Humayun MS, de Juan E, et al. Outcomes of 140 consecutive cases of 25-gauge transconjunctival surgery for posterior segment disease. Ophthalmology. 2005;112(5):817-24.

CHAPTER 23

Microincisional Vitrectomy Surgery

Lingam Gopal, Mohammed Naseer, Tengku Ain Kamalden

INTRODUCTION

Vitreoretinal surgery has come a long way since the introduction of pars plana approach by Robert Machemer.[1] In the past five decades, it has developed into a major subspecialty with well-structured fellowship programs. The indications for vitreoretinal surgery have expanded to include many hitherto untreatable conditions. Rapid strides in the technology have resulted in new instrumentation to assist the surgeon.[2] The most important development has been in the reduction of the dimensions of the instruments. In this chapter, we will cover the subject of microincisional vitrectomy surgery (MIVS) as it stands today.

RELEVANT ANATOMY

The vitreous base and the vitreoretinal relationship are perhaps the most important anatomical issues that dictate several aspects of vitreoretinal disease and surgery. Hence, a brief review of the same is not out of place. The vitreous base straddles the ora serrata and is the area of strongest vitreoretinal attachment. The vitreous is adherent firmly to the optic disk, the retina near the macula, to edges of lattice degeneration, and to sites of vitreoretinal abnormalities such as retinal tufts, etc. The vitreous detaches from the retina with age but this can occur earlier in high myopia, trauma, and inflammation of the posterior segment. While the expected event is a clean separation of the vitreous gel—initiating from posterior pole and subsequently proceeding anteriorly up to the posterior vitreous base, this happy occurrence can be marred by several factors. At the sites of abnormal vitreoretinal adhesions, the vitreous can tear the retina instead of cleanly separating from it. The vitreous can also split into layers (schisis) with part of vitreous remaining adherent to the retina while the rest separates out. Fibrosis is sequelae of many vitreoretinal diseases. At the minimum, it can result in epiretinal membranes producing distortion of the macula. More extensive fibrosis is seen in proliferative vascular retinopathies such as advanced diabetic retinopathy, and proliferative vitreoretinopathy that complicates retinal detachment.

HISTORY OF EVOLUTION OF VITREOUS INSTRUMENTATION

Kasner[3] first broke the concept of inviolability of vitreous in 1962 and intentionally removed the vitreous through open sky approach. It was Robert Machemer who developed the first instrumentation that could be used through small openings in the pars plana.[1] The prototype vitreous-infusion-suction-cutter had multiple functions including infusion, suction, cutter, and optionally a light pipe that could be added on top of it. By today's standards, it is an unwieldy and bulky instrument. Very quickly, it was realized that the size of the opening in the eye matters, in terms of ease of surgery as well as creation of complications. Connor O' Malley introduced the split function system, the "Ocutome".[4,5] This involved 20-gauge instrumentation using three ports—one for infusion, one for active instruments like cutter, scissors, forceps, etc., and one for light pipe. This has remained the standard of care in vitreoretinal surgery for over two decades. Machemer used the trocar–cannula system with the 20-gauge instruments.

With the advent of sutureless phacoemulsification for cataract surgery, the concept of sutureless vitreous surgery caught the imagination of the vitreoretinal surgeons. Chen[6] described the first sutureless 20-gauge vitrectomy in 1996. Self-sealing scleral tunnels were fashioned but did have significant complications including wound leaks, vitreous incarceration, and retinal tears.

It was Eugene de Juan who first developed a 25-gauge system,[7] while Claus Eckardt developed the 23-gauge system.[8] Several improvements in technology and techniques have made it possible to adopt the small gauge systems into routine practice, so much so that currently majority of vitreoretinal surgeries are conducted with the small gauge systems.

INSTRUMENTATION AND FLUIDICS IN MICROINCISIONAL VITRECTOMY SURGERY

Size of the Cutter

The outer diameter is 0.9 mm in a 20-gauge versus 0.6 mm in a 23-gauge, 0.5 mm in 25-gauge, and 0.4 mm in 27-gauge. Reduction in size of the cutter has a number of implications.[9,10]

Flow Rate

According to Poiseuille's law, the volume flow rate along a pipe is directly proportional to the fourth power of its radius. Hence, as the gauge of the vitrectomy cutter is reduced, the flow is also reduced unless it is compensated by an increase in suction and infusion pressure. At 600-mm Hg vacuum level, the flow rate in 23-gauge cutter is similar to that of 20-gauge, provided the infusion pressure is able to deliver the required amount of fluid. The balance between infusion pressure and suction is important to maintain safe intraocular pressure at all times. Too low an infusion pressure can result in collapse of the globe when high suction is applied since enough fluid is not being driven into the eye. On the other hand, high infusion pressure can have deleterious effect on retinal and optic disk function especially during the time when no active suction is being performed. Reduced flow rate due to smaller aperture of infusion cannulas is to some extent compensated by the reduced outflow from the cutters.

Duty Cycle

This is the percentage of the time the port is open in the entire cycle. In electrical cutters, the duty cycle remains fixed at 50% of the time while with pneumatic cutters, it varies with the cut rate.

T/C Delta

This refers to the difference between the outer diameter of the trocar and the inner diameter of the cannula. A large T/C delta means the aperture caused by the trocar in the tissue has to enlarge significantly to accommodate the cannula and there is a risk of tissue getting caught between the trocar and the cannula. While with too small a T/C delta, the introduction of the cannula is smooth but the removal of the trocar could be especially difficult.

Illumination

Since the diameter of the fiber optic carrying the light from the light source is thinner, proper coupling should be present to ensure efficient transmission of light. Systems designed for 20-gauge would not suffice for 23- or 25-gauge because of the coupling issues.

Instrument Rigidity

The main reason it took time for the small gauge instruments to gain wide acceptance is because of the rigidity issues. The initial instruments were rather flimsy and tended to bend when the eye was turned with the help of the instruments. Improved materials and improved design have increased the stiffness. The use of wide-angle system also reduced the need to turn the eye to reach the periphery, thus making it easy to use the small gauge instruments without bending them.

Disposable versus Reusable Instruments

In MIVS, damage to the instruments is a very high possibility in view of their slender diameter. Hence, disposable instruments are more preferred. Most of the important instruments such as forceps, scissors, diathermy tips, and aspiration silicone-tipped needles are available in small gauge. However, ultrasonic fragmentor is not available in 23-/25-gauge. Therefore, the use of this instrument entails enlargement of one sclerotomy to 20-gauge dimension.

Visualization

Wide-angle viewing systems have almost replaced the Lander's contact lens systems as the primary modality of visualization.[11] However, most surgeons prefer the contact lens for macular surgery. The value of wide-angle visualization in reducing the need for turning the eyeball has already been mentioned.

Cut Rate

Although not specific to small gauge instruments, technology to have high cut rates has developed almost along with the small gauge instrumentation. In general, high cut rates are safer than low cut rates. With low cut rates, the duration of time for which the port remains open is longer, and hence the traction on the vitreous and retina is increased.[10] High cut rates (2,500, 5,000, or 7,500 cuts/min) have enabled surgeons to get closer to the retina with reduced risk of iatrogenic retinal breaks. Some machines come with "shaving mode," which is a combination of low suction and high cutting rate, thereby literally enabling shaving of the peripheral vitreous very close to the retinal surface.

Port Location

The newer cutters also come with the port located closer to the tip of the shaft than in the 20-gauge cutters. This permits the surgeon to cut the membranes very close to the retinal surface and thus effectively reduces the dependence on the scissors during vitrectomy for proliferative vascular retinopathy.

Cannula with Valves

Valved cannulas are available that do not permit leakage of fluid when the instruments are removed from the eye.[12] This facilitates better maintenance of intraocular pressure and avoidance of hypotony-related complications. However, valved cannulas could pose a problem while injecting silicone oil. The egress of air in the eye may not take place due to the fact that the valve and intraocular pressure can shoot up. Appropriate measures are needed to vent the air out. This becomes an issue when oil is injected through the infusion sleeve.

Chandelier Light

To permit four-port vitrectomy for bimanual surgery, 25-gauge light pipes are available that can be placed through a separate opening superiorly or inferiorly. These work best with xenon light source and provide enough illumination for bimanual surgery.

Sclerotomies

A routine 20-gauge sclerotomy is meant to be sutured and is made perpendicular to the sclera. The orientation of the MVR blade can be limbus parallel or limbus perpendicular. Twenty-gauge sclerotomies use the MVR blade directly, and the active instruments as well as the infusion cannula are placed in the scleral opening without any cannula. In contrast, both 23- and 25-gauge sclerotomies are made with a trocar–cannula system wherein a cannula is left in place through which the instruments for vitreoretinal procedures including the infusion cannula are placed.

A 23-gauge sclerotomy is transconjunctival and meant to be sutureless (Fig. 23.1). Hence, various techniques are adopted to prevent the collapse of globe and to ensure the watertight closure of scleral openings once the instrument is removed.

PROCEDURES

Two-Step Procedure

As a first step, the blade is introduced 30°–35° to the sclera, and once the cannula edge is reached, the trocar is rotated to a more perpendicular position and the cannula is pushed into place.

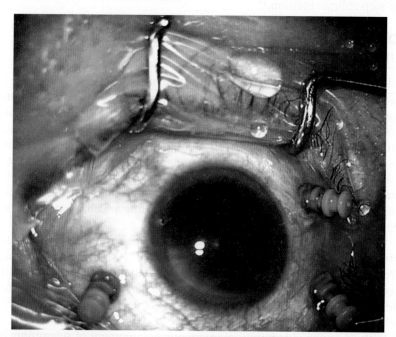

Fig. 23.1: External intraoperative photograph showing the three sclerotomies made for 23-gauge vitrectomy. Note the protrusion of the cannulas and the potential to bump against the lid margin. In eyes with narrow palpebral fissure, this could be a problem and one has to make all sclerotomies clustered close to the horizontal meridian.

Steve Charles Technique

Here the initial entry is tangential to the sclera, and once the sclera is cleared by the trocar, the angle is changed to 30° or more.[13] The incision is not biplanar since the sclera is incised in one sweep and the change in direction is to avoid accidental injury to the retina.

Radially Oriented versus Circumferentially Oriented Blade Entry

While piercing the sclera with a blade, some fibers are cut and some are separated. Considering the orientation of scleral fibers, a limbus parallel incision is likely to cut across less of scleral fibers compared to one radially oriented and has a better chance of closure without leakage. The flip side is that a limbus parallel incision in an oblique fashion will result in inner and scleral openings to be not at the same distance from the limbus. Depending upon which direction the trocar is pointing (toward limbus or away from limbus), the internal opening will be closer to the lens or to the ora serrata compared to the scleral opening. Twenty-five-gauge sclerotomies were initially placed perpendicular to the sclera but resulted in significant leakage and hypotonia. Currently, 25-gauge sclerotomies are also made at an angle to the sclera. Hypotony risk after 25-gauge vitrectomy has been shown to reduce after a two-step oblique incision.[14]

ADVANTAGES OF MICROINCISIONAL VITRECTOMY SURGERY

Reducing the aperture size in wall of the eye has obvious advantages for the overall safety of the eye. The small aperture, the presence of the trocar–cannula system, and the use of the wide-angle system have definitely reduced the risk of retinal breaks related to sclerotomy site. This is because of the more thorough vitrectomy that is made possible with wide-angle visualization as well as due to less traction on vitreous base when instruments are introduced and withdrawn in the cannula system. The eyes without sutures look quiet even on the first postoperative day and the patients are very comfortable. The relative lack of conjunctival scarring is a boon for eyes needing antiglaucoma surgery or those that already have a filtering bleb.

Eyes with fresh retinal detachment that are candidates for primary vitrectomy are most elegantly managed using the sutureless small gauge vitrectomy systems. Even in eyes where a buckle or band is placed in addition to pars plana vitrectomy, one can resort to small gauge vitrectomy, although these sclerotomies would need closure with sutures due to disturbed conjunctiva and tenons capsule.

With 20-gauge vitrectomy, spontaneous enlargement of sclerotomy is a potential risk in eyes with thin sclera. This results in leakage of fluid around the instrument shafts resulting in hypotony as well as potential incarceration of peripheral retina and vitreous in the sclerotomy. This risk is very much reduced with the trocar–cannula system of the smaller gauge instrumentations of MIVS.

LIMITATIONS OF MICROINCISIONAL VITRECTOMY SURGERY

Eyes with cataract surgery misadventure requiring retrieval of cortex, epinucleus, or nuclear fragments (Fig. 23.2) can be managed with small gauge vitrectomy at the same sitting. However, as has been indicated earlier, a hard dislocated nucleus would need a 20-gauge fragmatome. This can be managed by enlarging one sclerotomy to accommodate the instrument but one must be conscious of the fact that there is a mismatch between the inflow of fluid and the outflow of fluid. This can result in sudden collapse of the eye unless the suction is suitably controlled. If one tries to avoid the use of 20-gauge fragmatome, and uses small gauge cutters for the removal of epinucleus or relatively soft nucleus, it could sometimes be time consuming.

In eyes with severe diabetic retinopathy and extensive traction or combined retinal detachment, a 20-gauge scissors may sometimes be needed to make rapid dissection of thick fibrovascular tissue (Fig. 23.3). With improved efficiency of the 23-gauge scissors, the number of cases needing 20-gauge vitrectomy (even with severe diabetic retinopathy) has declined. The cutters with the port close to the tip have enabled the shaving of the tissue from the retinal surface in most cases, thus avoiding the use of scissors.

Silicone oil injection could become slightly problematic with smaller gauge instruments. However, with the use of machine injectors, even 5,000 centistokes oil can be injected through the fine ports. It is, however, a good practice to close these sclerotomies. Slow seepage of oil into subconjunctival space can result

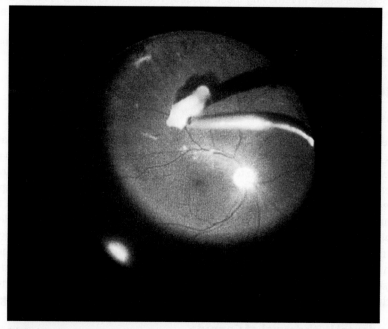

Fig. 23.2: Intraoperative fundus photograph showing dropped nucleus fragment. A hard nucleus would need enlargement of one sclerotomy to accommodate 20-gauge fragmatome.

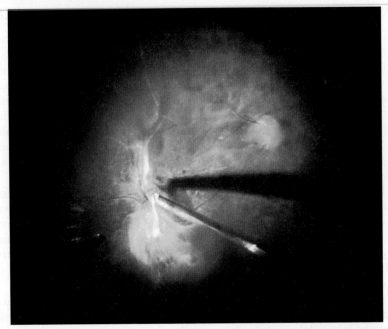

Fig. 23.3: Intraoperative fundus photograph showing the removal of preretinal fibrovascular tissue with the cutter. Small gauge cutters have reduced the need for scissors usage in removing these tissues. The closer to the tip location of the ports enables the removal of the fibrovascular tissue comfortably with the cutter.

in suboptimal fill in the early postoperative period and conjunctival cysts in the late postoperative period.

PROBLEMS WITH SMALL GAUGE VITRECTOMY

Unsutured Infusion Cannula

Twenty-gauge infusion cannulas are sutured with absorbable or nonabsorbable silk sutures that go across the flanges so that they are firmly anchored to the sclera. The trocar–cannula system does not permit suturing, and hence there is a real risk of the cannula slipping out of the eye during surgery. This can happen due to the assistant's hand accidentally yanking the tubing out or when the cannula keeps bumping into eyelid speculum, especially in eyes with a deep orbital socket. The consequences of slippage of infusion cannula would depend on the infusate. With fluid flowing into the eye, serous choroidal detachment can occur. If air is flowing in, the sudden transfer of the flow from intravitreal to subretinal or suprachoroidal space can have disastrous consequences including subretinal air, suprachoroidal air, or suprachoroidal hemorrhage.

Accidental Withdrawal of Cannula

Sometimes the instruments get stuck in the cannulas and can pull the cannula out with them. This is not a serious issue. The cannula can be reintroduced by threading it first on the trocar. Sometimes, however, the conjunctiva balloons out due to fluid seepage from the patent sclerotomy. This may make identification of the sclerotomy difficult for the reintroduction of the trocar. A conjunctival incision may be needed to locate the same, in which case the sclerotomy would ultimately need suturing.

Problems with Protruding Cannulas

All cannulas protrude from the surface of the eye—some to a greater extent than others (Bausch and Lomb). The three sclerotomies are usually grouped around the horizontal meridian to give maximum ease of mobility for the eyeball. Protruding cannulas can, however, pose problems in placing the sclerotomies in nonstandard locations (e.g. closer to the vertical meridian). The need to place sclerotomies in nonstandard locations arises in eyes with severe trauma, extensive scleral wounds, the presence of glaucoma drainage valves, or filtering blebs.

Suturing of Sclerotomy

In most of the cases, the removal of cannula would collapse the sclerotomy site resulting in its closure. However, there are several situations where the sclerotomy continues to leak that ultimately leads to hypotonia. Potential reasons for persistent leakage of sclerotomy are as follows:

- Thin sclera as in high myopia.
- Sclerotomy that has been manipulated vigorously, for example, when vitreous base excision is performed. The rotation of instruments within the sclerotomy in all directions will tend to make the sclerotomy less amenable to collapse and self-sealing.
- Aggressive vitreous base excision, as is indicated in eyes with retinal detachment and proliferative vitreoretinopathy, would not leave enough residual gel vitreous in the periphery to plug the internal lip of the sclerotomy.
- Opening the conjunctiva, as in cases of combined vitrectomy and scleral buckling, where encircling band or buckle is placed along with vitrectomy. In eyes when the conjunctiva is undisturbed, the adhesion of Tenon's capsule around the sclerotomy permits faster collapse of the sclerotomy.
- Surgeons have used partial air fill to try and reduce the chances of leaky sclerotomy. The surface tension of air can close the internal lip of sclerotomy better than the fluid.

Intraoperatively, the conjunctiva balloons up some time obscuring the site of sclerotomy. Where the surgeon has not displaced the conjunctiva much while making the sclerotomy, the fluid or air can be seen to leak out through the conjunctival opening. If attempts at collapsing the scleral opening with pressure have not succeeded, one should not hesitate to close the sclerotomy with suture. In most cases where the conjunctiva has not ballooned out, the sclerotomy can be closed with a single suture placed transconjunctivally. If conjunctival ballooning obscures the sclerotomy site, one would need to incise the conjunctiva, expose the sclerotomy, and close it. The sclerotomy for the infusion cannula is less likely to leak, since this site is least manipulated and there is no active infusion of fluid or air when this cannula is removed. In general, it is better to err on the side of placing a suture rather than to leave an eye sutureless and soft.

Postoperative Hypotonia

It is not unusual to see relatively soft eyes on the first postoperative day but most often the pressure builds up by second day. Gupta et al.[15] have reported that the incidence of postoperative hypotony is higher with fluid-filled eyes in comparison to air- or gas-filled eyes after 25-gauge vitrectomy. In eyes filled with silicone oil, most surgeons would prefer to close the sclerotomies with a suture to prevent subconjunctival migration of silicone oil leading to large cysts postoperatively.

Clear Corneal Cataract Surgery and 23- or 25-Gauge Vitrectomy

Wong et al.[16] highlighted the risk of corneal wound leak during the manipulations that are needed in the placement of the cannula in eyes that have recently underwent clear corneal cataract surgery. These eyes need suturing of the wound (Fig. 23.4) before any force is applied on the eye.

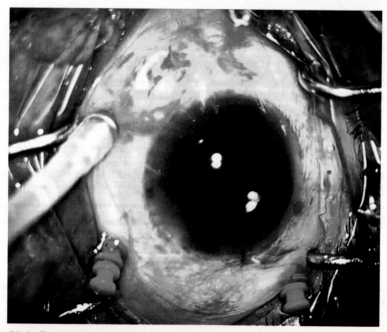

Fig. 23.4: External intraoperative photograph showing the 23-gauge cannulas in place. Note a single suture placed across the clear corneal wound. This suture (placed before sclerotomies are made) secures the wound and the force used to make the sclerotomies not result in prolapse of intraocular contents.

Corneal wound leak can potentially lead to iris prolapse, vitreous prolapse, and choroidal hemorrhage.

REFERENCES

1. Machemer R, Buettner H, Norton EW, et al. Vitrectomy: a pars plana approach. Trans Am Acad Ophthalmol Otolaryngol. 1971;75:813-20.
2. Charles S. An engineering approach to vitreoretinal surgery. Retina. 2004;24(3):435-4.
3. Kasner D. A new approach to the management of the vitreous. Highlights Ophthalmol. 1968;11:304-9.
4. Boyd B. Modern ophthalmology: highlights: the account of a master witnessing 60 yr epoch of Evolution and progress. Miami: Jaypee- Highlights Medical publishers INC; 2011. pp. 131.
5. O'Malley C, Heintz RM. Vitrectomy with an alternative instrument system. Ann Ophthalmol. 1975;7(4):585-8, 591-4.
6. Chen JC. Sutureless pars plana vitrectomy through self-sealing sclerotomies. Arch Ophthalmol. 1996;114:1273-5.
7. de Juan E Jr, Hickingbotham D. Refinements in microinstrumentation for vitreous surgery. Am J Ophthalmol. 1990;109(2):218-20.
8. Eckardt C. Transconjunctival sutureless 23-gauge vitrectomy. Retina. 2005;25(2):208-11.
9. Magalhaes O Jr, Chong L, DeBoer C, et al. Vitreous dynamics: vitreous flow analysis in 20-, 23-, and 25-gauge cutters. Retina. 2008;28(2):236-41.
10. Hubschman JP, Bourges JL, Tsui I, et al. Effect of cutting phases on flow rate in 20-, 23-, and 25-gauge vitreous cutters. Retina. 2008;29(9):1290-3.
11. Chalam KV, Shah VA. Optics of wide-angle panoramic viewing system-assisted vitreous surgery. Surv Ophthalmol. 2004;49(4):437-45.
12. Esmaili DD. Valved cannula systems. Wayne: Bryn Mawr Communications LLC; 2012. pp. 41
13. Krieglstein GK, Weinreb RN. Vitreo-retinal surgery: progress III In: Rizzo S, Patelli F, Chow DR (Eds). Essentials in Ophthalmology. Berlin: Springer; 2009. pp. 31.
14. Inoue M, Shinoda K, Shinoda H, et al. Two-step oblique incision during 25-gauge vitrectomy reduces incidence of postoperative hypotony. Clin Experiment Ophthalmol. 2007;35(8):693-6.
15. Gupta OP, Weichel ED, Regillo CD, et al. Postoperative complications associated with 25-gauge pars plana vitrectomy. Ophthalmic Surg Lasers Imaging. 2007;38(4):270-5.
16. Wong RW, Kokame GT, Mahmoud TH, et al. Complications associated with clear corneal cataract wounds during vitrectomy. Retina. 2010;30(6):850-5.

CHAPTER 24

Retinal Cyst: Management

Yog Raj Sharma, Soman Nair

INTRODUCTION

Retinal cyst is not a rare entity. It may occur in isolation or in association with diverse retinal pathologies. It may be developmental in origin or acquired. Developmental or congenital retinal cysts are uncommon. Among acquired, parasitic cysts of retina, especially cysticercosis, are relatively common in countries of South-East Asia and South America. Retinal cysts are of great clinical importance because they can lead to serious visual impairment or even to irretrievable blindness. In this chapter, a brief description of etiology, diagnosis, and management of various types of retinal cysts is presented.

CLASSIFICATION OF RETINAL CYSTS

Retinal cysts can be classified into two broad groups: congenital and acquired. Congenital cysts of retina may be primary or secondary in origin. The acquired retinal cysts are usually of the following types:

1. Parasitic cysts
   - Retinal cysticercosis
   - Retinal echinococcosis.
2. Retinal cyst associated with chronic retinal detachment
3. Retinal cyst associated with retinoschisis
4. Peripheral retinal cysts
5. Traumatic retinal cysts
6. Neoplastic retinal cysts.

CONGENITAL RETINAL CYSTS

Primary Congenital

Primary retinal cysts are bilateral, symmetrical, and most often located in the periphery of retina. The primary peripheral cysts may lead to retinal dialysis and retinoschisis. Congenital retinoschisis may be hereditary and present with bilateral peripheral giant cysts. Cibis[1] had extensively studied a number of cases of retinoschisis both clinically and histopathologically and reported a combination of multilocular retinal giant cysts, unilateral open-angle glaucoma, and unilateral retinal detachment. The giant cysts were found in the lower temporal quadrant of the eyes. Most of the patients were juveniles and presented mirror symmetry of the lesions suggesting a genetic developmental anomaly. Multiple bilateral cysts of the retina of unknown etiology were also reported by Paul.[2]

Secondary Congenital

Secondary congenital cysts of the retina may be associated with other congenital ocular anomalies such as microphthalmos and retinal dysplasia. Microphthalmos with cyst is a unilateral condition. The anomaly may be found associated with partial 18 monosomy syndrome. Occasionally, it is massive and may obscure the eye. The cyst may be lined by gliotic retina or filled with proliferated glial tissue.[3]

ACQUIRED RETINAL CYSTS

Parasitic Cysts

Retinal Cysticercosis

Cysticercosis, the most common ocular platyhelminth infestation in human, is caused by the larvae of the tapeworm *Taenia solium*.[4] Humans are the definitive hosts and pigs the intermediate hosts for *T. solium*. In ocular cysticercosis, humans become the intermediate host by ingesting eggs of *parasite* from contaminated food or water. After penetrating the intestinal wall, the embryo invades the bloodstream and can lodge in various organs, such as brain, skeletal muscles, eye, and subcutaneous tissue.[5] Ocular involvement in cysticercosis is seen in 13–46% of infected patients. The embryo possibly enters the eye via the choroidal circulation. From the choroid, it migrates into the subretinal space and then shifts into the vitreous cavity through a break in the retina (Figs. 24.1A and B). The parasite incites an inflammatory reaction in the retina which seals the retinal break and leaves behind a small chorioretinal scar. Occasionally, the cyst may enter the vitreous cavity from the retinal arteries, optic nerve head, or ciliary body.

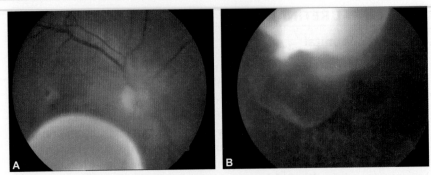

Figs. 24.1A and B: Intraocular retinal cysticercosis.

The diagnosis of cysticercosis can be made on history, clinical features, imaging, and histopathological examination. Clinical features of the disease include decrease in vision, floaters, occasionally pain, and injection. When the cyst is in the vitreous, it can be visualized by ophthalmoscope. It presents characteristic undulating expansion and contraction, which has earned the name of "living mobile pearl." Subretinal cysticercosis manifests as a white opalescent cystic lesion with the scolex attached to the cyst wall within. The presence of scolex confirms the diagnosis. It may be associated with retinal detachment (63%).[6] The ocular inflammatory response to degenerating cysts manifests as vitritis and occasionally spills over into the anterior segment. Traction retinal detachment may also ensue. Intraocular cysticercosis may simulate retinoblastoma in a child.[7]

The imaging procedures such as ultrasound A- and B-scans may be employed to confirm the diagnosis. On B-scan, a circular curvilinear echo corresponding to the cyst wall is seen, with the scolex appearing as a round, high-density echo connected to this curvilinear structure. A-scan demonstrates two high-amplitude echoes corresponding to the cyst walls and a 100% high reflective echo when the beam passes through the scolex. Spontaneous movements of the live cyst can also be observed on B-scan. Contrast-enhanced computed tomography scan (CECT) is usually performed to diagnose concurrent neurocysticercosis which may be seen in up to 25% of cases. CECT demonstrates hyperdense cortical lesions with ring enhancement on contrast. In the absence of demonstrable scolex, ELISA for anticysticercal antibodies may be employed.[8]

Since anticysticercal agents can result in profound inflammatory responses around the cyst, their use is contraindicated in the treatment of subretinal cysticercosis. Surgical removal of the cyst is the treatment of choice for subretinal cysticercosis. The intraocular cysticerci may be removed either through pars plana vitrectomy or through a transscleral approach.[1] A standard three-port plana vitrectomy is performed. Posterior vitreous detachment is carried out. A retinotomy is made close to the cyst avoiding the major retinal vessels and the cyst is then brought into the vitreous cavity using a silicone tip either passively or via active suction. The cyst is then aspirated using a flute needle or the vitreous cutter. The cyst may also be delivered in toto after enlarging the sclerotomy. The retinotomy site is subsequently is sealed with laser and associated retinal detachment and proliferative changes are managed appropriately.

An external approach may be employed in cysts located anterior to the equator. In this technique, the cyst is localized with indirect ophthalmoscopy, and the exact site is marked with diathermy. A radial sclerotomy of adequate size is made at this site with preplaced 6-O polyglactin sutures. The choroid is exposed after the scleral fibers are separated and obvious blood vessels are cauterized. Just before the choroid was incised, indirect ophthalmoscopy is repeated to confirm that the parasite had not moved. The cyst is removed through the choroidal incision with gentle pressure on the globe. This area may subsequently be supported with a silicone tire. Caution is called that pars plana approach is the preferred choice now. The external approach described is not, in general, current use.

In a surgical series on intraocular cysticercosis, Sharma and Sinha[4] reported an overall anatomic success rate of 86.6% and the functional success rate of 67.5% with final BCVA greater than 20/20 at a mean follow-up of 10 months employing both techniques. Complications encountered during surgery included iatrogenic retinal breaks (27%), intravitreal rupture of cyst during removal (13%), epiretinal membrane formation, and postoperatively formation of cataract. It has been reported that the cyst during the removal with the vitreous cutter may release toxic contents, inducing postoperative inflammation.[9] However, other studies do not show any such inflammatory reaction in the surgical results.[4] Perhaps, an adequate vitrectomy with the infusion of balanced salt solution can wash out all the toxic products.

The prognostic significance of several preoperative variables has been studied.[4,10] A better anatomic outcome has been found in the age group of above 30 years, in eyes without preoperative retinal detachment, with retinal detachment less than two quadrants, and with a preoperative visual acuity of more than 5/200. The functional outcome was better in eyes with retinal detachment less than two quadrants and a preoperative vision of more than 5/200. The presence of anterior segment inflammation significantly affected the anatomic outcome, but not the functional success.

Retinal Echinococcosis

Ocular echinococcosis is caused by the larval forms of canine tapeworm and includes cystic hydatid disease caused by *Echinococcus granulosus* and alveolar hydatid disease caused by *E. multilocularis*. The ova which infest the canine intestines are discharged in the feces and ingested by intermediary hosts such as humans, sheep, or other animals. After ingestion, the early larval form called oncosphere emerges, penetrates the digestive tract, and is carried away by bloodstream to various organs of the host's body. After reaching the organs, this larval form undergoes further development and enlarges concentrically to form a hydatid cyst. The resultant cyst may be unilocular or multilocular depending upon the organism causing the disease.[11]

Classically, ocular hydatid disease affects the orbit causing proptosis, bony erosion, and impairment of extraocular mobility.[12] Intraocular hydatid disease rarely presents either as a retrolental intravitreal mass or a subretinal mass.[11] In this location, the cyst may rapidly assume large proportions replacing the entire ocular volume. Glaucoma is frequently associated with ocular hydatid disease and the patient may have a painful blind eye.[13]

Diagnosis is usually based on the clinical presentation and serology using the indirect hemagglutination (IHA) test. The IHA test may be positive in less than 50% of the cases. The diagnosis is confirmed by histopathologic examination which shows the bilaminar nature of the cyst wall (the ectocyst and the endocyst) and the characteristic scolex with hooklets. Thorough investigations should be performed to detect systemic involvement of other organs including liver, lung, extremities, spleen, and bones.

Surgical extirpation of the cystic mass is the treatment of choice in intraocular echinococcosis. Conventional pars plana vitrectomy should be performed and cyst contents should be aspirated by a flute needle after retinotomy and cystotomy. In cases of painful blind eye with massive enlargement of globe, enucleation may have to be performed.

Chronic Retinal Detachment with Retinal Macrocyst

Secondary retinal macrocysts may develop in long-standing retinal detachment usually of more than 1 year duration. They are often associated with chronic retinal detachment secondary to traumatic dialysis. These cysts usually arise from the outer plexiform layer (Fig. 24.2).[14]

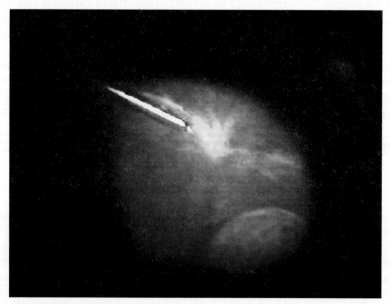

Fig. 24.2: Intraoperative view of chronic retinal detachment with retinal macrocyst.

Associated findings in chronic retinal detachment include pigmented demarcation line, retinal thinning, and intraretinal crystalline opacities.[15,16] Most of these retinal macrocysts do not require specific attention during retinal reattachment surgery because they undergo spontaneous regression following reattachment. If the cyst prevents closure of the primary break or is large enough to prevent macular reattachment, drainage may be carried out.

Retinoschisis

Retinoschisis is a splitting of the peripheral neurosensory retina into two layers.[16] This condition may be congenital or acquired. Two types of acquired or degenerative retinoschises have been described—typical and reticular. The eye with acquired or degenerative variant of retinoschisis usually occurs in hypermetropes beyond the age of 20 years. In this form, the splitting may occur at the outer plexiform layer (typical) or the nerve fiber layer (reticular). The reticular variant occurs primarily in the inferotemporal quadrant but may progress circumferentially until the entire retinal periphery is involved. This form may also be complicated by retinal and vitreous hemorrhages and retinal detachment when associated with inner and outer retinal breaks. Retinal macrocysts occur due to coalescence of intraretinal microcystoid degeneration. Coalescence of the schisis spaces may also lead to the formation of retinal macrocysts. Intracystic hemorrhages may occur due to rupture of blood vessels lining the schisis cavity.

Majority of acquired retinoschisis generally remains stable without causing significant functional impairment and only 13% of cases show any signs of progression. Treatment is recommended only in cases showing signs of progression or in patients with retinal detachment. In early cases of retinoschisis, laser or cryodelimitation of the affected area may be carried out. This may be combined with cryotherapy or laser ablation of the outer retina in the area of the schisis.[17] It is believed that the therapy decreases the fluid in the cystic spaces by either destroying the retinal elements secreting the fluid or by increasing the resorption of fluid from the choroidal circulation. In complicated cases with retinal detachment, a standard three-port pars plana vitrectomy with stripping of the posterior hyaloid should be carried out. It should be followed by the removal of the thick fluid using a silicone tip. Intraocular instillation of perfluorocarbon liquids may be performed to displace the fluid from within the cyst and flatten the retina.[18]

Peripheral Retinal Cysts

Cysts in the pars plana region have been reported in 16% of the general population.[19] They appear histologically as empty spaces between the ciliary pigment and nonpigment epithelium.[20] Histochemical studies show that these cysts possibly form due to an active secretion of hyaluronic acid by the nonpigment ciliary epithelium of the pars plana region.[21] Anteriorly, these cysts may extend variably over the pars plana toward the ciliary processes, and posteriorly they may continue with an area of retinal cystoid degeneration beyond the ora. These cysts are usually associated with peripheral degenerative retinoschisis and retinal cystoid changes.[20] Based on the internal wall profile as noted on ultrasound biomicroscopy,[22] these cysts have been classified as follows:

Isolated Cysts

These are either adjacent to each other or separated by intact areas of ciliary epithelium, presenting an internal wall with a smooth profile and a regular single convexity toward the vitreous body.

Confluent Cysts

They have an irregular profile of the internal wall which forms a double convexity toward the vitreous body.

Clustered Cysts

They are relatively the largest of the three types, are defined by a continuous but ragged internal lamina, and present multiple convexities toward the vitreous.

Pars plana cysts are commonly diagnosed during indirect ophthalmoscopy and Goldman's three-mirror examination. These cysts are usually innocuous and require no surgical intervention.[23]

Traumatic Retinal Cysts

Long-standing total retinal detachment with large holes and retinal macrocysts may occur. Mitamura[24] reported a case of macular hole which was accompanied with perifoveal cyst formation following 4 months after trauma.

Neoplastic Retinal Cysts

Some of the retinal neoplasms manifest as retinal cysts. Recently, a case of bilateral hemangioblastomatous cysts of retina associated with hemangioblastoma of the cerebellum has been reported.[25]

PSEUDOCYSTIC VITELLIFORM MACULAR DEGENERATION

Macular and extramacular cysts are usually found in the pseudocystic vitelliform macular degeneration (Best's disease). The cysts obstruct choroidal fluorescence during the early phase of FFA. Histopathological examination reveals a generalized enlargement of RPE which contains lipofuscin and melano-lipofuscin. Cystic lesions in retina may also be found in patients without Best's disease.[3]

REFERENCES

1. Cibis PA. Retinoshchisis—retinal cysts. Trans Am Ophthalmol Soc. 1965;63:417-53.
2. Paul SD. Multiple bilateral cysts of the retina. Ind J Ophthalmol. 1959;7(4):96-8.
3. Yanoff M, Fine BS. Ocular Pathology, 3rd edition. Philadelphia: Lippincott; 1989. pp. 427.

4. Sharma T, Sinha S. Intraocular cysticercosis: Clinical characteristics and visual outcome after vitreoretinal surgery. Ophthalmology. 1993;110(3):996-1004.
5. Earnest MP, Reller LB, Filley CM, et al. Neurocysticercosis in the United States: 35 cases and a review. Rev Inf Dis. 1987;9(5):961-79.
6. Cardenas F, Quiroz H, Plancarte A, et al. Taenia solium ocular cysticercosis: Findings in 30 cases. Ann Ophthalmol. 1992;24(1):25-8.
7. Agrawal B, Vemuganti GK, Honavar SG. Intraocular cysticercosis simulating retinoblastoma in a 5-year-old child. Eye. 2003;17:447-9.
8. Kaliaperumal S, Rao VA, Parija SC. Cysticercosis of the eye in South India--a case series. Indian J Med Microbiol. 2005;23(4):227-30.
9. Luger MH, Stilma JS, Ringens PJ, van Baarlen J. In-toto removal of subretinal Cysticercus cellulosae by pars plana vitrectomy. Br J Ophthalmol. 1991;75(9):561-3.
10. Messner KH, Kammerer WS. Intraocular cysticercosis. Arch Ophthalmol. 1979;97:1103-5.
11. Sen S, Venkatesh P, Chand M. Primary intraocular hydatid cyst with glaucoma. Jour Pediatric Ophthalmol Strab. 2003;40(5):312-3.
12. Nahri GE. A simplified technique for removal of orbital hydatid cyst. Br J Ophthalmol. 1991;75(12):743-5.
13. Litricin O. Echinococcus cyst of the eyeball. Arch Ophthalmol. 1953;50(4):506-9.
14. Marcus DF, Aaberg TM. Intraretinal macrocysts in retinal detachment. Arch Ophthalmol. 1997;97(7):1273-5.
15. Ahmed HR, McDonald H, Schatz RN, et al. Crystalline retinopathy associated with chronic retinal detachment. Arch Ophthalmol. 1998;116(11):1449-53.
16. Madjarov B, Hilton GF, Brinton DA, et al. A new classification of retinoschises. Retina. 1995;15(4):282-5.
17. Okun E, Cibis PA. The role of photocoagulation in the management of retinoschisis. Arch Ophthalmol. 1964;72:309-14.
18. Lomeo MD, Diaz-Rohena R. Use of perfluorocarbon liquid in the repair of retinoschisis retinal detachments. Ophthalmic Surg Lasers. 1996;27(9):778-81.
19. Oku E. Pathology in autopsy eyes. A J Ophthalmol. 1960;50:424.
20. Adams ST. Pars plana cysts. AMA Arch Ophthalmol. 1957;58:328.
21. Zimmerman LE, Fine BS. Production of hyaluronic acid by cysts and tumors of the ciliary body. Arch Ophthalmol. 1964;72:365-79.
22. Mannino G, Malagola R, Abdolrahimzadeh S, et al. Ultrasound biomicroscopy of the peripheral retina and the ciliary body in degenerative retinoschisis associated with pars plana cysts. Br J Ophthalmol. 2001;85(8):976-82.
23. Byer NE. Peripheral retinal lesions related to rhegmatogenous retinal detachment. In: Guyer DR, Yannuzzi LA, Chang S (Eds). Retina, Vitreous, Macula. Philadelphia: Saunders; 1999. pp. 1073-98.
24. Mitamura Y, Saito W, Ishida M, et al. Spontaneous closure of traumatic macular hole. Retina. 2001;21:385-9.
25. Robertson WJ. ANZ J Surg. 2008;4:45-62.

CHAPTER 25

Retinoblastoma

Fairooz P Manjandavida, Santosh G Honavar

INTRODUCTION

Retinoblastoma is the most common intraocular childhood malignancy that is completely curable if detected and treated early. It usually presents in children between 18 months and 36 months of age. Adult onset retinoblastoma is reported but rare. Retinoma or retinocytoma is considered the benign counterpart of retinoblastoma.[1]

The pathogenesis of retinoblastoma has been recently explained in terms of molecular genetics and stem cell biology. It is known to originate from the cells of neuroectodermal origin from the inner layer of the optic cup. The cell of origin of retinoblastoma is still debated. Earlier it was thought that retinoblastoma arises from the photoreceptors. They may have different cellular origin including retinal progenitor cells, cone precursor cells, and rod precursor cells. It is also hypothesized that retinoblastoma arising from retinal progenitor cells possess higher grades of anaplasia than those arising from cone rod cell origin.[2]

Incidence of retinoblastoma has wide geographical variation, so is the survival and prognosis. It occurs in 1 in every 15,000 to 20,000 live births. The estimated number of new cases of retinoblastoma diagnosed globally is 70,00–8,000 each year.[3] Outcome of retinoblastoma is favorable in countries like USA, Europe, Australia, New Zealand, and Japan, where mortality is less than 5%. In these countries, tremendous efforts are being made toward preserving vision with innovative treatments and also reducing treatment-related complications. In contrast, countries in Asia, Africa, and South America where the reported mortality rate is as high as 20%–60%, it is primarily a fight to save life.[4,5] It is estimated that 3,000–3,400 children die annually due to this eye cancer.[3,4]

GENETICS

Retinoblastoma gene (*RB1 gene*) is the first tumor suppressor gene to be identified. The genetics of retinoblastoma has been accepted as the prototype of numerous cancers in the human race. Two-step biallelic inactivation of human retinoblastoma susceptibility gene, *RB1* on chromosome 13q14 that codes for retinoblastoma protein, represents the key event in the pathogenesis of retinoblastoma.[6,7] According to Knudson's two-hit hypothesis, development of retinoblastoma requires mutation of both copies of *RB1* gene. It is also found that retinoblastoma can arise from MYC mutation in the absence of *RB1* mutation.[6] It was recently found that loss of both copies of *RB1* may lead to retinoma, but further genomic instability leads to the development of retinoma to retinoblastoma. It manifests as two forms, sporadic nonhereditary and familial hereditary due to somatic and germline mutations, respectively.[8,9] In the nonhereditary form (60%), the mutation occurs at the cellular level during the development of retina leading to unilateral sporadic form often presenting late after the first year of life. In hereditary retinoblastoma (40%), one allele is mutated in the germline and the other at the cellular level. The heritable form of retinoblastoma often has an early onset presenting as bilateral, multiple tumors and is transmitted to successive generations in an autosomal dominant fashion.[6,10-12] Approximately, 5–10% of patients have one or more affected member in the family. It also increases the risk of development of second nonocular cancers, namely, osteosarcoma in the long bones of arms and legs and soft tissue sarcomas of head and neck. Furthermore, patients undergoing radiotherapy before 1 year of age are at higher risk of developing the tumor of the irradiated field. More profound and lethal is the occurrence of primitive neuroectodermal tumors in the pineal gland—so-called trilateral retinoblastoma.[13,14] The prognosis of pinealoblastoma is invariably poor and children succumb to the disease. It is essential to identify the genetic mutation in retinoblastoma for the modification of management and identifying the generation at risk at an early stage. Genetic counseling is as important as treating the disease in a broader perspective. Molecular testing of the family members at risk allows for prompt management and screening of the disease. In the recent past, many centers in the developed world have successfully introduced genetic testing as a part of retinoblastoma management.[11,13] The breakthrough research in the genetics of retinoblastoma was the recent availability of preimplantation genetic diagnosis in combination with in vitro fertilization.[15,16] Apart from the established genetic mechanism, epigenetics also plays a role in the development of retinoblastoma, and is being explored. Yet another mechanism, named parental gonadal mosaicism, has been identified in children developing sporadic heritable retinoblastoma, and should be considered in suspected genetic disease with negative serum genetic analysis.[11,17,18]

CLASSIFICATION AND STAGING

The initial step in the management of retinoblastoma is categorizing the eyes depending on the clinical features to predict treatment success in terms of visual potential and eye salvage. The most popular classification proposed by Reese and Ellsworth[19] in 1963, four decades ago, was an initiative to predict globe salvage during the era of external beam radiotherapy, which is no more accurate in the contemporary era of chemoreduction and other advanced techniques. The Essen classification in 1983 by Hopping[20] tried to address the emerging newer treatment, but failed to be widely accepted. Shields et al.[21-23] evaluated the eyes undergoing chemoreduction using Reese–Ellsworth classification and showed erratic correlation with treatment success. Subsequently, it paved the way for the newer classification of intraocular retinoblastoma. The International Society of Retinoblastoma and Genetic Eye Disease in Paris (2003) formulated the current classification system—international classification of retinoblastoma that includes clinical grouping depending on the natural course and severity, emerging from the previous Philadelphia classification by Shields et al.,[23] and the Children's Hospital Los Angeles by Murphree et al. (Table 25.1).[24] Recently, the vitreous seeds were morphologically classified as spherules, clouds, and dusting.[25]

The recent international retinoblastoma staging system by Chantada et al.[26] is widely accepted and incorporates intraocular and extraocular disease under five distinct stages based on collective information on clinical evaluation, ocular imaging, histopathology, and systemic survey (Table 25.2). The staging system predicts life salvage and long-term survival. As in any other cancers, the TNM classification was applied to retinoblastoma by the International Union against Cancer and modified in 2010. The TNM is further subclassified as clinical TNM and pathological TNM classification.[27]

CLINICAL FEATURES

The most common symptom of retinoblastoma is white reflex (Fig. 25.1). Others include squint (exotropia or esotropia), redness, pain, and buphthalmos. In advanced stages with extraocular extension, children may present with proptosis or a protruding fungating mass. Ocular signs include white mass behind the lens. Clumps of tumors cells in the anterior chamber and

TABLE 25.1: International grouping of intraocular retinoblastoma.[22,24]	
Group	Clinical features
Group A	Any tumor <3 mm in size
Group B	Any tumor >3 mm Any tumor with subretinal fluid Any tumor in macular location
Group C	Any tumor >3 mm in size, occupying <50% of the globe with focal subretinal and vitreous seeds
Group D	Any tumor >3 mm in size, occupying <50% of the globe with diffuse subretinal and vitreous seeds
Group E	Any tumor >50% of globe, diffuse infiltrating, secondary glaucoma, hyphema, anterior segment seeds, vitreous hemorrhage, aseptic orbital cellulitis, and phthisis bulbi

TABLE 25.2: International staging system for retinoblastoma.[26]

Stage	Feature
Stage 0	No enucleation
Stage 1	Enucleation, tumor completely resected
Stage 2	Enucleation with microscopic residual tumor
Stage 3	Regional extension • Overt orbital disease • Preauricular or cervical lymph node extension

Stage 4	Metastatic disease
	• Hematogenous metastasis
	  – Single lesion
	  – Multiple lesion
	• Central nervous system (CNS) extension
	  – Prechiasmatic lesion
	  – CNS mass
	  – Leptomeningeal disease

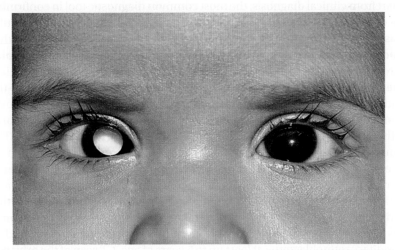

Fig. 25.1: The most common clinical feature is white reflex in retinoblastoma.

hypopyon are seen with anterior segment extension. Diffuse anterior segment retinoblastoma is a rare entity without the involvement of retina but only the anterior chamber. In the presence of secondary glaucoma, they may present with cloudy cornea, iris neovascularization, ectropion uveae and buphthalmos. Warning signs of RB include redness, buphthalmos, hyphema, hypopyon, iris neovascularization, vitreous hemorrhage, eyelid edema, proptosis, and unexplained phthisis bulbi.

On detailed fundus evaluation, retinoblastoma appears as a yellowish-white vascular retinal mass with associated calcification and subretinal fluid with dilated feeder vessels. It can be solitary or multiple. Sporadic retinoblastoma presents as solitary mass, whereas familial (germline) retinoblastoma is multifocal and bilateral. Tumor growth pattern incudes exophytic (tumor growing under the retina toward choroid associated with exudative retinal detachment), endophytic (tumor growing toward the vitreous), mixed (both exophytic and endophytic), diffuse infiltrating (grayish thickening of the retina), and anterior segment retinoblastoma (tumor involving the anterior segment structures with or without involvement of the peripheral retina). Subretinal seeds and vitreous seeds are frequent and these may be focal or diffuse.[1,2] Vitreous seeds are further morphologically classified as spherule, dust, and cloud. The benign counterpart of retinoblastoma, retinoma/retinocytoma, appears as regressed retinoblastoma, calcified or fleshy with surrounding choroidal atrophy and sheathing of vessels. The clinical differential diagnoses are Coats' disease, persistent fetal vasculature, vitreous hemorrhage, ocular toxocariasis, familial exudative vitreoretinopathy, coloboma, astrocytic hamartoma, and endogenous endophthalmitis.[1,2]

DIAGNOSIS

Apart from clinical diagnosis, the most common diagnostic tool in confirming the diagnosis is B-scan ultrasonography showing a characteristic intraocular mass with calcification as indicated by high internal reflectivity.[28] Other modalities that give supporting information are fluorescein angiography, autofluorescence, and optical coherence tomography.[29,30] Radiological imaging is indicated in identifying the extension of tumor outside the confines of the eyeball. Magnetic resonance imaging (MRI) is preferred over computerized tomography (CT) scan especially in patients of retinoblastoma with germline mutation.[31] MRI provides superior soft tissue details. The tumor characteristically appears hyperintense in T1 and hypointense in T2 whereas calcification remains markedly hypointense.[32] MRI is considered more valuable compared to CT scan in detecting optic nerve invasion and intracranial extension. In addition, it also helps in screening and detecting midline lesions associated with trilateral retinoblastoma—pinealoblastoma. It is wise to recommend yearly MRI in children harboring bilateral and or hereditary retinoblastoma at least up to 5 years of age. CT scan of the orbit can confirm intraocular calcification and delineate extraocular extension.

MANAGEMENT

Untreated retinoblastoma is uniformly fatal. The primary goal remains life salvage. The secondary and tertiary goals are eye salvage and vision salvage, respectively. Enucleation was considered the treatment of choice of retinoblastoma a century ago, and was replaced by more conservative external beam radiation with its well-recognized complications. Since the mid-1990s, the management of retinoblastoma has undergone a paradigm shift owing to better alternatives to save life, eye, and vision.[33] The introduction of systemic intravenous chemotherapy (IVC) was a breakthrough and to a larger extent has helped avoid enucleation in bilateral as well as unilateral retinoblastoma.[33,34]

Chemotherapy alone is not curable, without additional focal treatment such as cryotherapy and transpupillary thermotherapy. The more localized and targeted treatment involves plaque brachytherapy. The most recent additions to the armamentarium are intra-arterial and intravitreal chemotherapy.[35-38] In short, the management of retinoblastoma is highly individualized and requires a multidisciplinary team comprising trained ocular oncologist, oncopathologist, pediatric oncologist, radiation oncologist, interventional radiologist, neurosurgeon, and a geneticist. The available management modalities are briefly outlined here.

- Chemotherapy
  - Systemic
    - Intravenous chemotherapy
  - Local
    - Intra-arterial chemotherapy (IAC)
    - Intravitreal chemotherapy
    - Periocular subtenon's chemotherapy
- Radiotherapy
  - Plaque brachytherapy
  - External beam radiotherapy
  - Proton beam radiotherapy
- Focal therapy
  - Cryotherapy
  - Laser transpupillary thermotherapy
- Enucleation (with orbital implant).

Chemotherapy

Systemic Intravenous Chemotherapy

The introduction of IVC "chemoreduction" changed the outlook toward the dreadful childhood cancer, essentially increasing the survival rate and preserving the eye and vision. Chemoreduction reduces the size of the tumor and makes it amenable for focal treatment. IVC alone is not curative, but is used synergistically with intensive focal therapy with cryotherapy and laser treatment (Figs. 25.2A and B).[34,39,40] Though there exist many protocols, the most widely accepted is the triple drug regimen consisting of vincristine (1.5 mg/m^2), etoposide (150 mg/m^2), and carboplatin (560 mg/m^2) for six cycles, given 3–4 weeks apart. With this current protocol of chemoreduction and sequential consolidation with focal therapy, most eyes are salvageable with functional vision with excellent life salvage. It was observed that there was 100%, 93% and 90% tumor control in group A, B, and C eyes, respectively.[34] The eye salvage was less than 50% in advanced group D and E eyes; however, the use of high-dose IVC regimen with local delivery of subtenon's chemotherapy and low dose radiotherapy could still salvage about 83% of eyes.[41]

IVC is safe if administered under the supervision and care of pediatric oncologist. Most commonly identified complications are reversible myelosuppression, neurotoxicity, ototoxicity, and nonspecific gastrointestinal

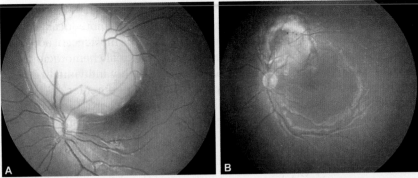

Figs. 25.2A and B: (A) Systemic intravenous chemotherapy in group B retinoblastoma showing a macular tumor overlying the fovea. (B) Chemoreduction and consolidation with laser therapy spared the fovea with 20/20 vision post-treatment.

toxicity. Apart from gaining control over the tumor, the major advantages of IVC lie in preventing the more devastating systemic micrometastasis, pinealoblastoma, and second malignant neoplasm.

Local

Periocular Subtenon's Chemotherapy

The major disadvantage of IVC is the poor penetration of the chemotherapeutic agents into the vitreous and not achieving higher drug concentration. Periocular chemotherapy was initially explored to achieve high drug concentration locally.[41] It is indicated in eyes with vitreous seeds. The drugs used are carboplatin (10–15 mg) and topotecan (1–2 mg). Most common complication is periocular edema and conjunctival scarring, and less common are extraocular muscle fibrosis and optic atrophy. Associated complications with topotecan are known to be less severe when compared to carboplatin and is therefore preferred.[41-45]

Intra-arterial Chemotherapy

Intra-arterial chemotherapy (IAC) is a targeted therapy of administering chemotherapeutic agent directly into the main blood vessel supplying the tumor.[36] IAC is currently used in many centers as the primary modality of treatment in advanced unilateral retinoblastoma. It is technologically challenging, requiring a highly skilled interventional radiologist or a neurosurgeon. The introduction of this technique dates back to 1955, when Reese and coworkers treated retinoblastoma with direct catheterization and infusion of triethylene melanamine into the internal carotid artery. Kaneko and Yamane developed a targeted approach of selective ophthalmic artery infusion (SOAI)—balloon occlusion technique using melphalan, in an effort to reduce complications.[46] But the authors failed to provide adequate data on tumor control and ocular complications. Abramson and Gobin further modified the technique into super-SOAI by directly entering the ophthalmic artery.[47] The drugs infused were topotecan, carboplatin, and melphalan. It is emerging as the treatment of choice in unilateral advanced retinoblastoma (Figs. 25.3A to D). The most common complications of IAC include periocular edema, mechanical ptosis, and forehead hyperemia. Major complications of IAC are related to vascular toxicity and or occlusion of ophthalmic artery and retinal and choroidal vessels, leading to central retinal artery occlusion, choroid atrophy, and vitreous hemorrhage.[36,48,49]

Intravitreal Chemotherapy

The outcome of advanced group D eyes with diffuse vitreous seeds remains a challenge, with high rate of recurrence and systemic chemotherapy failure, often requiring external beam radiotherapy. The globe salvage with EBRT is not more than 20%–30%, offering suboptimal control of the disease with associated complications especially in children with the only seeing eye in heritable bilateral retinoblastoma. The direct delivery of chemotherapeutic agents into the vitreous cavity was assumed to provide adequate tumor control.[38,50,51] Inomata and Kaneko found melphalan to be the most effective and relatively less toxic agent intravitreally as supported by the in vitro experiment in the rabbit model.[52] The most common chemotherapeutic drug used is melphalan,

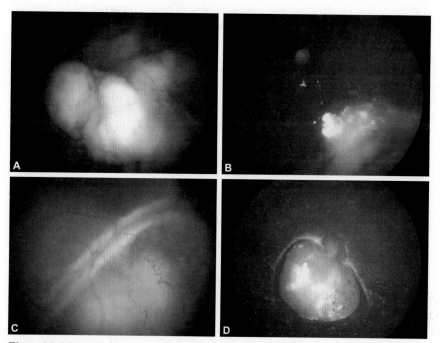

Figs. 25.3A to D: Intra-arterial chemotherapy in advanced retinoblastoma. (A) A group D eye with diffuse vitreous seeds; (B) After three cycles of intra-arterial chemotherapy; (C) A group E eye with a very large tumor and diffuse subretinal fluid; (D) After three cycles of intra-arterial chemotherapy.

although topotecan is also found to provide equally encouraging results.[38,50,51] The only complication observed was salt and pepper retinopathy noticed in 43% of eyes due to localized toxicity at the site of injection.[52] The initial results are encouraging; however, the results of a prospective phase II trial are still awaited and the long-term local and systemic complications are unknown. It was also observed that eyes receiving 8–10 µg showed suboptimal response and higher doses of greater than 50 µg led to phthisis bulbi.[53]

Radiotherapy

Plaque Brachytherapy

Focal application of radioactive device enables targeted treatment—delivery of radiation locally and reducing ocular side effects. Plaque brachytherapy is the method of placing a radioactive plaque on the sclera corresponding to the base of the tumor and rendering transscleral irradiation to the tumor. Most commonly used radioactive materials are Iodine 125 and Ruthenium 106. The main indication is recurrent or residual tumor following chemoreduction and focal treatment. Shields et al. analyzed the outcome of plaque brachytherapy as a primary treatment (29%) and secondary treatment (79%). The average tumor size was 8 mm in basal diameter and 4 mm in thickness. The dosage delivered to the tumor apex ranges from 3,500 cGy to 4,000 cGy, and mandates precise tumor localization and measurement of tumor dimensions for optimal treatment. The tumor control with Iodine 125 plaque brachytherapy has been reported as 95% at 5 years.[37,54]

External Beam Radiotherapy

The once popular modality is now less preferred owing to the short-term and long-term adverse effects. The most common complications include dry eye, radiation cataract, neovascular glaucoma, radiation retinopathy, and orbital and midfacial growth retardation. The most dreaded complication is the risk of development of second malignant neoplasm, especially in patients with hereditary forms of retinoblastoma and mostly radiation dose dependant.[55] The risk is as high as 50% in this group when compared to 6% in patients with nonheritable tumor. It is estimated that patients undergoing EBRT at less than 12 months of age are at greater risk when compared to those greater than 12 months.[56]

Focal Therapy

The cryotherapy and laser treatment are focal techniques, which are applied directly to the tumor either as a primary modality or most often as an adjunctive to chemoreduction for consolidation.[1,33]

Cryotherapy

Cryotherapy is effective in small equatorial and peripheral retinal tumors measuring up to 2 mm in thickness and 4 mm in basal diameter. The cryoprobe is applied trans-sclerally and classically triple freeze thaw protocol is used. Cryotherapy applied prior to chemotherapy has synergistic effect by increasing the delivery of chemotherapeutic agents across the blood retina barrier.[1,33,57]

Laser

Laser treatment plays a major role in tumor control. The use of diode laser transpupillary thermotherapy (TTT) is the most common and widely used technique with minimal complications. The focused heat generated by the infrared radiation is applied over the tumor at a subphotocoagulation level to induce tumor cell apoptosis sparing damage to the retinal vessels. The laser is applied with a 1,300-μm spot until the tumor turns subtle gray in color. This technique provides satisfactory control for small tumors with less than 2 mm in thickness. Multiple sessions are administered, until the tumor is reduced to a flat chorioretinal scar. Major advantage is its adjunctive role during chemoreduction, where the heat amplifies the cytotoxic effect of systemic carboplatin—the term known as chemothermotherapy. The known complications are focal iris atrophy, peripheral lens opacification, retinal traction, retinal vascular obstruction, and transient localized serous detachment.[58]

Enucleation

Despite the several advancements in the management of retinoblastoma as mentioned and discussed, enucleation is still considered the primary treatment of advanced retinoblastoma and is life-saving. In the last few decades, the frequency of enucleation has steadily decreased in favor of conservative modalities and because of relatively early detection of tumors. It is not uncommon in the developing countries where greater than 50% of children present with advanced retinoblastoma requiring primary enucleation.[59] The indications of enucleation are eyes belonging to group E, anterior chamber tumor seeding, neovascular glaucoma and hyphema, necrotic tumor with secondary orbital inflammation, and vitreous hemorrhage precluding visualization of the tumor. The technique requires modification to avoid the risk of accidental perforation and orbital tumor seeding. The preferred method is minimal manipulation enucleation with long optic nerve stump, ideally greater than 15 mm. Placement of an orbital implant is advised in all children undergoing enucleation, primarily to stimulate orbital growth and thereby improving cosmesis and enable fitting a custom-made prosthesis.[1,2]

Enucleation is not the end of retinoblastoma management and does not imply that the life is saved. The eyes undergoing enucleation may carry histopathological high-risk factors for systemic metastasis (Box 25.1). Histopathological high-risk factors in enucleated eyes are retrolaminar optic nerve invasion, choroidal invasion of 3 mm or greater, anterior segment invasion, any degree of optic nerve plus choroidal invasion, scleral invasion, and extrascleral extension (Box 25.1).[60,61] In the presence of high-risk features,

> **BOX 25.1:** Postenucleation histopathological high-risk features in retinoblastoma.[1,2,61]
>
> *Histopathological high-risk features*
> - Postlaminar optic nerve invasion
> - Choroidal invasion ≥3 mm in diameter or thickness
> - Anterior segment invasion
> - Any degree of optic nerve + choroidal invasion
> - Optic nerve transection involvement
> - Extrascleral extension

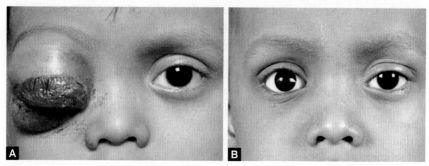

Figs. 25.4A and B: Intensive multimodal treatment protocol in orbital retinoblastoma. (A) Right eye showing secondary orbital recurrence of retinoblastoma after enucleation; (B) After completion of high-dose neoadjuvant chemotherapy, followed by radiation and adjuvant chemotherapy, the tumor is seen to have completely regressed, thereby preventing exenteration with optimal cosmesis and improved survival.

patients undergo adjuvant chemotherapy to reduce the risk of systemic metastasis.

Multimodal treatment protocol is followed in advanced cases with orbital extension of intraocular tumor. It includes initial neoadjuvant chemotherapy, enucleation, followed by radiation and adjuvant chemotherapy. This has improved the survival in locally advanced disease (Figs. 25.4A and B). Metastatic retinoblastoma has poor prognosis, especially central nervous system metastasis, and is the major cause of death in retinoblastoma.[62]

CONCLUSION

To summarize, retinoblastoma is curable if recognized early and managed appropriately. The choice of chemotherapeutic agents and route of administration continue to evolve. However, the management varies from patient to patient, depending on the stage of the disease, availability of technical skills, and optimal cost-effective therapeutic modalities. The art of management lies in early detection, selection of appropriate management strategy, and long-term follow-up to assess recurrence and treatment-related complications. Above all, it is the family whom we treat, not the patient alone.

REFERENCES

1. Ramasubramanian A, Shields CL. Epidemiology and magnitude of the problem. In: Ramasubramanian A, Shields CL (Eds). Retinoblastoma. New Delhi: Jaypee Brothers Medical Publishers (P) Ltd.; 2012, pp. 10-5.
2. Grossniklaus HE. Retinoblastoma. Fifty years of progress. The LXXI Edward Jackson Memorial Lecture. Am J Ophthalmol. 2014;158(5):875-91.
3. Kivela T. The epidemiological challenge of the most frequent eye cancer: retinoblastoma, an issue of birth and death. Br J Ophthalmol. 2009;93:1129-31.
4. Dimaras H, Dimba EAO, Gallie BL. Challenging global retinoblastoma survival. Br J Ophthalmol. 2010;95:1451-52.
5. Chantada GL, Qaddoumi I, Cantruk S, et al. Strategies to manage retinoblastoma in developing countries. Pediatr Blood Cancer. 2011;56:341-8.
6. Knudson AG. Mutation and cancer: statistical study of retinoblastoma. Proc Natl Acad Sci USA. 1971;68:820-3.
7. Friend SH, Bernards R, Rogelj S, et al. A human DNA segment with properties of the gene that predisposes to retinoblastoma and osteosarcoma. Nature.1986;323:643-46.
8. Gianciati C, Giordiano A. RB and cell cycle progression. Oncogene. 2006;25:5220-7.
9. Dimaras H, Khetan V, Halliday W, et al. Loss of RB1 induces non-proliferative retinoma: increasing genomic instability correlates with progression to retinoblastoma. Hum Mol Genet. 2008;17(10):1363-72.
10. Ganguly A, Shileds CL. Differential gene expression profile of retinoblastoma compared to normal retina. Mol Vis. 2010;16:1292-303.
11. Chakraborthy S, Khare S, Dorairaj SK, et al. Identification of genes associated with tumorigenesis of retinoblastoma by microarray analysis. Genomics 2007;90(3):344-53.
12. Reis AH, Vargas FR, Lemos B. More epigenetic hits than meets the eye: micro RNAs and genes associated with tumorigenesis of retinoblastoma. Front Genet. 2012;3:284.
13. Lohman DR, Gallie BL. Retinoblastoma: revisiting the model prototype of inherited cancer. Am J Med Genet C Semin Med Genet. 2004;129:23-8.
14. Meadows AT, Leahey AM. More about second cancers after retinoblastoma. J Natl Cancer Inst. 2008;100:1743-5.
15. Gallie BL, Hei YJ, Dunn JM. Retinoblastoma treatment in premature infants diagnosed prenataly by the ultrasound and molecular diagnosis. Am J Hum Genet Suppl. 65:A62.
16. Xu K, Rosenwaks Z, Beaverson K, et al. Preimplantation genetic diagnosis for retinoblastoma: the first reported live born. Am J Ophthalmol. 2004;137:18-23.
17. Murphree AL, Triche TJ. An epigenomic mechanism in retinoblastoma: the end of the story? Genome Med. 2012;4:15.
18. Livide G, Epistolato MC, Amenduni M, et al. Epigenetic and copy number variation analysis in retinoblastoma by MS-MLPA. Pathol Oncol Res. 2012;18:703-12.
19. Reese AB, Ellsworth RM. The evaluation and current concept of retinoblastoma therapy. Trans Am Acad Ophthalmol Otolaryngol. 1963;67:164-72.
20. Hopping W. The new Essen prognosis classification for conservative sight-saving treatment of retinoblastoma. In: Lommatzsch PK, Blodi FC (Eds). Intraocular Tumors: International Symposium Under the Auspices of the European Ophthalmological Society. Berlin: Springer-Verlag; 1983. pp. 497-505.
21. Shields CL, Mashayakhi A, Demirci H, et al. Practical approach to management of retinoblastoma. Arch Ophthalmol. 2004;122(5):729-35.

22. Shields CL, Shields JA. Basic understanding of current classification and management of retinoblastoma. Curr Opin Ophthalmol. 2006;17:228-34.
23. Shields CL, Mashayakhi A, Au AK, et al. The International Classification of Retinoblastoma predicts chemoreduction success. Ophthalmology. 2006;113:2276-80.
24. Murphree AL. Intraocular retinoblastoma: the case for a new group classification. Ophthalmol Clin North Am. 2005;18:41-53.
25. Munier FL. Classification and management of seeds in retinoblastoma. Ellsworth Lecture Ghent August 24th 2013. Ophthalmic Genet. 2014;35(4):193-207.
26. Chantada G, Doz F, Antoneli CB, et al. A proposal for an international retinoblastoma staging system. Pediatr Blood Cancer. 2006;47:801-5.
27. Edge SB, Byrd DR, Compton CC, et al. AJCC Cancer Staging Manual and Handbook, 7th edition. New York: Springer; 2010. pp. 623-9.
28. Shields JA, Shields CL. Diagnostic approaches to Retinoblastoma. In: Shields JA, Shields CL (Eds). Intraocular Tumors: A Text and Atlas. Philadelphia: WB Saunders; 1992. pp. 363-76.
29. Sony P, Garg SP. Optical coherence tomography in children with retinoblastoma. J Pediatr Ophthalmol Strabismus. 2005;42:134.
30. Bianciotto C, Shields CL, Iturralde JC, et al. Fluorescein angiographic findings after intra-arterial chemotherapy for retinoblastoma. Ophthalmology. 2012;119(4):843-9.
31. Pearce MS, Salotti JA, Little MP, et al. Radiation exposure from CT scans in childhood and subsequent risk of leukemia and brain tumours: a retrospective cohort study. Lancet. 2012;380:499-505.
32. De Potter, Shields CL, Shields JA, et al. The role of MR imaging in children with intraocular tumors and simulating lesions. Ophthalmology. 1996;103:1774-83.
33. Shields CL, Fulco EM, Arias JD, et al. Retinoblastoma frontiers with intravenous, intra-arterial, periocular, and intravitreal chemotherapy. Eye. 2012;27:253-64.
34. Shields JA, Shields CL, Meadows AT. Chemoreduction in the management of retinoblastoma. Am J Ophthalmol. 2005;140:505-6.
35. Abramson DH, Dunkel IJ, Brodie SE, et al. A phase I/II study of direct intra-arterial (ophthalmic artery) chemotherapy with melphalan for intraocular retinoblastoma initial results. Ophthalmology. 2008;115(8):1398-404, 1404.e1.
36. Shields CL, Manjandavida FP, Lally SE, et al. Intra-arterial chemotherapy for retinoblastoma in 70 eyes: outcomes based on the international classification of retinoblastoma. Ophthalmology. 2014;121(7):1453-60.
37. Shields CL, Shields JA, Cater J, et al. Plaque radiotherapy for retinoblastoma, long term tumor control and treatment complications in 208 tumors. Ophthalmology. 2001;108:2116-21.
38. Munier F, Gaillard MC, Balmer A, et al. Intravitreal chemotherapy for vitreous disease in retinoblastoma revisited: from prohibition to conditional indications. Br J Ophthalmol. 2012;96:1078-83.
39. Leahey AM. Systemic chemotherapy: a pediatric oncology perspective. In: Ramasubramanian A, Shields CL (Eds). Retinoblastoma. New Delhi: Jaypee Brothers Medical Publishers (P) Ltd.; 2012, pp. 81-5.
40. Gombos DS, Kelly A, Coen PG, et al. Retinoblastoma treated with primary chemotherapy alone: the significance of tumor size, location and age. Br J Ophthalmol. 2002;86:80-3.
41. Manjandavida FP, Honavar SG, Reddy VA, et al. Management and outcome of retinoblastoma with vitreous seeds. Ophthalmology. 2014;121(2):517-24.
42. Abramson DH, Frank CM, Dunkel IJ. A phase I/II study of subconjunctival carboplatin for intraocular retinoblastoma. Ophthalmology. 1999;106:1947-50.

43. Shome D, Honavar SG, Reddy VA. The role of periocular carboplatin as an adjunctive therapy in advanced intraocular retinoblastoma. In: Proceedings of the Annual Meeting of the American Academy of Ophthalmology, Chicago. 2005.
44. Carcaboso AM, Chiappetta DA, Opezzo JA, et al. Episcleral implants for topotecan delivery to the posterior segment of the eye. Invest Ophthalmol Vis Sci. 2010;51(4):2126-34.
45. Chantada GL, Fandino AC, Carcaboso AM, et al. A phase I study of periocular topotecan in children with intraocular retinoblastoma. Invest Ophthalmol Vis Sci. 2009;50:1492-6.
46. Yamane T, Kaneko A, Mohri M. The technique of ophthalmic arterial infusion therapy for patients with intraocular retinoblastoma. Int J Clin Oncol. 2004;9(2):69-73.
47. Gobin YP, Dunkel IJ, Marr BP, et al. Intra-arterial chemotherapy for the management of retinoblastoma: four-year experience. Arch Ophthalmol. 2011;129:732-37.
48. Shields CL, Bianciotto CG, Jabbour P, et al. Intra-arterial chemotherapy for retinoblastoma: report No. 2, treatment complications. Arch Ophthalmol. 2011;129:1407-15.
49. Eagle RC Jr, Shields CL, Bianciotto C, et al. Histopathologic observations after intra-arterial chemotherapy for retinoblastoma. Arch Ophthalmol. 2011;129:1416-50.
50. Manjandavida FP, Shields CL. The role of intravitreal chemotherapy for retinoblastoma. Indian J Ophthalmol. 2015;63(2):141-5.
51. Shields CL, Manjandavida FP, Arepalli S, et al. Intravitreal melphalan for persistent or recurrent retinoblastoma vitreous seeds: preliminary results. JAMA Ophthalmol. 2014;132(3):319-25.
52. Ueda M, Tanabe J, Inomata M, et al. Study on conservative treatment of retinoblastoma—effect of intravitreal injection of melphalan on the rabbit retina. Nippon Ganka Gakkai Zasshi. 1995;99:1230-5.
53. Ghassemi F, Shields CL. Intravitreal melphalan for refractory or recurrent vitreous seeding from retinoblastoma. Arch Ophthalmol. 2012;130:1268-71.
54. Shields CL, Shields JA, De Potter P, et al. Plaque radiotherapy in the management of retinoblastoma. Use as a primary and secondary treatment. Ophthalmology. 1993;100:216-24.
55. Choi SY, Kim MS, Yoo S, et al. Long term follow-up results of external beam radiotherapy as primary treatment for retinoblastoma. J Korean Med Sci. 2010;25:546-5
56. Abramson DH, Frank CM. Second non-ocular tumors in survivors of bilateral retinoblastoma; a possible age effect on radiation-related risk. Ophthalmology. 1998;105:573-80.
57. Wilson TW, Chan HS, Moselhy GM, et al. Penetration of chemotherapy into vitreous is increased by cryotherapy and cyclosporine in rabbits. Arch Ophthalmol. 1996;114:1390-5.
58. Shields CL, Santos MC, Diniz W, et al. Thermotherapy for retinoblastoma. Arch Ophthalmol. 1999;117:885-93.
59. Gupta R, Vemuganti GK, Reddy VA, et al. Histopathologic risk factors in retinoblastoma in India. Arch Pathol Lab Med. 2009;133:1210-4.
60. Eagle RC Jr. High-risk features and tumor differentiation in retinoblastoma: a retrospective histopathologic study. Arch Pathol Lab Med. 2009;133:1203-9.
61. Honavar SG, Singh AD, Shields CL, et al. Post-enucleation adjuvant therapy in high-risk retinoblastoma. Arch Ophthalmol. 2002;120:923-31.
62. Honavar SG, Singh AD. Management of advanced retinoblastoma. Ophthalmol Clin North Am. 2005;18:65-73.

CHAPTER 26

Radiation Retinopathy

Karobi Lahiri Coutinho

INTRODUCTION

Radiation retinopathy is a predictable complication following exposure to any source of radiation. It was first described in 1933 by Stallard following treatment of retinoblastoma. Radiation retinopathy is a slowly progressive occlusive vasculopathy characterized by radiation-induced endothelial damage. It appears clinically as microaneurysms, telangiectases, neovascularization, retinal hemorrhage, hard exudates, cotton-wool spots, and macular edema.

ETIOLOGY

Exposure to any radiation source including external beam and plaque brachytherapy specifically, external beam radiation as treatment for nasopharyngeal, paranasal sinus or orbital tumors, where there is limited protection for the eye, can often lead to clinically significant radiation retinopathy.[1] Plaque brachytherapy in the treatment of intraocular tumors can also cause severe damage to the immediate retina and choroid. Radiation retinopathy is seen following radiation for ocular tumors like retinoblastoma, choroid melanoma, angioma, head and neck cancers, optic nerve sheath meningioma, Hodgkin's lymphoma, and ill-defined choroidal neovascular membranes. Head and neck irradiation can cause ophthalmic complications like cataracts, optic neuropathy, and radiation retinopathy.

RADIATION THERAPY

Radiation Timing and Modality

The optimum timing of therapy (before, during, or after visual changes) and the optimum radiation strategy—lateral port external beam, fractionated conformal, fractionated stereotactic, and intensity-modulated radiation therapy—remain evolving concepts.

Effects of Radiation Treatment

Most systemic side effects are transient and self-limited. They include nausea, vomiting, focal alopecia, swelling, pain, and mild erythematous skin changes. Ocular side effects are less frequent and often delayed; they include radiation retinopathy, optic neuropathy, cataract formation, and dry eye. Cranial nerve dysfunction, pituitary dysfunction, brain necrosis, hearing loss, and new tumor induction can develop after decades.

Recent advances in achieving greater precision for delivering higher isodose levels to smaller volumes of tissue (thereby reducing the dosage to uninvolved tissue) should theoretically reduce side effects to the surrounding tissues.

The duration of follow-up in published cases that detail new techniques is more limited, and the future side effect incidence rate should be determined with a longitudinal follow-up.

RISK FACTORS

Higher total radiation dose has been shown to increase the risk of radiation retinopathy. The fractionation, field design, type, and rate of administration of radiation should also be accounted for. While there are no definite thresholds, estimates for external beam radiation range from 15 Gy to 60 Gy. The incidence of retinopathy increases steadily at doses greater than 45 Gy.[2] Radiation retinopathy has been reported in doses as low as 11 Gy but infrequent below 45 Gy dose. The risk of induction of retinopathy increases with dose used from 25 Gy to 35 Gy. The external beam irradiation is more likely to induce changes.

Hyperfractionation has been associated with a decreased incidence of radiation retinopathy.[3] Patients who receive less than 25 Gy in fractions of 2 Gy or less are unlikely to develop significant retinopathy.

With local or external beam irradiation, patients develop retinopathy 6 months to 3 years after treatment.

With plaque brachytherapy, the risk of radiation retinopathy is related to the total radiation dose. In the treatment of uveal melanoma, therapeutic apical doses range from 80 Gy to 100 Gy. Factors that affect total radiation dose such as tumor height and location also increase the risk of retinopathy. Tumor thickness greater than 4 mm has been associated with a greater risk for radiation maculopathy.[4] A decreased distance to the fovea has also been associated with decreased time to maculopathy.[5] Increased fraction size is correlated with the increase in retinal complications.

COMORBIDITIES

Comorbidities such as diabetes, hypertension, autoimmune disorders, concurrent chemotherapy, and pregnancy are associated with an increased risk of radiation retinopathy.[6] Risk factors for developing proliferative radiation retinopathy include younger age, preexisting diabetes mellitus, and shorter tumor distance from the optic disk.[7] Patients with preexisting vascular diseases such as collagen vascular disease, hypertension, or previous chemotherapy have also been reported to develop radiation retinopathy at even lower doses of radiation.

PATHOGENESIS

Radiation can cause both acute and chronic effects on retina.

Acute changes occur within 6 hours of radiation and show nuclear pyknosis among rods, and edema in the outer retinal layers.

Chronic changes occur due to endothelial cell injury owing to retinal ischemia resulting in necrosis of the nerve tissue, and fibrovascular proliferation. Exposure of radiation is thought to cause preferential loss of vascular endothelial cells with relative sparing of the pericytes.[8] It is hypothesized that differential sensitivity between endothelial cells and pericytes is the result of direct exposure of the endothelial cells to high ambient oxygen and iron found in the blood which generates free radicals and leads to cell membrane damage.[9] This damage leads to the occlusion of capillary beds and microaneurysm formation. The retinal ischemia from areas of retinal nonperfusion ultimately leads to macular edema, neovascularization, vitreous hemorrhage, and tractional retinal detachment.

DIAGNOSIS

History

Patients will have a history of radiation exposure or radiotherapy few months to years ago. Intelligent patients often remember the nature of the disease and mode of therapy. They may give history of malignant melanoma for which radiation therapy, brachytherapy, or cobalt plaque therapy was instituted.[10-14] It has been reported that radiation retinopathy can develop anywhere from 1 month to 15 years. However, it most commonly occurs between 6 months and 3 years.[6] Attempts have been made to attenuate the ill effects of radiotherapy by vitreous substitution[15] or by injecting periocular triamcinolone.[16]

Physical Examination

Evaluation for radiation retinopathy includes a complete ophthalmologic examination including a dilated funduscopy to look for pathologic features of retinopathy described later.

Symptoms

Patients with early or mild retinopathy may be asymptomatic but advanced disease can present with decreased vision or floaters. Sudden loss of vision after radiation is not rare. Chronic blurring of vision, distorted vision, and defective color vision are common.

Signs

Dilated funduscopic examination (Fig. 26.1) may reveals the following features:

- Retinal microaneurysms
- Retinal hemorrhages
- Retinal telangiectatic vessels
- Retinal hard exudates
- Macular edema
- Cotton-wool spots
- Retinal neovascularization
- Vitreous hemorrhage
- Tractional retinal detachment
- Capillary dilation
- Capillary closure
- Perivascular sheathing
- Retinal pigment epithelium (RPE) atrophy
- Central retinal artery or vein occlusion.

Optic disk edema, neovascularization of the iris, neovascularization of the angle, neovascular glaucoma, and cataract are associated features of the radiation retinopathy.

Visual impairment ranges from mild to severe and is secondary to macular ischemia or edema. The most severe change is a progressive development of capillary nonperfusion areas in periphery and posterior pole. These features are similar to changes in diabetic retinopathy with exception that microaneurysms are less frequent in radiation retinopathy. RPE atrophy due to vaso-obliteration is seen in radiation retinopathy.

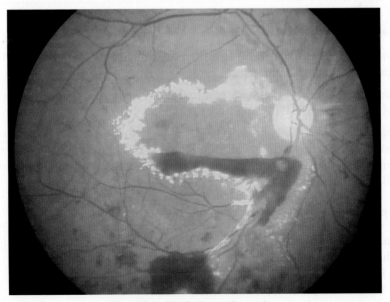

Fig. 26.1: Radiation retinopathy.

In proliferative retinopathy, ischemia is seen in area that receives the highest dose of radiation as compared to nasal location and diabetic retinopathy. Latency by radiation exposure and clinical manifestations of vascular changes may range either from 3 weeks to 7 years or 6 months to 3 years.

Macular changes include hard exudates, cystoid and noncystoid edema, and serous detachment that can lead to significant visual loss.

Optic neuropathy occurs in the acute phase which is marked by disk edema, intraretinal hemorrhages, hard exudates, and the presence of subretinal fluid. The optic nerve appears progressively pale and atrophic with variable visual acuity during a few weeks or months.

Biomicroscopy

Biomicroscopic examination may show conjunctival hemorrhage, conjunctival scars, signs of dry eye, symblepharon, corneal aberrations, corneal opacification, anterior uveitis, and cataract.

Finger Classification

Radiation retinopathy is classified according to Finger into four stages.
- Stage 1: It is located outside the macula and visual acuity is good.
- Stage 2: It is located at the macula and has guarded prognosis.
- Stage 3: It presents some vision loss and carries a severe risk of neovascularization, macular edema, and retinal ischemia.
- Stage 4: Any of the above combination with vitreous hemorrhage and retinal ischemia can affect vitreous, macula, and extra macular area (> or = to 5 DA).

Diagnostic Procedures

Fundus fluorescein angiogram can be helpful in highlighting the microvascular features of radiation retinopathy.

Indocyanine green angiography can reveal precapillary arteriolar occlusion and areas of choroidal hypoperfusion.

Optical coherence tomography (OCT) can be helpful in evaluating macular edema. A study by Horgan et al. found that OCT was able to detect evidence of macular edema approximately 5 months earlier than clinically detectable radiation maculopathy.[17]

DIFFERENTIAL DIAGNOSIS

The following conditions should be considered in the differential diagnosis of radiation retinopathy:
- Diabetic retinopathy
- Branch retinal vein occlusion
- Central retinal vein occlusion

- Hypertensive retinopathy
- Coats' disease
- Perifoveal telangiectasia.

MANAGEMENT

Medical

Anti-vascular Endothelial Growth Factor Therapy

Vascular endothelial growth factor (VEGF) is a secreted protein that promotes vascular leakage and angiogenesis.[18] Bevacizumab is a humanized monoclonal antibody to VEGF. Several studies have examined the use of intravitreal bevacizumab (1.25 mg in 0.05 mL) in the treatment of radiation retinopathy and maculopathy;[18-21] and demonstrated an improvement in macular edema following intravitreal bevacizumab though a sustained decrease often required multiple injections. However, visual acuity was not found to improve significantly in most of the studies. Anti-VEGF agents can decrease edema, hemorrhages, exudates, and microaneurysms and may improve the visual acuity with a decrease in macular edema.

Finger[19] reported on a series of 21 patients in which intravitreal bevacizumab (1.25 mg/0.05 mL) was injected every 6–12 weeks. At a mean follow-up of 7.8 months, 18 patients (86%) had improvement or stabilization of visual acuity, and 3 (14%) improved by two or more lines of vision. The authors also reported improvement in vascular leakage as determined by fluorescein angiography. Another report by the same group[20] investigated the use of ranibizumab for radiation retinopathy in five patients. A mean of 8.2 injections of ranibizumab (0.5 mg) was given over a mean follow-up of 8 months. Visual acuity improved by a mean of six letters, with four patients showing a modest improvement on average of 9.5 letters, and one patient losing seven letters. A decrease in vascular leakage and macular edema was seen, and CMT thickness decreased from 416 µm to 270 µm, a 35% reduction. Adverse effects were minimal, including subconjunctival hemorrhage at the injection site and transient postinjection intraocular pressure elevations. These studies show that periodic dosing, such as is used in treatment of age-related macular degeneration, may be beneficial in sustaining a treatment effect.

At Bascom Palmer Eye Institute, a study[21] was performed on a series of patients who were given 5,496 intravitreal bevacizumab injections for radiation retinopathy. Based on the observations, it was concluded that early identification of radiation retinopathy (using OCT), followed by early treatment, results in stability and often improvement. It was also observed that combined therapy with triamcinolone and bevacizumab, in the radiation-induced macular edema, possibly has a synergistic effect. Contrary to earlier reports, a limited usefulness of anti-VEGF agents in radiation retinopathy was found on a longer follow-up. These preliminary reports and observations, therefore, warrant further studies to define the precise role of these agents in the management of radiation retinopathy.

Triamcinolone Acetonide Therapy

Triamcinolone acetonide is thought to downregulate various cytokines and regulate capillary permeability. It is used to treat macular edema secondary to various retinal pathologies and has similarly been used to treat radiation maculopathy. While the data are limited, some studies suggest that intravitreal triamcinolone acetonide (4 mg/0.1 mL) does transiently reduce macular edema and improve visual acuity.[22,23] Further studies are needed to determine whether these results are sustainable and whether the benefit of frequent injections outweighs the known risks of glaucoma, cataract, and endophthalmitis.

Laser

Grid Macular Laser Photocoagulation

Grid macular laser photocoagulation has been used to treat radiation maculopathy with variable success. Studies by Kinyoun et al.[24] and Hykin et al.[25] demonstrated a beneficial effect of photocoagulation in visual acuity. However, the effect was not sustained with longer follow-up in the study conducted by Hykin et al.[25]

Sector Scatter and Panretinal Laser Photocoagulation

Sector scatter and panretinal laser photocoagulation have also been used to treat nonproliferative and proliferative radiation retinopathy. In a study by Finger et al.,[26] patients received sector scatter laser photocoagulation at the first sign of retinopathy, proliferative or nonproliferative. Retinopathy regressed in 64% of their treated patients. Similarly, in a study by Bianciotto et al.,[7] panretinal photocoagulation was found to cause regression of neovascularization in 66% of eyes with proliferative radiation retinopathy. There are also case reports of successful treatment of radiation retinopathy using hyperbaric oxygen[27] and oral pentoxifylline.[28]

Surgery

Advanced proliferative radiation retinopathy complicated by vitreous hemorrhage and/or tractional retinal detachment may require pars plana vitrectomy.

CONCLUSION

Radiation is a time-honored treatment for intraocular tumors. The resultant radiation retinopathy is a well-known formidable complication, which has no effective treatment. The retinopathy with macular edema must be detected early. Currently, intravitreal triamcinolone, repetitive treatment with anti-VEGF drugs, a combined therapy, and laser photocoagulation are recommended to reduce macular edema and improve visual acuity. However, these modalities particularly anti-VEGF and corticosteroids warrant further evaluation.

Preventive platelet-rich plasma or Avastin injection is helpful in prevention of neovascularization of retina, vitreous hemorrhage, and neovascular glaucoma.

To date, there is no prevention of radiation retinopathy except to fractionate the doses and decrease the total cumulative dose of radiation.

REFERENCES

1. Yanoff M, Duker JS, Augsburger JJ. Ophthalmology, 2nd edition. St. Louis: Mosby; 2004.
2. Parsons JT, Bova FJ, Fitzgerald CR, et al. Radiation retinopathy after external-beam irradiation: analysis of time-dose factors. Int J Radiat Oncol Biol Phys. 1994;30(4):765-73.
3. Monroe AT, Bhandare N, Morris CG, et al. Preventing radiation retinopathy with hyperfractionation. Int J Radiat Oncol Biol Phys. 2005;61(3):856-64.
4. Stack R, Elder M, Abdelaal A, et al. New Zealand experience of I125 brachytherapy for choroidal melanoma. Clin Exp Ophthalmol. 2005;33(5):490-4.
5. Puusaari I, Heikkonen J, Kivela T. Ocular complications after iodine brachytherapy for large uveal melanomas. Ophthalmology. 2004;111(9):1768-77.
6. Durkin SR, Roos D, Higgs B, et al. Ophthalmic and adnexal complications of radiotherapy. Acta Ophthalmol Scand. 2007;85(3):240-50.
7. Bianciotto C, Shields CL, Pirondini C, et al. Proliferative radiation retinopathy after plaque radiotherapy for uveal melanoma. Ophthalmology. 117(5):1005-12.
8. Archer DB, Amoaku WM, Gardiner TA. Radiation retinopathy—clinical, histopathological, ultrastructural and experimental correlations. Eye. 1991;5(Pt 2):239-51.
9. Archer DB, Gardiner TA. Ionizing radiation and the retina. Curr Opin Ophthalmol. 1994;5(3):59-65.
10. Damato B, Patel I, Campbell IR, et al. Visual acuity after Ruthenium (106) brachytherapy of choroidal melanomas. Int J Radiat Oncol Biol Phys. 2005;63(2):392-400.
11. Puusaari I, Heikkonen J, Kivela T. Effect of radiation dose on ocular complications after iodine brachytherapy for large uveal melanoma: empirical data and simulation of collimating plaques. Invest Ophthalmol Vis Sci. 2004;45(10):3425-34.
12. Char DH, Lonn LI, Margolis LW. Complications of cobalt plaque therapy of choroidal malanomas. Am J Ophthalmol. 1977;84(4):536-41.
13. Stallard HB. Radiotherapy for malignant melanoma of the choroid. Br J Ophthalmol. 1966;50(3):147-55.
14. Horgan N, Shields CL, Mashayekhi A, et al. Early macular morphological changes following plaque radiotherapy for uveal melanoma. Retina. 2008;28(2):263-73.
15. Oliver SC, Leu MY, DeMarco JJ, et al. Attenuation of iodine 125 radiation with vitreous substitutes in the treatment of uveal melanoma. Arch Ophthalmol. 2010;128(7):888-93.
16. Horgan N, Shields CL, Mashayekhi A, et al. Periocular triamcinolone for prevention of macular edema after plaque radiotherapy of uveal melanoma: a randomized controlled trial. Ophthalmology. 2009;116(7):1383-90.
17. Mason JO III, Albert MA Jr., Persaud TO, et al. Intravitreal bevacizumab treatment for radiation macular edema after plaque radiotherapy for choroidal melanoma. Retina. 2007;27(7):903-7.
18. Finger PT, Chin K. Anti-vascular endothelial growth factor bevacizumab (Avastin) for radiation retinopathy. Arch Ophthalmol. 2007;125(6):751-6.

19. Finger PT. Radiation retinopathy is treatable with anti-vascular endothelial growth factor bevacizumab (Avastin). Int J Radiat Oncol Biol Phys. 2008;70(4):974-7.

20. Gupta A, Muecke JS. Treatment of radiation maculopathy with intravitreal injection of bevacizumab (Avastin). Retina. 2008;28(7):964-8.

21. Cavalcante LL, Cavalcante ML, Murray TG, et al. Intravitreal injection analysis at the Bascom Palmer Eye Institute: evaluation of clinical indications for the treatment and incidence rates of endophthalmitis. Clin Ophthalmol. 2010;4:519-24.

22. Shields CL, Demirci H, Dai V, et al. Intravitreal triamcinolone acetonide for radiation maculopathy after plaque radiotherapy for choroidal melanoma. Retina. 2005;25(7):868-74.

23. Sutter FK, Gillies MC. Intravitreal triamcinolone for radiation-induced macular edema. Arch Ophthalmol. 2003;121(10):1491-3.

24. Kinyoun JL, Zamber RW, Lawrence BS, et al. Photocoagulation treatment for clinically significant radiation macular oedema. Br J Ophthalmol. 1995;79(2):144-9.

25. Hykin PG, Shields CL, Shields JA, et al. The efficacy of focal laser therapy in radiation-induced macular edema. Ophthalmology. 1998;105(8):1425-9.

26. Finger PT, Kurli M. Laser photocoagulation for radiation retinopathy after ophthalmic plaque radiation therapy. Br J Ophthalmol. 2005;89(6):730-8.

27. Gall N, Leiba H, Handzel R, et al. Severe radiation retinopathy and optic neuropathy after brachytherapy for choroidal melanoma, treated by hyperbaric oxygen. Eye. 2007;21(7):1010-12.

28. Gupta P, Meisenberg B, Amin P, et al. Radiation retinopathy: the role of pentoxifylline. Retina. 2001;21(5):545-7.

Index